Recent Advances in Autoimmune Rheumatic Diseases: 2nd Edition

Recent Advances in Autoimmune Rheumatic Diseases: 2nd Edition

Guest Editor

Diana Mieliauskaitė

Basel • Beijing • Wuhan • Barcelona • Belgrade • Novi Sad • Cluj • Manchester

Guest Editor
Diana Mieliauskaitė
Department of Personalised Medicine
State Research Institute Centre for
Innovative Medicine
Vilnius
Lithuania

Editorial Office
MDPI AG
Grosspeteranlage 5
4052 Basel, Switzerland

This is a reprint of the Special Issue, published open access by the journal *Medicina* (ISSN 1648-9144), freely accessible at: https://www.mdpi.com/journal/medicina/special_issues/89JBL5G205.

For citation purposes, cite each article independently as indicated on the article page online and as indicated below:

Lastname, A.A.; Lastname, B.B. Article Title. *Journal Name* **Year**, *Volume Number*, Page Range.

ISBN 978-3-7258-5905-4 (Hbk)
ISBN 978-3-7258-5906-1 (PDF)
https://doi.org/10.3390/books978-3-7258-5906-1

Contents

About the Editor

Diana Mieliauskaitė

Diana Mieliauskaitė, MD, PhD, is a chief researcher and head of the Personalized Medicine Department at the State Research Institute Center for Innovative Medicine. She is also chair of the Institute's Scientific Council. D. Mieliauskaitė's main areas of scientific interest are autoimmunity and Sjögren's disease.

Preface

This reprint of the Special Issue of *Medicina* entitled "Recent Advances in Autoimmune Rheumatic Diseases" is dedicated to the state of the art in autoimmune rheumatic diseases, and aims to be highly beneficial in clinical practice, enhance public health, and provide the latest information on innovations in the field of autoimmune rheumatic diseases.

Diana Mieliauskaitė
Guest Editor

medicina

MDPI

Editorial

Editorial for Recent Advances in Autoimmune Rheumatic Diseases: 2nd Edition

Diana Mieliauskaitė

Department of Personalised Medicine, State Research Institute Centre for Innovative Medicine, Santariškių St. 5, LT-08406 Vilnius, Lithuania; diana.mieliauskaite@imcentras.lt

This Special Issue of *Medicina*, entitled "Recent Advances in Autoimmune Rheumatic Diseases", is dedicated to the state of the art in autoimmune rheumatic diseases, with the expectation that it will be highly beneficial in clinical practice and enhance public health, and provide the latest information on innovations in the field of autoimmune rheumatic diseases.

Autoimmune rheumatic diseases (ARD) are a major global health problem with increasing prevalence. In addition, these diseases are linked to high morbidity, mortality, and disability rates. Autoimmune rheumatic diseases do not have diagnostic criteria and are guided by classification criteria, so the confirmation of the diagnosis is often delayed. These diseases as highly heterogeneous diseases involve complex pathophysiological mechanisms, resulting in variations in treatment response among individuals [1,2]. This heterogeneity underscores the need for individualized and precise treatment strategies and encourages patient-centered collaboration between clinicians and researchers.

We present the latest research advances in rheumatoid arthritis, vasculitis, SLE, and other autoimmune rheumatic diseases in this Special Issue. In parallel, the latest research advances in the field of autoimmune rheumatic diseases are summarized in reviews. Therefore, I would like to briefly review the contents of this Issue.

The introduction of Janus kinase inhibitors (JAKIs) for the treatment of rheumatoid arthritis (RA) has significantly changed treatment options. When using Janus kinase inhibitors (JAKIs), it is important to consider the safety of the drug, especially the risk of cardiovascular disease and cancer, and so additional studies are conducted in real clinical conditions. Priora M et al. evaluated the long-term efficacy of Janus kinase inhibitor Tofacitinib (TOFA) and predictors of responses to treatment in two RA patient subpopulations stratified according to different cardiovascular risk profiles. Summarizing the results, the authors conclude that tofacitinib showed similar efficacy in RA patients with both high- and low-risk cardiovascular subgroups, and disease activity decreased significantly both after six months and after one year. TOFA remained an effective treatment for all patients, and remission or LDA rates were reasonable despite safety considerations regarding the risk of cardiovascular events. Age had a negative impact on treatment response. This highlights the role of immunosenescence in the treatment of RA. The study results confirm the use of TOFA as an individualized approach to RA treatment, emphasizing the importance of carefully assessing cardiovascular and age-related risk factors when making clinical decisions [3].

The relationship between the use of rehabilitation services (RS) and changes in inflammatory responses in patients with RA has not yet been sufficiently investigated, although the effectiveness of rehabilitation services (RS) is supported by evidence. Huang HJ et al.

sought to evaluate changes in inflammatory markers before and after long-term rehabilitation. The authors conclude that integrating RS into routine care may be beneficial for controlling inflammation in RA patients. Further studies should be conducted using randomized controlled trials to confirm the effectiveness of RS [4].

In chronic autoimmune rheumatic diseases such as rheumatoid arthritis, self-efficacy is an important element of successful disease management. However, there is little information available on self-efficacy and its influencing factors among RA patients. Hsiao I-Y et al. assessed the level of self-efficacy and its corresponding prognostic factors among RA patients. Summarizing the results of the study, the authors state that healthcare providers need to assess the level of self-efficacy—a feature that seems to be related to a few medical characteristics—to facilitate the adaptation of healthcare regimens [5].

Anti-neutrophil cytoplasmic antibody (ANCA)-associated vasculitis (AAV) targets small and medium-sized blood vessels and is hallmarked by ANCA production. The term "ANCA-negative" is applied if a person fulfills the criteria for AAV but has negative serological ANCA test findings. Deresevičienė G. et al. conducted a cross-sectional study at a tertiary university hospital involving 73 patients diagnosed with anti-neutrophil cytoplasmic antibody (ANCA)-associated vasculitis (AAV) to evaluate clinical features of ANCA-positive and ANCA-negative vasculitis patients. The results of the study showed that the clinical condition of ANCA-positive patients is more severe in terms of organ damage and laboratory changes [6].

Children with juvenile idiopathic arthritis (JIA) suffer from a reduced quality of life due to their illness, and there is little research on child and parent satisfaction with disease management. Using symptom status acceptable to parents of children with juvenile arthritis (JA-PASS), demographic characteristics, disease course, and treatment, Romano F et al. conducted a cross-sectional study of 63 children diagnosed with JIA to investigate factors influencing parental satisfaction with the management of their children's JIA. Summarizing the results of the study, the authors conclude that JA-PASS provides useful information on how parents see the disease progressing and how well treatments work, and they suggest adding it to patient management [7].

There is insufficient data on immune disorders in systemic lupus erythematosus (SLE), especially those associated with disease flares. Kosałka-Węgiel J et al. revealed significant links between different B cell subsets and SLE disease activity. The authors emphasize an individualized approach to SLE patients in order to identify those at higher risk of SLE flare-ups [8].

Viral infections, including coronavirus disease 2019 (COVID-19), tend to cause more severe disease in patients with autoimmune rheumatic diseases (AIRD). Rutskaya-Moroshan K et al. examined the clinical characteristics of rheumatology patients and risk factors for severe infection. AIRDs of the study included rheumatoid arthritis, ankylosing spondylitis, systemic lupus erythematosus, and systemic sclerosis. This study showed that patients with AIRD were more likely to experience joint pain, depression, and shortness of breath. Patients with AIRD tended to have more severe diseases. Patients with arterial hypertension, diabetes mellitus, chronic kidney and lung diseases, receiving corticosteroid treatment, had longer illnesses, and highly active autoimmune disease increased the chance of getting a more severe form of COVID-19 [9].

Review by Vaduva O-A et al. demonstrated that dietary choices can lead to significant modification Psoriasis Area and Severity Index (PASI) scores. Low-calorie diets rich in antioxidants are effective, especially when the focus is on vegetables and animal proteins are restricted. The Mediterranean diet and possibly the ketogenic diet are beneficial because they provide omega-3 fatty acids and may alter the gut microbiome. Topical vitamin D and its analogs, together with corticosteroids, can alleviate psoriasis symptoms at the skin level. Low-calorie diets containing antioxidants are very powerful in this regard, especially when the focus is on vegetables and the consumption of animal-derived proteins is limited. Oral vitamin D supplements have a positive effect on psoriatic arthritis and may reduce the risk of related complications [10].

In order to properly assess the systemic manifestations of Sjögren's disease and to individualize the treatment of Sjögren's disease, the article by Mieliauskaitė D and Kontenis V presented evidence-based links between Sjögren's disease and gastroesophageal reflux disease (GERD). In general, there is a limited number of evidence-based studies evaluating the relationship between GERD and Sjögren's disease and GERD-related alterations in the microbiota in a multidisciplinary context. Future studies are necessary to improve the timely diagnosis and individualized treatment of Sjögren's disease [11].

Fibroblast-like synoviocytes (FLS) are one of the main factors in most cases of arthritis. Kirdaite G. et al. review the hallmarks and therapeutic challenges at the time of arthritis course, and review novel treatment targets, including surface biomarkers and intracellular proteins, non-coding ribonucleic acids (RNA) [12].

The review by Alexandru C et al. attracted considerable interest. This review examines the role of anti-receptor recognition particle (anti-SRP) antibodies in the diagnosis and treatment of collagen diseases with cardiac damage.

Rare reports of overlap syndrome between systemic sclerosis and immune-mediated necrotizing myositis have been reported. It is known that myositis can be a sign of scleroderma, and it is important to diagnose the overlap syndrome of these two diseases, as they can be interpreted as separate diseases, although specific treatment and monitoring should be applied. Anti-signal recognition particle (anti-SRP) antibodies act on skeletal muscle fibers and suppress myoblast regeneration, which leads to muscle fiber atrophy and necrosis. Anti-SRP antibodies are characteristic of immune-mediated necrotizing myopathies, which are characterized by muscle necrosis and minimum inflammatory response, with weakness of proximal muscles and representative external muscle symptoms. There is conflicting evidence regarding the link between cardiac symptoms and the presence of these antibodies, and the latest studies cannot prove a meaningful relationship between these two factors. Myocarditis is a condition with unpredictable and possibly serious consequences, ranging from heart failure and dilated cardiomyopathy to death. Diagnosing this disease is difficult because myocardial biopsy is an invasive procedure, so the results of cardiac magnetic resonance imaging are usually evaluated to make assumptions. This article addressed issues related to the management of collagen diseases by investigating the role of anti-SRP antibodies in the pathogenesis of cardiac damage [13].

Challenges remain in the field of rheumatology due to an aging population and the complexity of diseases, the need to manage comorbidity, the need to address health disparities between different population groups, and the challenges associated with the effective and appropriate integration of new technologies into the management of autoimmune rheumatic diseases.

Conflicts of Interest: The author declares no conflict of interest.

References

1. Choi, M.Y.; Costenbader, K.H.; Fritzler, M.J. Environment and systemic autoimmune rheumatic diseases: An overview and future directions. *Front. Immunol.* **2024**, *15*, 1456145. [CrossRef]
2. Hassan, R.; Faruqui, H.; Alquraa, R.; Eissa, A.; Alshaiki, F.; Cheikhet, M. Classification Criteria and Clinical Practice Guidelines for Rheumatic Diseases. In *Skills in Rheumatology*; Almoallim, H., Cheikh, M., Eds.; Springer: Singapore, 2021; Chapter 25. [CrossRef]

3. Priora, M.; Becciolini, A.; Celletti, E.; Di Penta, M.; Lo Gullo, A.; Paroli, M.; Bravi, E.; Andracco, R.; Nucera, V.; Ometto, F.; et al. Effectiveness and Predictors of Long-Term Treatment Response to Tofacitinib in Rheumatoid Arthritis Cohort: General Analysis and Focus on High-Cardiovascular-Risk Subgroup—A Multicenter Study. *Medicina* **2024**, *60*, 1982. [CrossRef]
4. Huang, H.-J.; Chen, W.-J.; Livneh, H.; Huang, H.-L.; Lu, M.-C.; Tsai, T.-Y. Integrating Rehabilitation Services into Routine Care of Rheumatoid Arthritis May Reduce the Inflammatory Response: A Hospital-Based Follow-Up Study in Taiwan. *Medicina* **2024**, *60*, 1938. [CrossRef] [PubMed]
5. Hsiao, I.-Y.; Livneh, H.; Chen, W.-J.; Lu, M.-C.; Tsai, T.-Y. An Exploration of Self-Efficacy and Its Associated Factors among Rheumatoid Arthritis Patients in Taiwan. *Medicina* **2024**, *60*, 1653. [CrossRef] [PubMed]
6. Dereseviciene, G.; Dadoniene, J.; Miltiniene, D. Similarities and Differences Between Patients Diagnosed with ANCA-Associated Vasculitis Who Are Positive and Negative for ANCA: University Clinic Practice and Expertise. *Medicina* **2025**, *61*, 1369. [CrossRef] [PubMed]
7. Romano, F.; Mombasi, P.; Garofalo, F.; Namarvari, N.; Franco, F.; Defabianis, P.; Berta, G.N. Parents' Satisfaction with Juvenile Idiopathic Arthritis Care: Findings from a Cohort of Italian Children Using the JAMAR Questionnaire. *Medicina* **2025**, *61*, 1115. [CrossRef] [PubMed]
8. Kosałka-Wegiel, J.; Jakieła, B.; Dziedzic, R.; Milewski, M.; Siwiec-Koźlik, A.; Zareba, L.; Bazan-Socha, S.; Sanak, M.; Musiał, J.; Korkosz, M. Circulating B Lymphocyte Subsets in Patients with Systemic Lupus Erythematosus. *Medicina* **2024**, *60*, 1994. [CrossRef] [PubMed]
9. Rutskaya-Moroshan, K.; Abisheva, S.; Abisheva, A.; Amangeldiyeva, Z.; Vinnik, T.; Batyrkhan, T. Clinical Characteristics, Prognostic Factors, and Outcomes of COVID-19 in Autoimmune Rheumatic Disease Patients: A Retrospective Case–Control Study from Astana, Kazakhstan. *Medicina* **2024**, *60*, 1377. [CrossRef]
10. Vaduva, O.-G.; Periferakis, A.-T.; Doncu, R.E.; Voiculescu, V.M.; Giurcaneanu, C. Dietary Principles, Interventions and Oxidative Stress in Psoriasis Management: Current and Future Perspectives. *Medicina* **2025**, *61*, 1296. [CrossRef]
11. Mieliauskaite, D.; Kontenis, V. Sjögren's Disease and Gastroesophageal Reflux Disease: What Is Their Evidence-Based Link? *Medicina* **2024**, *60*, 1894. [CrossRef]
12. Kirdaite, G.; Denkovskij, J.; Mieliauskaite, D.; Pachaleva, J.; Bernotiene, E. The Challenges of Local Intra-Articular Therapy. *Medicina* **2024**, *60*, 1819. [CrossRef] [PubMed]
13. Alexandru, C.; Donisa, A.; Bobirca, F.; Dascalu, A.M.; Dumitrescu, D.; Ancuta, I.; Bojinca, M.; Balahura, A.M.; Manea, C.; Belaconi, I.; et al. Anti-SRP Antibodies and Myocarditis in Systemic Sclerosis Overlap Syndrome with Immune-Mediated Necrotizing Myositis (IMNM). *Medicina* **2024**, *60*, 1756. [CrossRef] [PubMed]

medicina

MDPI

Article

Clinical Characteristics, Prognostic Factors, and Outcomes of COVID-19 in Autoimmune Rheumatic Disease Patients: A Retrospective Case–Control Study from Astana, Kazakhstan

Kristina Rutskaya-Moroshan [1], Saule Abisheva [1,*], Anilim Abisheva [1], Zhadra Amangeldiyeva [1], Tatyana Vinnik [1,2] and Tansholpan Batyrkhan [1]

[1] Department of Family Medicine №1, NJSC «Astana Medical University», Astana 010000, Kazakhstan; rutskayakristina@gmail.com (K.R.-M.); aanelim@bk.ru (A.A.); zhadra_82@mail.ru (Z.A.); tatyanavinnik15@gmail.com (T.V.); tansholpan.batyrkhan@gmail.com (T.B.)

[2] Department of Molecular Biology, Ariel University, Ariel 40700, Israel

* Correspondence: saule_tabisheva@mail.ru

Abstract: *Background:* Viral infections, including coronavirus disease 2019 (COVID-19), in patients with autoimmune rheumatic diseases (AIRDs) tend to present more severe disease. This study aims to investigate the clinical characteristics and risk factors for severe infection in rheumatologic patients. *Methods:* We included patients with a diagnosis of AIRD and COVID-19 infection between January 2022 and July 2023. Patients with AIRDs infected with SARS-CoV-2 were matched with control patients of the general population according to age (±5 years) and sex in a 1:1 ratio. Confirmed infection was defined if a patient had a positive polymerase chain reaction (PCR) test. The severity was divided into mild, moderate, severe, and critical according to the guidelines of the United States National Institutes of Health (NIH). *Results:* A total of 140 individuals (37 males, 103 females; mean age 56.1 ± 11.3 years) with rheumatic disease diagnosed with COVID-19 infection were enrolled in the study. AIRDs included rheumatoid arthritis (RA) (n = 63, 45%), ankylosing spondylitis (AS) (n – 35, 25%), systemic lupus erythematosus (SLE) (n = 26, 8.6%), and systemic sclerosis (SSc) (n = 16, 11.4%). The AIRDs group had more SARS-CoV-2-related dyspnea (38.6%), arthralgia (45.7%), and depression (27.1%) than the control group (p = 0.004). The rate of lung infiltration on radiographic examination was higher in 58 (41.4%, p = 0.005) patients with rheumatic diseases than in those without them. Severe SARS-CoV-2 infection was more common in the AIRDs group than in the control group (22% vs. 12%; p = 0.043). *Conclusions:* Patients with AIRDs experienced more symptoms of arthralgia, depression, and dyspnea. There was a trend towards an increased severity of the disease in patients with AIRDs. Patients with arterial hypertension, diabetes, chronic lung, and kidney disease, treated with corticosteroids, had a longer duration, and high activity of autoimmune disease had an increased risk of severe COVID-19.

Keywords: SARS-CoV-2 infection; autoimmune diseases; disease course; prognostic factors; disease-modifying antirheumatic drugs

1. Introduction

The COVID-19 pandemic is the result of the SARS-CoV-2 virus, which has presented significant challenges throughout the world and has affected societies and healthcare systems around the world. To date, almost 775 million cases worldwide have been surpassed, with more than seven million deaths [1]. Protecting high-risk individuals has been an essential public health focus, although identifying these high-risk groups has been somewhat complex due to the novel nature of SARS-CoV-2. In general, patients with AIRDs are more likely to be susceptible to infections [2], including SARS-CoV-2 [3]. In these cohorts, the worse outcomes of SARS-CoV-2 have been associated with immunological alterations, damage to vital organs, and the indirect impact of the drug received [4–6]. However, several medications used in the routine of rheumatologists, e.g., hydroxychloroquine [7], glucocorticoids (GCs) [8], IL-6 [9], and anti-TNF inhibitors [10], have been repurposed for the potential treatment of SARS-CoV-2.

During the pandemic, the practice of health care in Kazakhstan has undergone some profound difficulties. In addition to the existing risks of severe infection, patients with AIRD found themselves in a zone of "increased vulnerability". This was explained by the inability of local health authorities to provide diagnostic investigations and procure antirheumatic drugs due to a shortage of supplies. Patients with rheumatological conditions experiencing exacerbations and those requiring regular infusions of biological antirheumatic drugs encountered significant challenges with hospitalisation and access to specialized care. These difficulties were particularly pronounced in remote areas of the country, where access to well-equipped hospitals and medical care was more limited [11]. Along with the implementation of the distance from consultation [12], the availability of national diagnostic–therapeutic disease-specific protocols (based on international guidelines even before the pandemic), contributed, to some extent, to reducing the negative consequences for individuals affected by rheumatic diseases in Kazakhstan.

In recent years, large cohort and multicentral studies have investigated how patients with AIRDs have fared with respect to COVID-19. On the contrary, there is still a paucity of research data from Central Asian countries, particularly from Kazakhstan, on the pandemic influence on rheumatology patients. Studying the clinical features and prognostic factors of SARS-CoV-2 in rheumatological patients in our region will help fill a specific gap in national research, contribute to the development of national guidelines, and support the effective clinical management of rheumatological patients during and after the pandemic. This research investigated the SARS-CoV-2 characteristics of the four most prevalent AIRDs in Kazakhstan, including RA and AS, followed by SLE and SSc [13]. The primary objective was to compare the clinical characteristics, hospitalisation rates, and outcomes of COVID-19 patients with those of healthy controls. Secondary analyses focused on determining risk factors associated with the severity of the infection.

2. Materials and Methods

2.1. Study Design

The multi-centre retrospective observational case–control study was conducted to evaluate whether patients with AIRDs and infected with COVID-19 are at a higher risk of more severe clinical manifestations than those without an AIRDs. The research was carried out in city medical clinics in the capital of Kazakhstan, Astana city, in the period from January 2022 to July 2023.

2.2. Settings

In Kazakhstan, the first case of COVID-19 infection was recorded in March 2020, and the cases were considerably elevated from April 2020 [14]. The first vaccine was implemented on 1 February with the Russian Gam-COVID-Vac vaccine (Sputnik V) vaccine. Since 26 April 2021 the, Kazakhstan-made QazCovid-In vaccine (QazVac) has been administered after the third phase of clinical trials [15]. During the wave of pandemics, the local health system has provided free vaccination, testing systems, and COVID-19 treatment to all residents. The public vaccine programme succeeded in vaccinating 70% of the 20 million people living in Kazakhstan by 26 November 2023, and 36% were vaccinated with at least one booster dose. The Delta variant of SARS-CoV-2 was predominant in the country after July 2021. As of March 2024, Kazakhstan had surpassed more than 1.5 million SARS-CoV-2 cases, resulting in almost 19 thousand deaths.

2.3. Participant Selection

Inclusion and exclusion criteria were established to determine the patient's eligibility for the study. The inclusion criteria consisted of the following factors:

- Patients 18 years of age and older.

- Patients tested with a positive reverse transcription RNA PCR test against SARS-CoV-2.
- Patients with confirmed rheumatic diseases such as SLE, RA, AS, and SSC before SARS-CoV-2 infection. The recruited diagnoses were explained by these four most prevalent AIRDs in Kazakhstan [13].
- Patients who have filled out the information consent for the processing of personal data and participation in the survey.

The following exclusion criteria were applied:

- Patients with an unclear diagnosis purely on the basis of symptoms and other rheumatic diseases.
- Patients under the age of 18.
- Patients residing outside of Astana city. The place of residence is indicated on the title page of the case note. The study did not include patients with registered residence in other cities or regions of Kazakhstan.
- Patients who died from SARS-CoV-2.

The final sample consisted of 140 individuals with AIRDs in Astana city. We used the online sample size calculator to determine the minimum number of subjects to enrol in a study for adequate power. Gender distribution was considered irrespective of gender identity, while the age criteria set the minimum age at 18.

Control group: adult participants who did not receive immunosuppressive therapy from the general population and who were positive for the SARS-CoV-2 PCR test (n = 140). The control group was matched 1 to 1 with rheumatologic patients of age and sex.

2.4. Registration of COVID-19 Patients and Results

During the research period, we used the comprehensive patient self-reporting questionnaire for the initial recruitment of outpatient rheumatological patients. The questionnaire validation procedure consisted of the following stages: development, discussion with experts, translation, and pilot testing. The questionnaire was developed according to international standards under the direct control of the research supervisor. The questionnaire consisted of a total of 20 questions: 6 questions about personal data, 7 questions related to the clinical characteristics of AIRD, and 7 questions based on COVID-19 infection. Details on demographics, background and comorbidities, treatment and vaccination status, diagnostic tests for COVID-19, rheumatic disease activity at the beginning and after infection, symptoms, and patient-reported outcome measures of COVID-19 were also included. Demonstration of the original version of the questionnaire took place at the extended meeting of the Department of Family Medicine No1 NJSC 'Astana Medical University' (2021-19-10-EXP-3). At the next stage, we translated the version No. 1 into Kazakh language with the assistance of professional medical interpreters and created the pilot version of the questionnaire. For providing the free of biases and effective in collecting the intended data, the survey was tested in a pilot regime on a limited sample size (n = 20) in the period from November 2022 to December 2023.

The percentage of unanswered questions allowed us to evaluate how accessible the questions were for the participants to understand. In addition, the interviewees provided feedback for more precise and accurate wording of the questions. Following the pilot phase, the final version of the questionnaire was launched in January 2022. Informed consent was obtained from each patient individually before data collection.

Participants were instructed to complete the sections only if they had accurate information. Before the analysis, we contacted the patients to clarify any inaccuracies. For the mitigation of potential biases from self-reporting method, the received answers were checked manually by cross-referencing of medical records.

Additionally, we analysed patients' electronic medical cards to gather accurate information about comorbidities, autoimmune diseases, and characteristics of COVID-19. COVID-19 characteristics included information on diagnosis, treatment, hospitalisation, and complications. Data on rheumatic diseases included clarification of diagnosis, duration, and prior AIRD activity (categorised as remission, low/moderate, severe, and unknown).

At the start of COVID-19 treatment, details of GCs in prednisone equivalent doses (up to or more than 10 mg, unknown, without therapy), disease-modifying conventional synthetic antirheumatic drugs (csDMARDs) or biologic antirheumatic drugs (bDMARD) were collected. The history of comorbidities included chronic lung disease (asthma, obstructive or interstitial lung disease) and kidney disease, hypertension, cardiovascular and cerebrovascular pathology, diabetes, obesity, cancer, hepatitis, psoriasis, inflammatory bowel disease, and thyroid pathology.

We used the updated United States NIH COVID-19 treatment guidelines to categorise severity into mild, moderate, severe, or critical disease, according to clinical and radiological criteria [16]. SARS-CoV-2 reported outcomes included outpatient management, hospitalisation without oxygen requirements, hospitalisation with oxygen requirements or invasive mechanical ventilation, admission to the intensive care unit (ICU), and the development of complications.

2.5. The Sample Size Calculation

The main endpoint in the sample calculation was the occurrence of COVID-19-associated pneumonia and the development of severe COVID-19-associated pneumonia in patients with AIRD compared to those without AIRDS (control group). Initial study of the relevant literature revealed that severe pneumonia occurs in 14–15% of patients with COVID-19 [17–19]. Based on the expert opinion, we calculated that severe pneumonia would occur approximately about 2 times more often, i.e., 30%, in patients with AIRDs. Based on these figures, we calculated the minimum required sample size (Table 1).

Table 1. The sample size calculation for the case–control study.

For:			
	Two-sided confidence level (1-alpha)	95	
	Power (% chance of detecting)	80	
	Ratio of Controls to Cases	1	
	Hypothetical proportion of controls with exposure	15	
	Hypothetical proportion of cases with exposure:	30	
	Least extreme Odds Ratio to be detected:	2.43	
	Kelsey [20]	Fleiss [21]	Fleiss with CC
Sample Size-Cases	122	121	134
Sample Size-Controls	122	121	134
Total sample size:	244	242	268
CC = continuity correction			
Results are rounded up to the nearest integer.			
Results from OpenEpi, Version 3, open-source calculator—SSCC			

Using the Fleiss formula [21] with continuity correction, it was determined that the minimum sample size required for each group was 134 observations. Rounding it up, we recruited 140 patients in each sample in case of dropout from the study or possible incomplete records.

2.6. Statistical Analysis

Rheumatological patients were matched according to age (±5 years) and sex, with SARS-CoV-2-positive results without AIRDs. Numbers and percentages were used to summarize categorical data. Continuous data were presented as medians or means ± SD, as appropriate. The Shapiro–Wilk test was employed to determine whether continuous numerical variables followed a normal distribution. Differences between categorical variables were evaluated using the chi-square test or Fisher's exact test. For comparisons of continuous variables related to disease-specific characteristics between cases and controls, either Student's *t*-test or the Mann–Whitney test was used, as appropriate. Binary logistic regression analysis was conducted to explore the association between the binary dependent variable (severe infection) and independent factors, using a logit model. A p-value < 0.05 was considered statistically significant in all tests. Statistical analyses were performed using IBM SPSS software (version 19).

2.7. Ethical Statement

The study received approval from the Ethics Committee of the NJSC Astana Medical University (2022-31-01-EXP-5). The study was not funded. This research was carried out in compliance with the ethical principles outlined in the Declaration of Helsinki.

3. Results

3.1. Demographic and Baseline Clinical Characteristics

During the study period, 140 patients with AIRDs and confirmed SARS-CoV-2 infection were registered. We also included 140 COVID-19-matched individuals without AIRD from the general population. Both study groups were balanced in terms of baseline characteristics, including age and sex. The average age of the patients in the case group was 56.1 years (±11.3), and in the control group, it was 51.5 years (±13.6). Both groups were predominantly female, with 73.6% (n = 103) in the case group and 69.3% (n = 97) in the control group. Smoking was observed in 16% of patients with AIRD compared to 23% in the control group.

Arterial hypertension was notably more frequent in AIRD patients than in the control group (32.1% vs. 20%, p = 0.021). There were no significant differences in other comorbidities. In the case group, 15.7% had lung disease, 14.3% had thyroid problems, 10% had diabetes, and 8.6% had cardiovascular disease. In the control group, 20% had hypertension, 10.7% had thyroid disease, 9.3% had lung disease, 6.4% had diabetes, and 5.7% had cardiovascular disease. Table 2 summarises the baseline demographic and clinical characteristics of the research groups.

Table 2. The primary demographic and clinical characteristics of the research groups.

	AIRDS	Control Group
SEX n (%)		
Female	103 (73.6%)	97 (69.3%)
Male	37 (26.4%)	43 (30.7%)
Age, mean (SD)	56.1 ± 11.3	51.5 ± 13.6
18–44	46	50
45–59	64	69
60–74	24	19
75–90	6	2
Smoker	22	32
Comorbidities		
Hypertension	45 (32.1%)	28 (20%)
Diabetes	14 (10%)	9 (6.4%)
Cardiovascular disease	12 (8.6)	8 (5.7%)
Cerebrovascular disease	6 (4.3%)	4 (2.9%)
Chronic lung disease	22 (15.7%)	13 (9.3%)
Chronic kidney disease	4 (2.9%)	2 (1.4%)
Cancer	5 (3.6%)	3 (2.1%)
Psoriasis	3 (2.1%)	6 (4.3%)
Hepatitis	4 (2.9%)	3 (2.1%)
Inflammatory bowel disease	10 (7.1%)	4 (2.9%)
Hypo/hyperthyroidism	20 (14.3%)	15 (10.7%)
Nationality		
Kazakh	103	100
Russian	22	18
Tatars	6	7
Ukrainian	3	4
Poles	3	6

Table 2. Cont.

	AIRDS	Control Group
Germans	2	5
Greeks	1	0

3.1.1. AIRDs Baseline Characteristics

The most prevalent rheumatic disease was RA, consisting of 63 patients (45%), followed by AS with 35 patients (25%) and SLE with 26 patients (18.6%). The SSc subgroup represented 11.4% of the cases (n = 16). The duration of rheumatic disease was classified as follows: 20 (14.3%) patients had a diagnosis under five years, 45 (32.1%) patients between five and nine years, and 75 (53.6%) for ten years or more. At the onset of infection, most patients (37.1%) had low or moderate disease activity, 33.6% were in remission, while 22.9% had high disease activity. The status of the disease activity was unknown in 6.4% of the individuals.

At the beginning of COVID-19, 72.1% of the patients (n = 101) were receiving treatment with at least one conventional DMARD. Methotrexate and leflunomide were the most commonly used Cs-DMARDs in 52 (37.1%) and 19 (13.6%) patients, followed by azathioprine (n = 12, 8.6%). Biological DMARDs were used in 40 patients (28.6%), with golimumab being most commonly used (n = 23, 16.4%). None of the patients were taking rituximab. A considerable number of patients received baseline oral glucocorticoids (n = 80, 42.9%). More details on the underlying diseases and immunosuppressive therapy are provided in Table 3.

Table 3. Details on immunosuppressive therapy for underlying diseases.

Therapy	Diagnosis							
	RA		AS		SSc		SLE	
No NSAIDs (regular)	50	79.4%	24	68.6%	6	100.0%	25	96.2%
NSAIDs (regular)	13	20.6%	11	31.4%	0	0.0%	1	3.8%
No csDMARDs therapy	15	23.8%	14	40.0%	7	43.8%	3	11.5%
Metotrexate	31	49.2%	17	48.6%	4	25.0%	0	0.0%
Leflunomide	10	15.9%	4	11.4%	3	18.8%	2	7.7%
Mycophenolatmophetil	0	0.0%	0	0.0%	0	0.0%	7	26.9%
Sulfasalazine	0	0.0%	1	6.3%	0	0.0%	0	0.0%
Hydroxychloroquine	7	11.1%	0	0.0%	0	0.0%	3	11.5%
Azathioprine	0	0.0%	0	0.0%	1	6.3%	11	42.3%
No steroids	40	63.5%	35	100.0%	2	12.5%	3	11.5%
Up to 5 mg	12	19.0%	0	0.0%	8	50.0%	7	26.9%
5–10 mg	11	17.5%	0	0.0%	6	37.5%	6	23.1%
More than 10 mg	0	0.0%	0	0.0%	0	0.0%	10	38.5%
No bDMARDs therapy	48	76.2%	10	28.6%	16	100.0%	26	100.0%
Golimumab	9	14.3%	14	40.0%	0	0.0%	0	0.0%
Adalimumab	1	1.6%	6	17.1%	0	0.0%	0	0.0%
Tocilizumab	5	7.9%	2	5.7%	0	0.0%	0	0.0%
Infliximab	0	0.0%	3	8.6%	0	0.0%	0	0.0%

Notes: NSAIDs: non-steroidal anti-inflammatory drugs, csDMARD: conventional synthetic disease-modifying antirheumatic drug, bDMARDs: biologic disease-modifying antirheumatic drugs.

3.1.2. SARS-CoV-2 Infection Characteristics of the Study Groups and Results

In both groups, the majority of patients (n = 215, 76.8%) showed symptoms related to SARS-CoV-2, while the remaining were asymptomatic. Before SARS-CoV-2 identification, only 32 individuals with AIRDs (22.9%) had no symptoms. The most commonly reported symptoms in both groups were fever (48.9%) and headache (40.4%), followed by cough (39%) and fatigue (38.6%). The prevalence of arthralgia, shortness of breath, and depression symptoms was statistically higher in the AIRDs' group (45.7% vs. 26.4%, p = 0.001; 38.6% vs.

22.9%, $p = 0.004$; 27.1% vs. 8.6%, $p < 0.001$, respectively). Headache, dysgeusia, and anosmia were higher in the control group; however, these differences did not achieve statistical significance. The presence of gastrointestinal symptoms was minimal, with vomiting and nausea observed in 7.5% of the patients. Table 4 provides a comparison of the clinical characteristics of SARS-CoV-2 infection between the study cohorts.

Table 4. Clinical features of SARS-CoV-2 infection in the study groups.

Indicators		Study Group				*p*
		Case		Controls		
		N	%	N	%	
SARS-CoV-2 pneumonia	No	82	58.6%	104	74.3%	0.006
	Yes	58	41.4%	36	25.7%	
CT-stages	>25%	20	33.9%	16	45.7%	0.681
	25–50%	22	37.3%	10	28.6%	
	50–75%	14	23.7%	7	20.0%	
	>75%	2	3.4%	2	5.7%	
Fever	No	79	56.4%	64	45.7%	0.073
	Yes	61	43.6%	76	54.3%	
Cough	No	79	56.4%	92	65.7%	0.111
	Yes	61	43.6%	48	34.3%	
Headache	No	84	60.0%	83	59.3%	0.903
	Yes	56	40.0%	57	40.7%	
Dyspnoea	No	86	61.4%	108	77.1%	0.004
	Yes	54	38.6%	32	22.9%	
Throat pain	No	102	72.9%	110	78.6%	0.265
	Yes	38	27.1%	30	21.4%	
Arthralgia	No	76	54.3%	103	73.6%	0.001
	Yes	64	45.7%	37	26.4%	
Myalgia	No	89	63.6%	91	65.0%	0.803
	Yes	51	36.4%	49	35.0%	
Dysgeusia	No	105	75.0%	96	68.6%	0.232
	Yes	35	25.0%	44	31.4%	
Anosmia	No	92	65.7%	83	59.3%	0.267
	Yes	48	34.3%	57	40.7%	
Irritability/Depression	No	102	72.9%	128	91.4%	<0.001
	Yes	38	27.1%	12	8.6%	
Asthenia/Fatigue	No	79	56.4%	93	66.4%	0.086
	Yes	61	43.6%	47	33.6%	
Diarrhoea/vomiting	No	130	92.9%	129	92.1%	0.821
	Yes	10	7.1%	11	7.9%	
Thorax pain	No	118	84.9%	120	85.7%	0.846
	Yes	21	15.1%	20	14.3%	

The prevalence of CT pneumonia associated with SARS-CoV-2 was significantly higher in AIRD patients ($n = 58$, 41.4%) compared to controls ($n = 36$, 25.7%, $p = 0.05$). No statistical differences were found in the CT stages of pneumonia between the study cohorts ($p = 0.638$). In the control group, 12 (8.6%) patients met the guidance criteria for severe COVID-19, while 22 patients (15.7%) with AIRDs had evidence of the severe course of infection. Other data on the severity of the disease are shown in Figure 1.

During the study period, 11 (7.8%) admissions occurred in the general population (mean age: 57.3 ± 6.6 years, 7 (63.6%) females). Among patients with AIRD, 104 (74.3%) (mean age: 48.8 ± 13.0 years, 73 (70.3%) female) did not require hospitalisation, while 36 (25.7%) (mean age: 53.9 ± 9.9 years, 30 (83.3%) female) were hospitalised. As shown, AIRDs were associated with an increased rate of hospitalisation hazard (4.1 95% CI: 2.0–8.4, $p < 0.001$). According to the prevalence of RA in the main group, the majority of the latter were patients with RA ($n = 13$, 36.1%). Among the hospitalised, 58.3% had hypertension, 41.7% had glucocorticoids at a dose of 5–10 mg daily, and 38.9% had methotrexate. Only two patients (5.6%) used bDMARDs (golimumab). Other characteristics of hospitalised patients from the case and control groups are presented in Tables 5 and 6.

Table 5. Characteristics of hospitalised patients with AIRDs.

Patients with AIRDs		Hospitalisation				*p*
		Yes		No		
		N	%	N	%	
Gender	Male	6	16.7%	31	29.8%	0.123
	Female	30	83.3%	73	70.2%	
Age	18–44	5	13.9%	41	39.4%	0.007
	45–59	21	58.3%	43	41.3%	
	60–74	10	27.8%	14	13.5%	
	75–90	0	0.0%	6	5.8%	
Diagnosis	RA	13	36.1%	50	48.1%	0.042
	AS	6	16.7%	29	27.9%	
	SLE	9	25.0%	17	16.3%	
	SSc	8	22.2%	8	7.7%	
Duration of the disease	<5 years	4	11.1%	16	15.4%	0.153
	5–10 years	7	19.4%	38	36.5%	
	11–20 years	20	55.6%	42	40.4%	
	>20 years	5	13.9%	8	7.7%	
Comorbidity	No	5	13.9%	53	51.0%	<0.001
	Yes	31	86.1%	51	49.0%	
Smoking	No	27	75.0%	75	72.1%	0.793
	Yes	6	16.7%	16	15.4%	
	Past smokers	3	8.3%	13	12.5%	
GCS (doses)	No	7	19.4%	73	70.2%	<0.001
	<5 mg	9	25.0%	18	17.3%	
	5–10 mg	15	41.7%	8	7.7%	
	>10 mg	5	13.9%	5	4.8%	
GCs therapy duration	<5 years	9	25.0%	16	15.4%	<0.001
	5–10 years	13	36.1%	14	13.5%	
	>10 years	7	19.4%	0	0.0%	
NSAIDs (regular)	No	28	77.8%	87	83.7%	0.428
	Yes	8	22.2%	17	16.3%	
csDMARDs	No immunosuppressive therapy	9	25.0%	30	28.8%	0.492
	Metotrexate	14	38.9%	38	36.5%	
	Leflunomide	3	8.3%	16	15.4%	
	Mycophenolatmophetil	2	5.6%	5	4.8%	
	Sulfasalazine	0	0.0%	1	1.0%	
	Hydroxychloroquine	2	5.6%	8	7.7%	
	Azathioprine	6	16.7%	6	5.8%	
duration csDMARDs duration	<5 years	10	27.8%	36	34.6%	0.119
	5–10 years	10	27.8%	37	35.6%	
	>10 years	15	41.7%	27	26.0%	
bDMARDs	No biological therapy	34	94.4%	66	63.5%	0.011
	Golimumab	2	5.6%	21	20.2%	
	Adalimumab	0	0.0%	7	6.7%	
	Tocilizumab	0	0.0%	7	6.7%	
	Infliximab	0	0.0%	3	2.9%	

Notes: RA: rheumatoid arthritis; AS: ankylosing spondylitis; SLE: systemic lupus erythematosus; SSc: systemic sclerosis; GCS: glucocorticosteroids; NSAIDs non-steroidal anti-inflammatory drugs; csDMARDs: conventional synthetic disease-modifying antirheumatic drugs; bDMARDs: biologic disease-modifying antirheumatic drugs.

Among patients with AIRD, 30 (83.3%) were treated on the ward, and 6 (16.7%) were treated in the intensive care unit (ICU). The percentage of patients who required oxygen therapy was significantly higher in the AIRD group compared to the control group (23 (16.4%) vs. 5 (3.5%), $p = 0.004$). Invasive mechanical ventilation was necessary for five patients (3.5%) treated in the ICU, most of whom were women ($n = 4$) and used baseline DMARDs such as methotrexate, leflunomide, azathioprine, and sulfasalazine, all of which were discontinued during the infection period. In comparison, in the control group, three patients (2%) were treated in the ICU, with two (1.4%) requiring invasive mechanical ventilation. A statistical analysis of the results comparing patients with AIRDs with controls is presented in Figure 2.

When analysing complications, 25 cases (n = 17.8%) were recorded in patients in the AIRD group, while only 14 people (n = 10%) in the control group had unfavourable consequences of infection. There were no statistically significant differences between the two groups ($p = 0.147$). As shown in Figure 2, these were respiratory failure in nine patients, pericarditis in three, acute heart failure in two, and ischemic stroke, deep vein thrombosis, ulcer, and pancreatic necrosis in one patient. Acute respiratory distress syndrome possibly associated with underlying SSc was recorded in one woman. More than two complications had five patients with AIRDs. The comparison of complications in the study groups is shown in Figure 3.

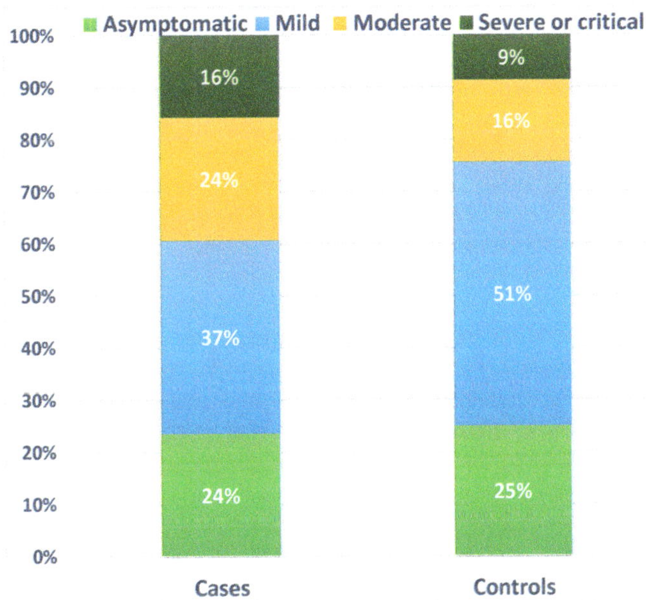

Figure 1. Proportions of the severity of COVID-19 in the case and control groups.

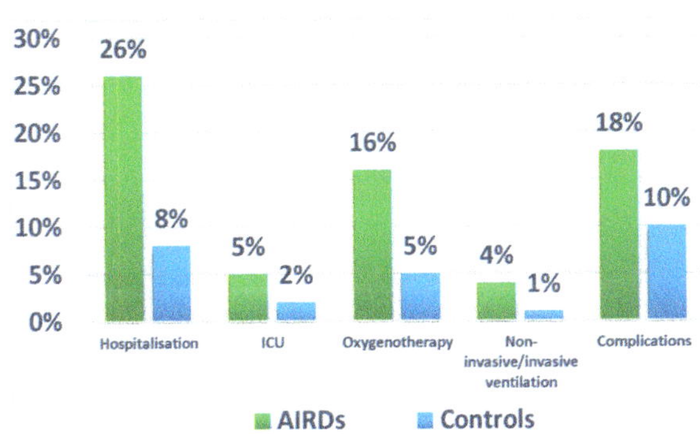

Figure 2. Comparison of COVID-19 outcomes between study groups.

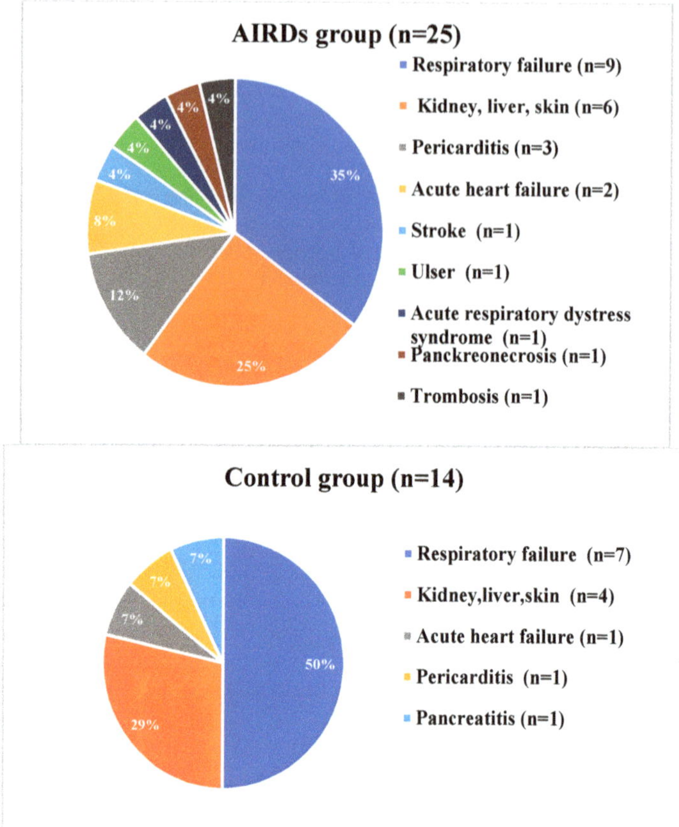

Figure 3. The comparison of COVID-19′s complications.

Table 6. Characteristics of hospitalised patients (control group).

Control Group		Hospitalisation				p
		Yes		No		
		N	%	N	%	
Gender	Male	4	36.4%	43	33.3%	0.838
	Female	7	63.6%	86	66.7%	
Age	18–44	0	0.0%	86	66.7%	<0.001
	45–59	1	9.1%	34	26.4%	
	60–74	8	72.7%	9	7.0%	
	75–90	2	18.2%	0	0.0%	
Comorbidity	No	0	0.0%	86	66.7%	<0.001
	Yes	11	100.0%	43	33.3%	
Smoking	No	6	54.5%	85	65.9%	0.719
	Yes	3	27.3%	29	22.5%	
	Past smokers	2	18.2%	15	11.6%	

3.2. Factors Related to Severe SARS-CoV-2 Infection in Patients with AIRDs

We compared the main characteristics of patients with AIRD who had a mild infection with SARS-CoV-2 with those who developed a severe infection with SARS-CoV-2 in Table 7. Patients with severe SARS-CoV-2 were more likely to have the following risk factors: age over 45 years, diabetes mellitus, hypertension, cardiovascular disease, cerebrovascular disease, and chronic kidney and lung disease. It is noteworthy that 50% of patients hospitalised with AIRD who had chronic obstructive or interstitial lung disease were smokers. The high disease activity at the onset of the infection, the long duration of the disease, the GCs therapy for more than 10 years, and the dose of steroids more than 10 mg in a prednisolone equivalent were also associated with a severe course of infection.

Table 7. Factors associated with severe and non-severe SARS-CoV-2 infection in 140 patients with autoimmune rheumatic diseases.

Factors		SARS-CoV-2 Severity				p
		Mild/Moderate		Severe/Critical		
		n	%	n	%	
Gender	Male	33	28.0%	4	18.2%	0.339
	Female	85	72.0%	18	81.8%	
Age	18–44	44	37.3%	2	9.1%	0.019
	45–59	51	43.2%	13	59.1%	
	60–74	17	14.4%	7	31.8%	
	75–90	6	5.1%	0	0.0%	
Diagnosis	RA	53	44.9%	10	45.5%	0.840
	AS	31	26.3%	4	18.2%	
	SSc	13	11.0%	3	13.6%	
	SLE	21	17.8%	5	22.7%	
Comorbidity		61	51.7%	21	95.5%	0.000
Hypertension		28	23.7%	17	77.3%	0.000
Cardiovascular pathology		7	5.9%	5	22.7%	0.010
Diabetes mellitus		3	2.5%	11	50.0%	0.000
Chronic obstructive/interstitial lung disease		12	10.2%	10	45.5%	0.000
Cerebrovascular pathology		3	2.5%	3	13.6%	0.018
Cancer		3	2.5%	2	9.1%	0.129
Obesity		7	5.9%	4	18.2%	0.050
Psoriasis		3	2.5%	0	.0%	0.450
Hepatitis		3	2.5%	1	4.5%	0.605
Chronic kidney disease		0	0.0%	4	18.2%	0.000
Hypo/hyperthyroidism		7	5.9%	3	13.6%	0.198
Inflammatory bowel disease		13	11.0%	7	31.8%	0.010
Smoking	No	85	72.0%	17	77.3%	0.144
	Yes	17	14.4%	5	22.7%	
	Past smokers	16	13.6%	0	0%	
Disease activity at the time of infection	Remission	46	39.0%	1	4.5%	0.000
	Low/moderate	47	39.8%	5	22.7%	
	High activity	19	16.1%	13	59.1%	
	Unknown	6	5.1%	3	13.6%	
GCS (doses)	No	75	63.6%	5	22.7%	0.000
	<5 mg	24	20.3%	3	13.6%	
	5–10 mg	13	11.0%	10	45.5%	
	>10 mg	6	5.1%	4	18.2%	
AIRD duration	<5 years	18	15.3%	2	9.1%	0.011
	5–10 years	43	36.4%	2	9.1%	
	11–20 years	49	41.5%	13	59.1%	
	>20 years	8	6.8%	5	22.7%	
GCS therapy duration	No	76	64.4%	5	22.7%	0.000
	1–5 years	23	19.5%	2	9.1%	
	<5 years	19	16.1%	15	68.2%	
Duration csDMARDs	5–10 years	45	38.1%	6	27.3%	0.082
	>10 years	42	35.6%	5	22.7%	
	>10 years	31	26.3%	11	50.0%	

Table 7. *Cont.*

Factors		SARS-CoV-2 Severity				*p*
		Mild/Moderate		Severe/Critical		
		n	%	n	%	
csDMARDs	No immunosuppressive therapy	34	28.8%	5	22.7%	0.955
	Metotrexate	43	36.4%	9	40.9%	
	Leflunomide	16	13.6%	3	13.6%	
	Mycophenolatmophetil	6	5.1%	1	4.5%	
	Sulfasalazine	1	0.8%	0	0.0%	
	Hydroxychloroquine	9	7.6%	1	4.5%	
	Azathioprine	9	7.6%	3	13.6%	
NSAIDs (regular)		17	14.4%	8	36.4%	0.014
bDMARDs	No biological therapy	79	66.9%	21	95.5%	0.111
	Golimumab	22	18.6%	1	4.5%	
	Adalimumab	7	5.9%	0	0.0%	
	Tocilizumab	7	5.9%	0	0.0%	
	Infliximab	3	2.5%	0	0.0%	

Notes: GCS: glucocorticosteroids; NSAIDs: non-steroidal anti-inflammatory drugs; csDMARDs: conventional synthetic disease-modifying antirheumatic drugs; bDMARDs: biologic disease-modifying antirheumatic drugs.

These severity factors are also demonstrated in Figure 4, in which the *p*-values and the unadjusted odds ratios for each factor have been calculated. Although the confidence intervals were wide due to the small sample, the highest OR was found in the presence of diabetes (OR = 38.3 (9.28–158.36)) and high autoimmune activity (OR = 31.47 (3.84–257.79)).

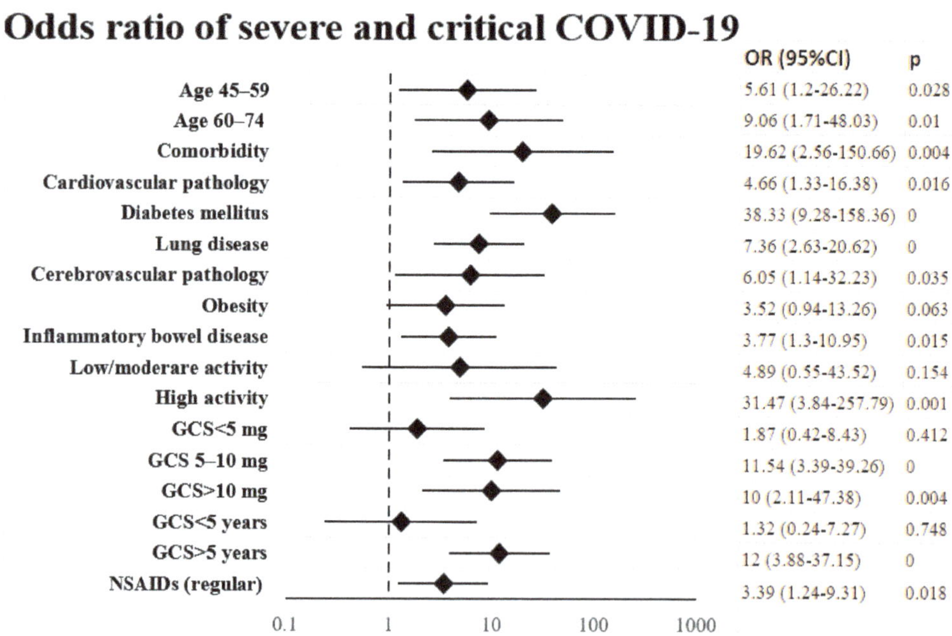

Figure 4. Predictive severity factors of COVID-19 in 140 patients with autoimmune rheumatic diseases.

4. Discussion

Patients with AIRDs have increased risks of COVID-19 infection [16,22] and severe forms of COVID-19 with mortality [23–25]. The "vulnerability" of this cohort can be explained for a number of reasons.

First, immune dysregulation as a result of AIRD can affect innate immune responses, which play a crucial role in preventing virus replication and developing an adaptive immune response [26]. Disability to reduce viral load in the early stages of the disease can lead to a hyperinflammatory reaction leading to tissue damage and multiple organ failure [27]. In patients with AIRD and verified COVID-19, a more severe degree of respiratory failure was observed compared to patients without a background disease [28]. Secondly, COVID-19 per se affects both the course of AIRD and antirheumatic therapeutic options. Contrary to that, the drugs used to treat AIRDs can affect the outcomes of COVID-19. Along with the studied factors of unfavourable prognosis in patients with AIRDs, the severe course of COVID-19 was associated with the use of GCS, anti-B-cell therapy [6,29], and Janus-kinase inhibitors (JAK) [30]. Thirdly, the peculiarities of the COVID-19 in patients with AIRDs echoed the issues of short-term infection or persistent neurological, respiratory, cardiovascular, endocrine consequences (including the post-COVID syndrome), or consequences of vaccination against COVID-19, with the need to study the frequency of this manifestations as well as their further impact on the course of the systemic disease. It is important to highlight that the increased exposure of rheumatological patients to COVID-19 has significant public health implications, particularly regarding their ability to work. This situation results in economic strain not only for individual families, but also on a broader social scale [31].

Our research shows that people with AIRDs had a higher susceptibility to severe SARS-CoV-2. More patients in the AIRDs group required hospitalisation, oxygen, and mechanical ventilation. These findings are consistent with those of a report on a large national cohort study in Denmark [32], in which patients diagnosed with AIRD were more likely to suffer from severe COVID-19 with a substantial increased risk of and mechanical ventilation. In a recent retrospective study conducted in Poland [33], patients with AIRDs required considerably more high-flow nasal oxygen and/or noninvasive ventilation. Interestingly, some previous studies have not identified significant differences in hospitalisation requirements [34] and admission to the ICU [35] between cohorts. However, a metanalysis showed [22] that the incidence of hospitalisation and serious clinical treatment (ICU admission and mechanical ventilation) was significantly higher in rheumatological patients.

It is crucial to clarify the clinical data and the factors that impact the prognosis of individuals with autoimmune diseases during the SARS-CoV-2 era, especially regarding the course of the disease [36]. Recent matched case–control studies have indicated that COVID-19 infection affects individuals with and without rheumatic disease in a similar way. In Nas's research [37], rheumatologic patients had higher rates of anosmia, ageusia, dyspnoea, myalgia, arthralgia, and gastrointestinal symptoms. In our study, arthralgia, shortness of breath, and depression symptoms were statistically higher in the AIRDs group. In contrast, patients in the control group were more likely to have headaches, dysgeusia, and anosmia.

The COVID-19 Global Rheumatology Alliance (C19-GRA) established a physician-reported registry for individuals with rheumatic diseases and COVID-19 at the start of the pandemic. This registry has offered valuable insights into the outcomes of COVID-19 for those with rheumatic conditions [38]. The C19-GRA reported [29] that cardiovascular disease, combined with hypertension and chronic lung and kidney disease, were associated with higher odds of death. This may be explained by the pathogenetic characteristics of SARS-CoV-2 viruses, of which the cytotoxic effect is mediated by tropism to the ACE-2 receptor, expressed mainly in the heart, lungs and kidneys [39–41]. Additionally, factors related to an increased risk of hospitalisation included advanced age, high disease activity, and treatment with GCs greater than 10 mg per day [42]. In the study, we identified risk factors for severe COVID-19 infection in rheumatological patients and confirmed that older age, hypertension, diabetes, cardiovascular, chronic lung and kidney disease, and high disease activity were positively correlated with the severity of COVID-19. These results are consistent with those reported in the existing literature [29,42,43].

Pablos et al. [34] found a higher prevalence of obesity and cardiovascular disorders in people with COVID-19 and AIRD. In particular, the prevalence of comorbidity background in our cohort consisted of 44%. We found no significant disparity between the research groups in terms of incidence and type of comorbidity, except for arterial hypertension.

In line with comorbidities, age was associated with hospitalisation during the COVID-19 pandemic in further studies [22,40]. In the study Fonseca D. et al. [44], the severity of COVID-19 correlated with an age-related increasing of the titres of autoantibodies to cardiolipin, claudine, and platelet glycoprotein, which were identified as stratification markers of severe COVID-19 patients aged ≥50 years. The severe course of COVID-19 in the elderly can also be explained by the "ageing" phenomenon of the immune system with a decrease in physiological reserves [45]. Interestingly, in our study, patients with severe infection were more likely to have an age younger than 45 years. The severe course of infection was correlated with the male sex [46,47]. We did not find a statistical significance between the sex and the severity of the COVID-19 infection, which was probably due to the small sample size, and this is one of the limitations of our study.

There is an increasing amount of literature highlighting racial and ethnic health disparities related to COVID-19. Some studies have shown that racial and ethnic minorities, particularly Asians, experience worse COVID-19 outcomes compared to others [48,49]. The C19-GRA study found that Asian, African American, and Latin patients had higher odds of hospitalisation compared to White patients [50]. Additionally, racial and ethnic minority patients with rheumatic conditions tend to face a greater burden of disease [51], with higher disease activity, poorer functional status, and lower quality of life compared to White patients [52]. Unfortunately, the small sample size in our study limited the ability to examine racial predisposition to severe outcomes of COVID-19. More research is needed to understand and address the underlying causes of these disparities, especially those related to socioeconomic status and healthcare access.

Strangfeld A. et al. have shown [29] that treatment with rituximab, azathioprine, sulfasalazine, mycophenolate mofetil, cyclosporine, tacrolimus, and GCs at an equivalent dose of prednisolone of 10 mg/day was also associated with increased mortality risks compared to methotrexate monotherapy. According to data from the French cohort of rheumatological COVID-19, rheumatological drugs associated with severe infection were corticosteroids, mycophenolate mofetil, and rituximab [53]. On the contrary, b-DMARDs, such as antitumor necrosis factor α, were not associated with severe COVID-19 infection and appear to lead to a reduction in the risk of severe COVID-19 [10]. In our study, 101 patients used cs-DMARD, and 40 patients used b/DMARD. Some associations between cs-DMARDs and the severity of infection were not detected in our study. Conversely, the proportion of b/DMARD-received patients among non-hospitalised cohort was significantly higher. This circumstance allows one to consider the use of b/DMARD as a protective factor of the course of the severe infection. Previous evidence obtained from other studies showed an increased severity of the disease in patients receiving rituximab [54,55], which could lead to persistent viremia without low viral clearance [56,57]. Notably, none of the patients in our study received anti-B cell therapy.

Other unique risk factors for patients with ARDs with a possible impact on the severity of SARS-CoV-2 infection were the use of oral GCs. Corticosteroid treatment was associated with a more severe course of the disease, and the negative impact of oral corticosteroids, regardless of the indication, has been well proved in recent studies [6,29,58,59]. Treatment with higher dosages of glucocorticoids (>10 mg/day prednisolone-equivalent dose vs. no use) was also found to be associated with hospitalisation and mortality [29]. The probable reasons for this are the high activity of AIRD, which requires increasing the dose of GCS [29], as well as the potentially negative effect of steroid therapy on the process of viral replication [43]. In our rheumatic disease group, more than 42% were on baseline

GCs therapy, of whom 62.5% used low doses (≤10 mg/day). As we found, GCS in a dose > 10 mg/day was significantly associated with severe SARS-CoV-2. In contrast, the efficacy of high-dose GCs for the treatment of SARS-CoV-2 was shown in the RECOVERY study [60]. The cause of this discrepancy may be explained by the timing of use in relation to the diagnosis of SARS-CoV-2 [43].

In our study, we found significant differences in terms of infection development and AIRD duration; however, no clear relationship between these aspects has been observed in the literature.

Limitations and Strengths of the Study

Our study has some limitations that should be considered when interpreting the results, including the lack of laboratory parameters, such as C-reactive protein, ferritin, and interleukins levels. In this retrospective design, data collection could be subject to potential biases and affect all groups of patients, both cases and controls, in the same way. In particular, there was a rapid development of scientific knowledge around COVID-19, including the development of COVID-19 vaccines and the mutation of virus variants. Unfortunately, our data were collected over a long period of time and may not reflect the current situation. Interpreting the prevalence of depression symptoms in the main group of our study could introduce bias, as these symptoms are generally more common in individuals with AIRDs than in the general population. Additionally, a significant limitation of our research was the exclusion of deceased COVID-19 patients from the outcome measures, which could lead to bias, particularly in underestimating the impact of COVID-19 on the AIRD population in our region. This exclusion may also affect the results by hindering a comprehensive understanding of the full spectrum of disease severity. Lastly, the sample size was insufficient to include a broader range of diagnoses, limiting our ability to extrapolate the effects of rare specific diagnoses or less commonly used DMARDs on COVID-19 infection.

However, our study has several strengths. We manually recruited the patient sample evaluated within multiple medical centres in a single city. Subsequently, using the online DAMUMED database, we were able to conduct a case–control study matched with propensity score, adjusted for age, sex, and comorbidities commonly associated with the severity of COVID-19. These factors were well balanced between the two groups. Free access to patient medical records allowed us to verify information on the diagnosis of underlying AIRDs, comorbidities, treatment, and outcomes. The study population was from a single centre with a unified management protocol for COVID-19 infection, which eliminated inconsistencies in quality of care between study subjects. The included outcomes measures for oxygen therapy and ventilation support were objective guided by objective clinical measures and were not affected by caregiver decisions or pandemic circumstances. On the contrary, due to the limitations of resources during pandemic peaks, hospitalisation criteria could change, affecting study outcomes. Our definition of severe SARS-CoV-2 infection was compatible with the WHO definition and recommended in the updated WHO guidelines for September 2020. All SARS-CoV-2 cases were confirmed by PCR tests in medical centres, which were providers of COVID-19 care in Astana during the pandemic. Importantly, the extensive tracking and testing strategy applied in Kazakhstan allowed us to identify cases with mild or no symptoms. Therefore, our study reflects the true rate of severe COVID-19 infection. Finally, to our knowledge, this is the first study in our region that has provided global data on the prognostic factors of this infection in individuals with rheumatic diseases.

5. Conclusions

In this study, we extracted data from Astana, Kazakhstan, on the baseline characteristics, outcomes, and risk factors of COVID-19 in patients with AIRDs. Compared to non-AIRD controls, AIRD patients required hospitalisation, oxygen therapy, and invasive mechanical ventilation more frequently. The age over 45 years, diabetes mellitus, hypertension, cardiovascular and cerebrovascular disease, and chronic kidney and chronic lung disease were identified as risk factors for the severe SARS-CoV-2. The AIRD-mediated factors, as the high disease activity, the duration of the disease, the GCs therapy for more than 10 years, and the dose more than 10 mg in a prednisolone equivalent were also associated with a severe course of infection.

The authors hope that the results contribute to the growing volume of evidence on the clinical characteristics and outcomes of SARS-CoV-2 in this cohort of patients. In summary, our study had serious limitations of the small sample size, retrospective design, potential biases in terms of using self-report data, and exclusion of COVID-19-associated death from the outcome measures. Therefore, more research with larger sample sizes is needed to further characterise the infection process in patients with AIRDs. Realising regional guidelines and research can help accumulate personal experience and knowledge on aspects of SARS-CoV-2 and rheumatology, as well as optimising the treatment of rheumatological patients in the post-pandemic era.

Author Contributions: Conceptualization, K.R.-M. and S.A.; methodology, K.R.-M.; software, A.A.; validation, K.R.-M., S.A. and Z.A.; formal analysis, T.V.; investigation, Z.A.; resources, T.B.; data curation, Z.A.; writing—original draft preparation, K.R.-M.; writing—review and editing, S.A.; visualization, Z.A.; supervision, T.V. All authors have read and agreed to the published version of the manuscript.

Funding: This research received no external funding.

Institutional Review Board Statement: The study was conducted in accordance with the Declaration of Helsinki, and approved by the Institutional Review Board (or Ethics Committee) of NJSC Astana Medical University (EXP-5-2022-31-01).

Informed Consent Statement: Informed consent was obtained from all subjects involved in the study.

Data Availability Statement: The original contributions presented in the study are included in the article, further inquiries can be directed to the corresponding authors.

Conflicts of Interest: The authors declare no conflicts of interest.

References

1. COVID-19 Cases | WHO COVID-19 Dashboard. Available online: https://data.who.int/dashboards/covid19/cases (accessed on 29 June 2024).
2. Maddur, M.S.; Vani, J.; Lacroix-Desmazes, S.; Kaveri, S.; Bayry, J. Autoimmunity as a Predisposition for Infectious Diseases. *PLoS Pathog.* **2010**, *6*, e1001077. [CrossRef] [PubMed]
3. Cordtz, R.; Lindhardsen, J.; Soussi, B.G.; Vela, J.; Uhrenholt, L.; Westermann, R.; Kristensen, S.; Nielsen, H.; Torp-Pedersen, C.; Dreyer, L. Incidence and Severeness of COVID-19 Hospitalisation in Patients with Inflammatory Rheumatic Disease: A Nationwide Cohort Study from Denmark. *Rheumatology* **2020**, *60*, SI59–SI67. [CrossRef]
4. Amigues, I.; Pearlman, A.H.; Patel, A.; Reid, P.; Robinson, P.C.; Sinha, R.; Kim, A.H.; Youngstein, T.; Jayatilleke, A.; Konig, M. Coronavirus Disease 2019: Investigational Therapies in the Prevention and Treatment of Hyperinflammation. *Expert. Rev. Clin. Immunol.* **2020**, *16*, 1185–1204. [CrossRef]
5. Williamson, E.J.; Walker, A.J.; Bhaskaran, K.; Bacon, S.; Bates, C.; Morton, C.E.; Curtis, H.J.; Mehrkar, A.; Evans, D.; Inglesby, P.; et al. Factors Associated with COVID-19-Related Death Using OpenSAFELY. *Nature* **2020**, *584*, 430–436. [CrossRef] [PubMed]
6. Gianfrancesco, M.; Hyrich, K.L.; Al-Adely, S.; Carmona, L.; Danila, M.I.; Gossec, L.; Izadi, Z.; Jacobsohn, L.; Katz, P.; Lawson-Tovey, S.; et al. Characteristics Associated with Hospitalisation for COVID-19 in People with Rheumatic Disease: Data from the COVID-19 Global Rheumatology Alliance Physician-Reported Registry. *Ann. Rheum. Dis.* **2020**, *79*, 859–866. [CrossRef]
7. Yao, X.; Ye, F.; Zhang, M.; Cui, C.; Huang, B.; Niu, P.; Liu, X.; Zhao, L.; Dong, E.; Song, C.; et al. In Vitro Antiviral Activity and Projection of Optimized Dosing Design of Hydroxychloroquine for the Treatment of Severe Acute Respiratory Syndrome Coronavirus 2 (SARS-CoV-2). *Clin. Infect. Dis.* **2020**, *71*, 732–739. [CrossRef]
8. Sinha, S.; Rosin, N.L.; Arora, R.; Labit, E.; Jaffer, A.; Cao, L.; Farias, R.; Nguyen, A.P.; de Almeida, L.G.N.; Dufour, A.; et al. Dexamethasone Modulates Immature Neutrophils and Interferon Programming in Severe COVID-19. *Nat. Med.* **2022**, *28*, 201–211. [CrossRef]
9. Wei, Q.; Lin, H.; Wei, R.-G.; Chen, N.; He, F.; Zou, D.-H.; Wei, J.-R. Tocilizumab Treatment for COVID-19 Patients: A Systematic Review and Meta-Analysis. *Infect. Dis. Poverty* **2021**, *10*, 71. [CrossRef]

10. Kokkotis, G.; Kitsou, K.; Xynogalas, I.; Spoulou, V.; Magiorkinis, G.; Trontzas, I.; Trontzas, P.; Poulakou, G.; Syrigos, K.; Bamias, G. Systematic Review with Meta-Analysis: COVID-19 Outcomes in Patients Receiving Anti-TNF Treatments. *Aliment. Pharmacol. Ther.* **2022**, *55*, 154–167. [CrossRef] [PubMed]
11. Mukusheva, Z.; Assylbekova, M.; Poddighe, D. Management of pediatric rheumatic patients in Kazakhstan during the coronavirus disease 2019 (COVID-19) pandemic. *Rheumatol. Int.* **2020**, *40*, 1351–1352. [CrossRef]
12. Battakova, Z.; Imasheva, B.; Slazhneva, T.; Imashev, M.; Beloussov, V.; Pignatelli, M.; Tursynkhan, A.; Askarov, A.; Abdrakhmanova, S.; Adayeva, A.; et al. Public Health Response Measures for COVID-19 in Kazakhstan. *Disaster Med. Public Health Prep.* **2023**, *17*, e524. [CrossRef] [PubMed]
13. Agency for Strategic Planning and Reforms of the Republic of Kazakhstan Bureau of National Statistics—Main. Available online: https://stat.gov.kz/en/ (accessed on 29 June 2024).
14. Balakrishnan, V.S. COVID-19 response in central Asia. *Lancet Microbe* **2020**, *1*, e281. [CrossRef] [PubMed] [PubMed Central]
15. Rutskaya-Moroshan, K.; Abisheva, S.; Sarsenova, M.; Ogay, V.; Vinnik, T.; Aubakirova, B.; Abisheva, A. Autoimmune Rheumatic Diseases and COVID-19 Vaccination: A Retrospective Cross-Sectional Study from Astana. *Reumatologia* **2024**, *62*, 26–34. [CrossRef] [PubMed]
16. Wang, Q.; Liu, J.; Shao, R.; Han, X.; Su, C.; Lu, W. Risk and clinical outcomes of COVID-19 in patients with rheumatic diseases compared with the general population: A systematic review and meta-analysis. *Rheumatol. Int.* **2021**, *41*, 851–861. [CrossRef] [PubMed] [PubMed Central]
17. Mahendra, M.; Nuchin, A.; Kumar, R.; Shreedhar, S.; Mahesh, P.A. Predictors of mortality in patients with severe COVID-19 pneumonia—A retrospective study. *Adv. Respir. Med.* **2021**, *89*, 135–144. [CrossRef]
18. Wu, Z.; McGoogan, J.M. Characteristics of and Important Lessons From the Coronavirus Disease 2019 (COVID-19) Outbreak in China: Summary of a Report of 72 314 Cases From the Chinese Center for Disease Control and Prevention. *JAMA* **2020**, *323*, 1239–1242. [CrossRef]
19. Flook, M.; Jackson, C.; Vasileiou, E.; Simpson, C.R.; Muckian, M.D.; Agrawal, U.; McCowan, C.; Jia, Y.; Murray, J.L.K.; Ritchie, L.D.; et al. Informing the public health response to COVID-19: A systematic review of risk factors for disease, severity, and mortality. *BMC Infect. Dis.* **2021**, *21*, 342. [CrossRef]
20. Kelsey, J.L.; Evans, A.S.; Alice, S. *Methods in Observational Epidemiology*, 2nd ed.; Oxford University Press: Oxford, UK, 1996.
21. *Fleiss, Statistical Methods for Rates and Proportions, Formulas 3.18 &3.19*; John Wiley & Sons: Hoboken, NJ, USA, 2003.
22. Wang, F.; Ma, Y.; Xu, S.; Liu, H.; Chen, Y.; Yang, H.; Shao, M.; Xu, W.; Kong, J.; Chen, L.; et al. Prevalence and risk of COVID-19 in patients with rheumatic diseases: A systematic review and meta-analysis. *Clin. Rheumatol.* **2022**, *41*, 2213–2223. [CrossRef]
23. Lu, W.; Chen, X.; Ho, D.C.W.; Wang, H. Autoimmune inflammatory rheumatic diseases and COVID-19 outcomes in South Korea: A nationwide cohort study. *Lancet Rheumatol.* **2021**, *3*, e698–e706. [CrossRef]
24. Xu, C.; Yi, Z.; Cai, R.; Chen, R.; Thong, B.Y.; Mu, R. Clinical outcomes of COVID-19 in patients with rheumatic diseases: A systematic review and meta-analysis of global data. *Autoimmun. Rev.* **2021**, *20*, 102778. [CrossRef]
25. Liu, M.; Gao, Y.; Zhang, Y.; Shi, S.; Chen, Y.; Tian, J. The association between severe or dead COVID-19 and autoimmune diseases: A systematic review and meta analysis. *J. Infect.* **2020**, *81*, e93–e95. [CrossRef] [PubMed]
26. Horwitz, D.A.; Fahmy, T.M.; Piccirillo, C.A.; La Cava, A. Rebalancing Immune Homeostasis to Treat Autoimmune Diseases. *Trends Immunol.* **2019**, *40*, 888–908. [CrossRef] [PubMed]
27. Dadras, O.; Afsahi, A.M.; Pashaei, Z.; Mojdeganlou, H.; Karimi, A.; Habibi, P.; Barzegary, A.; Fakhfouri, A.; Mirzapour, P.; Janfaza, N.; et al. The relationship between COVID-19 viral load and disease severity: A systematic review. *Immun. Inflamm. Dis.* **2022**, *10*, e580. [CrossRef] [PubMed]
28. Zhong, J.; Shen, G.; Yang, H.; Huang, A.; Chen, X.; Dong, L.; Wu, B.; Zhang, A.; Su, L.; Hou, X.; et al. COVID-19 in patients with rheumatic disease in Hubei province, China: A multicentre retrospective observational study. *Lancet Rheumatol.* **2020**, *2*, e557–e564. [CrossRef]
29. Strangfeld, A.; Schäfer, M.; Gianfrancesco, M.A.; Lawson-Tovey, S.; Liew, J.W.; Ljung, L.; Mateus, E.F.; Richez, C.; Santos, M.J.; Schmajuk, G.; et al. Factors associated with COVID-19-related death in people with rheumatic diseases: Results from the COVID-19 Global Rheumatology Alliance physician-reported registry. *Ann. Rheum. Dis.* **2021**, *80*, 930–942. [CrossRef] [PubMed] [PubMed Central]
30. Conway, R.; Grimshaw, A.; Konig, M.; Putman, M.; Duarte-García, A.; Tseng, L.; Cabrera, D.; Chock, Y.; Degirmenci, H.; Duff, E.; et al. SARS-CoV-2 Infection and COVID-19 Outcomes in Rheumatic Diseases: A Systematic Literature Review and Meta-Analysis. *Arthritis Rheumatol.* **2022**, *74*, 766–775. [CrossRef] [PubMed] [PubMed Central]
31. Gastelum-Strozzi, A.; Pascual, V.; Hernández-Garduño, A.; Moctezuma-Rios, J.F.; Guaracha-Basañez, G.A.; Sotelo, T.; Garcia-Garcia, C.; Contreras-Yañez, I.; Álvarez-Hernández, E.; Infante-Castañeda, C.; et al. Perception of risk and impact of the COVID-19 pandemic on patients with rheumatic diseases: A case-control study. *Clin. Rheumatol.* **2022**, *41*, 3211–3218. [CrossRef]
32. Outcomes Following SARS-CoV-2 Infection in Individuals with and without Inflammatory Rheumatic Diseases: A Danish Nationwide Cohort Study | Annals of the Rheumatic Diseases. Available online: https://ard.bmj.com/content/82/10/1359 (accessed on 29 June 2024).
33. Rorat, M.; Zarębska-Michaluk, D.; Kowalska, J.; Kujawa, K.; Rogalska, M.; Kozielewicz, D.; Lorenc, B.; Sikorska, K.; Czupryna, P.; Bolewska, B.; et al. The Course of COVID-19 in Patients with Systemic Autoimmune Rheumatic Diseases. *J. Clin. Med.* **2022**, *11*, 7342. [CrossRef]

34. Pablos, J.L.; Galindo, M.; Carmona, L.; Lledó, A.; Retuerto, M.; Blanco, R.; Gonzalez-Gay, M.A.; Martinez-Lopez, D.; Castrejón, I.; Alvaro-Gracia, J.M.; et al. Clinical Outcomes of Hospitalised Patients with COVID-19 and Chronic Inflammatory and Autoimmune Rheumatic Diseases: A Multicentric Matched Cohort Study. *Ann. Rheum. Dis.* **2020**, *79*, 1544–1549. [CrossRef]
35. Kastritis, E.; Kitas, G.D.; Vassilopoulos, D.; Giannopoulos, G.; Dimopoulos, M.A.; Sfikakis, P.P. Systemic Autoimmune Diseases, Anti-Rheumatic Therapies, COVID-19 Infection Risk and Patient Outcomes. *Rheumatol. Int.* **2020**, *40*, 1353–1360. [CrossRef]
36. Mikuls, T.R.; Johnson, S.R.; Fraenkel, L.; Arasaratnam, R.J.; Baden, L.R.; Bermas, B.L.; Chatham, W.; Cohen, S.; Costenbader, K.; Gravallese, E.M.; et al. American College of Rheumatology Guidance for the Management of Rheumatic Disease in Adult Patients During the COVID-19 Pandemic: Version 2. *Arthritis Rheumatol.* **2020**, *72*, e1–e12. [CrossRef] [PubMed]
37. Nas, K.; Güçlü, E.; Keskin, Y.; Dilek, G.; Kalçık Unan, M.; Can, N.; Tekeoğlu, İ.; Kamanlı, A. Clinical Course and Prognostic Factors of COVID-19 Infection in Patients with Chronic Inflammatory-Rheumatic Disease: A Retrospective, Case-Control Study. *Arch. Rheumatol.* **2023**, *38*, 44–55. [CrossRef]
38. Robinson, P.C.; Yazdany, J. The COVID-19 Global Rheumatology Alliance: Collecting data in a pandemic. *Nat. Rev. Rheumatol.* **2020**, *16*, 293–294. [CrossRef] [PubMed]
39. Hamming, I.; Timens, W.; Bulthuis, M.L.C.; Lely, A.T.; Navis, G.J.; van Goor, H. Tissue distribution of ACE2 protein, the functional receptor for SARS coronavirus. A first step in understanding SARS pathogenesis. *J. Pathol.* **2004**, *203*, 631–637. [CrossRef]
40. Rodriguez-Perez, A.I.; Labandeira, C.M.; Pedrosa, M.A.; Valenzuela, R.; Suarez-Quintanilla, J.A.; Cortes-Ayaso, M.; Mayán-Conesa, P.; Labandeira-Garcia, J.L. Autoantibodies against ACE2 and angiotensin type-1 receptors increase severity of COVID-19. *J. Autoimmun.* **2021**, *122*, 102683. [CrossRef] [PubMed]
41. Briquez, P.S.; Rouhani, S.J.; Yu, J.; Pyzer, A.R.; Trujillo, J.; Dugan, H.L.; Stamper, C.T.; Changrob, S.; Sperling, A.I.; Wilson, P.C.; et al. Severe COVID-19 induces autoantibodies against angiotensin II that correlate with blood pressure dysregulation and disease severity. *Sci. Adv.* **2022**, *8*, eabn3777. [CrossRef] [PubMed]
42. Haberman, R.H.; Castillo, R.; Chen, A.; Yan, D.; Ramirez, D.; Sekar, V.; Lesser, R.; Solomon, G.; Neimann, A.L.; Blank, R.B.; et al. COVID-19 in Patients With Inflammatory Arthritis: A Prospective Study on the Effects of Comorbidities and Disease-Modifying Antirheumatic Drugs on Clinical Outcomes. *Arthritis Rheumatol.* **2020**, *72*, 1981–1989. [CrossRef]
43. Robinson, P.C.; Morand, E. Divergent Effects of Acute versus Chronic Glucocorticoids in COVID-19. *Lancet Rheumatol.* **2021**, *3*, e168–e170. [CrossRef]
44. Fonseca, D.L.M.; Filgueiras, I.S.; Marques, A.H.C.; Vojdani, E.; Halpert, G.; Ostrinski, Y.; Baiocchi, G.C.; Plaça, D.R.; Freire, P.P.; Pour, S.Z.; et al. Severe COVID-19 patients exhibit elevated levels of autoantibodies targeting cardiolipin and platelet glycoprotein with age: A systems biology approach. *NPJ Aging.* **2023**, *9*, 21. [CrossRef]
45. Watson, A.; Wilkinson, T.M.A. Respiratory viral infections in the elderly. *Ther. Adv. Respir. Dis.* **2021**, *15*, 1753466621995050. [CrossRef]
46. Li, J.; Huang, D.Q.; Zou, B.; Yang, H.; Hui, W.Z.; Rui, F.; Yee, N.T.S.; Liu, C.; Nerurkar, S.N.; Kai, J.C.Y.; et al. Epidemiology of COVID-19: A systematic review and meta-analysis of clinical characteristics, risk factors, and outcomes. *J. Med. Virol.* **2021**, *93*, 1449–1458. [CrossRef]
47. Pijls, B.G.; Jolani, S.; Atherley, A.; Derckx, R.T.; Dijkstra, J.I.R.; Franssen, G.H.L.; Hendriks, S.; Richters, A.; Venemans-Jellema, A.; Zalpuri, S.; et al. Demographic risk factors for COVID-19 infection, severity, ICU admission and death: A meta-analysis of 59 studies. *BMJ Open.* **2021**, *11*, e044640. [CrossRef]
48. Lassale, C.; Gaye, B.; Hamer, M.; Gale, C.R.; Batty, G.D. Ethnic disparities in hospitalisation for COVID-19 in England: The role of socioeconomic factors, mental health, and inflammatory and pro-inflammatory factors in a community-based cohort study. *Brain Behav. Immun.* **2020**, *88*, 44–49. [CrossRef] [PubMed]
49. Yan, B.; Ng, F.; Nguyen, T. High Mortality from COVID-19 among Asian Americans in San Francisco. Asian American Research Center on Health. 2020. Available online: https://scholar.google.com/citations?view_op=view_citation&hl=en&user=SbnK3p8AAAAJ&citation_for_view=SbnK3p8AAAAJ:eQOLeE2rZwMC (accessed on 20 April 2024).
50. Gianfrancesco, M.A.; Leykina, L.A.; Izadi, Z.; Taylor, T.; Sparks, J.A.; Harrison, C.; Trupin, L.; Rush, S.; Schmajuk, G.; Katz, P.; et al. Association of Race and Ethnicity With COVID-19 Outcomes in Rheumatic Disease: Data From the COVID-19 Global Rheumatology Alliance Physician Registry. *Arthritis Rheumatol.* **2021**, *73*, 374–380. [CrossRef] [PubMed] [PubMed Central]
51. Bruce, B.; Fries, J.F.; Murtagh, K.N. Health status disparities in ethnic minority patients with rheumatoid arthritis: A cross-sectional study. *J. Rheumatol.* **2007**, *34*, 1475–1479. [PubMed]
52. Greenberg, J.D.; Spruill, T.M.; Shan, Y.; Reed, G.; Kremer, J.M.; Potter, J.; Yazici, Y.; Ogedegbe, G.; Harrold, L.R. Racial and ethnic disparities in disease activity in patients with rheumatoid arthritis. *Am. J. Med.* **2013**, *126*, 1089–1098. [CrossRef]
53. FAI2R/SFR/SNFMI/SOFREMIP/CRI/IMIDIATE consortium and contributors. Severity of COVID-19 and survival in patients with rheumatic and inflammatory diseases: Data from the French RMD COVID-19 cohort of 694 patients. *Ann. Rheum. Dis.* **2021**, *80*, 527–538. [CrossRef] [PubMed]
54. Jones, J.M.; Faruqi, A.J.; Sullivan, J.K.; Calabrese, C.; Calabrese, L.H. COVID-19 Outcomes in Patients Undergoing B Cell Depletion Therapy and Those with Humoral Immunodeficiency States: A Scoping Review. *Pathog. Immun.* **2021**, *6*, 76–103. [CrossRef]
55. Loarce-Martos, J.; García-Fernández, A.; López-Gutiérrez, F.; García-García, V.; Calvo-Sanz, L.; del Bosque-Granero, I.; Terán-Tinedo, M.A.; Boteanu, A.; Bachiller-Corral, J.; Vázquez-Díaz, M. High Rates of Severe Disease and Death Due to SARS-CoV-2 Infection in Rheumatic Disease Patients Treated with Rituximab: A Descriptive Study. *Rheumatol. Int.* **2020**, *40*, 2015–2021. [CrossRef]

56. Tepasse, P.-R.; Hafezi, W.; Lutz, M.; Kühn, J.; Wilms, C.; Wiewrodt, R.; Sackarnd, J.; Keller, M.; Schmidt, H.H.; Vollenberg, R. Persisting SARS-CoV-2 Viraemia after Rituximab Therapy: Two Cases with Fatal Outcome and a Review of the Literature. *Br. J. Haematol.* **2020**, *190*, 185–188. [CrossRef]
57. Leipe, J.; Wilke, E.L.; Ebert, M.P.; Teufel, A.; Reindl, W. Long, Relapsing, and Atypical Symptomatic Course of COVID-19 in a B-Cell-Depleted Patient after Rituximab. *Semin. Arthritis Rheum.* **2020**, *50*, 1087–1088. [CrossRef] [PubMed]
58. McKeigue, P.M.; Porter, D.; Hollick, R.J.; Ralston, S.H.; McAllister, D.A.; Colhoun, H.M. Risk of Severe COVID-19 in Patients with Inflammatory Rheumatic Diseases Treated with Immunosuppressive Therapy in Scotland. *Scand. J. Rheumatol.* **2023**, *52*, 412–417. [CrossRef]
59. Gao, Y.-D.; Ding, M.; Dong, X.; Zhang, J.-J.; Kursat Azkur, A.; Azkur, D.; Gan, H.; Sun, Y.-L.; Fu, W.; Li, W.; et al. Risk Factors for Severe and Critically Ill COVID-19 Patients: A Review. *Allergy* **2021**, *76*, 428–455. [CrossRef] [PubMed]
60. RECOVERY Collaborative Group; Horby, P.; Lim, W.S.; Emberson, J.R.; Mafham, M.; Bell, J.L.; Linsell, L.; Staplin, N.; Brightling, C.; Ustianowski, A.; et al. Dexamethasone in Hospitalized Patients with COVID-19. *N. Engl. J. Med.* **2021**, *384*, 693–704. [CrossRef]

medicina

MDPI

Article

An Exploration of Self-Efficacy and Its Associated Factors among Rheumatoid Arthritis Patients in Taiwan

I-Yu Hsiao [1,2,3,†], Hanoch Livneh [4,†], Wei-Jen Chen [5,6,7,8,†], Ming-Chi Lu [3,9,*] and Tzung-Yi Tsai [10,11,*]

1 Department of Nursing, Dalin Tzu Chi Hospital, Buddhist Tzu Chi Medical Foundation, Chiayi 62247, Taiwan; df383346@tzuchi.com.tw
2 Department of Psychology, National Chung Cheng University, Chiayi 621301, Taiwan
3 Division of Allergy, Immunology and Rheumatology, Dalin Tzu Chi Hospital, Buddhist Tzu Chi Medical Foundation, Chiayi 62247, Taiwan
4 Rehabilitation Counseling Program, Portland State University, Portland, OR 97207-0751, USA; livnehh@pdx.edu
5 Department of Chinese Medicine, Dalin Tzuchi Hospital, Buddhist Tzu Chi Medical Foundation, Chiayi 62247, Taiwan; tough2915@hotmail.com
6 Graduate Institute of Sports Science, National Taiwan Sport University, Taoyuan 333325, Taiwan
7 School of Post-Baccalaureate Chinese Medicine, Tzu Chi University, Hualien 97004, Taiwan
8 Center of Sports Medicine, Dalin Tzuchi Hospital, Buddhist Tzu Chi Medical Foundation, Chiayi 62247, Taiwan
9 School of Medicine, Tzu Chi University, Hualien 97004, Taiwan
10 Department of Environmental and Occupational Health, College of Medicine, National Cheng Kung University, Tainan 70428, Taiwan
11 Department of Medical Research, Dalin Tzu Chi Hospital, Buddhist Tzu Chi Medical Foundation, Chiayi 62247, Taiwan
* Correspondence: dm252940@tzuchi.com.tw (M.-C.L.); dm732024@tzuchi.com.tw (T.-Y.T.); Tel.: +886-5-2648000 (ext. 8713) (M.-C.L.); +886-5-2648000 (ext. 3209) (T.-Y.T.); Fax: +886-5-2648006 (M.-C.L. & T.-Y.T.)
† These authors contributed equally to this work.

Abstract: Self-efficacy is an important ingredient in successful disease management, especially in patients with chronic conditions such as rheumatoid arthritis (RA). However, the information on self-efficacy and its influencing factors among RA patients is scarce. This study investigated the level of self-efficacy and its pertinent predictors among RA patients in Taiwan. This cross-sectional study recruited patients with RA from a hospital in Taiwan between January and October 2023. A structured questionnaire was used to collect data on respondents' demographic and job characteristics and included a Chinese version of the Arthritis Self-Efficacy Scale (ASES). Multiple linear stepwise regression analysis was employed to identify predictors of self-efficacy. A total of 284 RA patients were enrolled during the study period. The mean ASES score among enrollees was 1607.1, indicating a moderate level of self-efficacy (score range of 200–2000). The regression model displayed that those with higher disease activity scores, Taiwanese Depression Questionnaire scores, fatigue level, shorter disease duration, swollen upper limb joints, and no regular exercise regimen reported lower ASES scores, accounted for 46% of the total variance. The study findings may be useful for healthcare providers in identifying RA patients with low self-efficacy attitudes, a trait that appears to be linked to several medical indicators, and thus facilitating the provision of future tailored healthcare regimens.

Keywords: self-efficacy; rheumatoid arthritis; arthritis self-efficacy scale; factors; Taiwan

1. Introduction

Rheumatoid arthritis (RA) is a chronic immune-mediated systemic disease that causes persistent joint inflammation. Because RA mainly affects persons of working age, this condition takes a heavy toll on physical functioning and work capacity [1]. Approximately 30% of the affected individuals become disabled within the first 3 years of RA onset, posing a high socioeconomic burden [2]. A recent study reports that the all-cause societal cost of RA annually is approximately USD 40 billion, and the per-capita healthcare costs for people with RA are equal to USD 20,919, triple that of those with no RA [3].

In addition to posing a profound economic burden, RA is a precursor of a wide array of comorbid conditions caused by chronic inflammation, including cancer, kidney dysfunction, lung disease, and cardiovascular disorder [4–7]. A recent study based on real-world data reports that the life expectancy of people with RA is 3–10 years shorter than the general population [8]. Successful adjustment to living with a debilitating chronic disorder, such as RA, requires that a patient possess sufficient knowledge, skills, and a positive attitude [9]. A concept developed by Albert Bandura's social cognitive theory, namely self-efficacy, represents an individual's belief in his or her capacity to effectively achieve specific performance attainments [10]. Since then, this concept has been viewed as a cornerstone in the field for managing chronic disease. Accumulating evidence these days shows that the higher the level of self-efficacy, the better a patient copes with the impact of a chronic illness [11,12]. One observational study of 3266 arthritis patients reports that baseline self-efficacy level significantly correlated with a higher frequency of physical activity per week and a lower self-reported pain level [13]. Hence, the rationale behind self-efficacy-based educational interventions can substantially improve individual self-management routines, which in turn would assist patients in coping successfully with subsequent manifestations of this disease [14,15]. On top of that, the topic of self-efficacy has been discussed and viewed as a priority in the recent recommendations by the European Alliance of Associations for Rheumatology (EULAR) for the management of inflammatory arthritis, as it profoundly boosts individual treatment adherence [16]. Therefore, to enable the use of tailored strategies geared at preventing or lessening the likelihood of poor prognosis, targeted assessment of self-efficacy among people with RA is of outmost importance.

Today, the global prevalence of persons living with RA is increasing. Based on the estimation from one recent review, the annual incidence of RA is 20–50 per 100,000 persons in European countries [17]; likewise, RA affects 0.6% to 1% of the adult population in the USA, with an incidence of 44 per 100,000 US adults per year [18]. In Taiwan, the estimated number per 100,000 persons living with RA has arisen from 57.7 in 2000 to 99.6 in 2007, with an increase of 73% [19]. In such a case, the majority of existing literature in Taiwanese rheumatology cohorts still focuses on epidemiological surveys [20], nursing interventions [21], and assessment of complementary therapies, like herbals and acupuncture [22,23]. Thus far, very few studies have explored the role of self-efficacy among RA patients, thus hampering the provision of appropriate rehabilitation at an early stage of the condition. To minimize this gap, the purpose of this study was to explore the self-efficacy and its associated factors among RA patients in Taiwan, with the goal of securing findings that could serve in helping patients to cope with and manage the sequelae of RA.

2. Materials and Methods

2.1. Study Design and Subjects

This cross-sectional study was conducted at a teaching hospital in Taiwan. Participants who visited the clinic of rheumatology and immunology between January and October 2023 were enrolled. The study cohort included persons who were: (1) over 20 years of age; (2) able to effectively express their opinions using oral and written communication skills; (3) able to speak Mandarin or Taiwanese; and (4) having RA diagnosis for more than 3 months and made by the rheumatologist in the target hospital using the 2010 classification criteria established by the American College of Rheumatology and the European League Against Rheumatism (EULAR) [24,25]. The excluded criteria included the following: having a serious cognitive impairment or disconinuning the participation at any phase of this study. The sample size needed in this survey was established by Cohen's methodology [26], where á was set to 0.05, power was set to 0.8, and the effect size was set to 0.15. In accordance with the aforesaid indices and the considerations of multivariate linear regression analysis and the number of predictors involved, a sample of at least 82 subjects was required for this investigation via G-POWER 3.1 analytical software (Heinrich Heine University, Dusseldorf, Germany).

2.2. Assessments

Patients' data were collected using the Chinese version of the Arthritis Self-Efficacy Scale (ASES) and an additional questionnaire that contained information on demographic and disease features. The ASES, developed by Lorig and colleagues in the late 1980s [27], assesses and classifies pain (5 items), physical function (9 items), and other symptoms (6 items), all of which are used to determine perceived self-efficacy during the past month. using the aforesaid domains. Respondents rank each item out of the total 20 items on a ten-point scale classification, ranging from 10 (very uncertain) to 100 (very certain), and overall scores are obtained by summing the scores for all answers, with higher scores indicating higher self-efficacy [27]. As of now, the scale has been so far proven acceptably reliable and valid for measuring self-efficacy across the rheumatic disease spectrum [11].

ASES has been translated into Chinese by Tsai and colleagues among Taiwanese patients with rheumatic diseases. They examined the validity of the Chinese version of ASES by comparing results with those of the Taiwanese Depression Questionnaire (TDQ) and reported a significant negative correlation coefficient of -0.69 ($p < 0.01$) [28]. In addition, they used principal factor analysis on data obtained from 258 rheumatology patients to assess the construct validity of the Chinese version of ASES. After using the Kaiser–Meyer–Olkin index, they applied principal component analysis with orthogonal rotations to extract three factors from these 20 items based on an eigenvalue greater than 1.0 and factor loading greater than 0.4; each item loaded on the 3 domains as expected, with 59.78% of the total variance explained. As for overall internal consistency, the findings showed Cronbach's alpha coefficients of 0.82, 0.84, and 0.89 for pain, other symptoms, and physical function, respectively [28]. Cronbach's alpha for the Chinese version of ASES was 0.94 in the current study.

The second part of the questionnaire contained information on demographic and disease characteristics, all of which were extracted from previous studies and clinical experience [29]. The demographic data collected included sex, age, marital status, education, monthly income, living status, religion, and lifestyle factors including smoking and exercising. Those who responded "currently" or "yes/past" to smoking were classified as smokers. Regular exercisers were defined if the subjects exercised for at least 20 min thrice weekly, including running, walking, stair climbing, swimming or cycling, etc. The disease characteristics included the accompanying chronic diseases (diabetes mellitus, hypertension, heart disease, stroke, or cancer), disease activity score in 28 joints (DAS28), duration of RA, body mass index (BMI), self-rating fatigue level, and depressive symptoms as assessed by the visual analog scale (0–10 scale) and TDQ, respectively. Additionally, the prescriptions of biological disease-modifying anti-rheumatic drugs (DMARDs) covered etanercept, adalimumab, infliximab, or rituximab. Participants were asked if they had ever taken biological DMARDs for more than 3 months after RA onset. All of the aforesaid clinical characteristics were confirmed by chart review.

2.3. Data Gathering Procedure

To safeguard enrollees' rights, the researchers explained the purpose of this study and its procedures. Informed consent was obtained after subjects understood and agreed to take part in this survey. During the survey administration period, the researchers were available to answer any inquiries regarding the questionnaires. Those who were unable to complete the questionnaires in the allotted time were given the questionnaires and a pre-stamped addressed envelope to take home and were asked to return them within one week. To ensure patients' anonymity, the questionnaires were returned with no identifying information on them. Throughout the study period, subjects had the option to withdraw from the study at any time. Before commencement of this study, approval was given by the Ethics Committee and Scientific Council of the Buddhist Dalin Tzu Chi Hospital on January 2023 (No. B11201014).

2.4. Data Analysis

All study variables were obtained during the initial entry into this study. The data normality was evaluated using the Kolmogorov–Smirnov criteria ($p > 0.05$ for all variables) and Q-Q normality plots. The data for all variables were reasonably normally distributed, allowing for analysis using parametric methods. Baseline characteristics are reported as the mean ± standard deviation (SD) for continuous variables and frequencies and percentages for categorical variables. Thereafter, the independent t test, analysis of variance (ANOVA), and Pearson correlation were used to analyze the bivariate relationships between baseline data and self-efficacy level. When applying ANOVA, a subsequent post hoc test with the Bonferroni procedure was performed for multiple comparisons. Variables that correlated significantly with the criterion measure (ASES scores) were entered into multiple linear stepwise regression analysis to determine significant predictors of self-efficacy. Meanwhile, to identify possible multicollinearity across self-efficacy predictive variables, we conducted collinearity analysis with the variance inflation factor (VIF) before conducting multiple regression analysis. Assumptions of normality, linearity, and homoscedasticity were tested as well. All analyses were conducted using SAS version 9.3 (SAS Institute Inc., Cary, NC, USA), and a p-value below 0.05 was considered statistically significant.

3. Results

3.1. Demographic Data and Disease Characteristics

Of the eligible subjects who were initially recruited as participants, a total of 284 questionnaires were returned within the study period. The mean age for the recruited patients was 54.1 years (SD = 15.4). The majority were females (78.9%), married (80.3%), had a lower educational level (below 9th grade) (54.2%), and were cohabitating (87.3%). More than two-thirds of the enrollees had a monthly income of ≤30,000 New Taiwan dollars (NTD) (70.1%) and reported having other concurrent comorbidities (60.9%). Slightly less than half reported regular exercising routines (48.2%), and approximately 80% were non-smokers. The mean TDQ in this group was 15.3 (SD = 9.1). The mean duration of RA was 9.7 years (SD, 5.6), and the average BMI, fatigue, and DAS28 were 24.1 (SD = 4.5), 3.3 (SD = 2.1), and 3.5 (SD = 1.3), respectively (Table 1).

Table 1. Demographic data and disease characteristics (N = 284).

Variables	Mean ± SD	*n* (%)
Demographic data		
Gender		
Male		60 (21.1)
Female		224 (78.9)
Marital status		
Single		56 (19.7)
Married		228 (80.3)
Educational level		
Low (below junior college)		154 (54.2)
High (above junior college)		130 (45.8)
Monthly income		
≤NTD 30,000 *		199 (70.1)
≥NTD 30,001		85 (29.9)
Living status		
Living alone		36 (12.7)
Cohabitating		248 (87.3)

Table 1. *Cont.*

Variables	Mean ± SD	n (%)
Cigarette smoking		
Yes		58 (20.4)
No		226 (79.6)
Regular exercise		
Yes		147 (51.8)
No		137 (48.2)
Age (years)	54.1 ± 15.4	
Disease characteristics		
Disease duration (years)	9.7 ± 5.6	
Swollen joint site		
Upper limbs		149 (52.5)
Lower limbs		120 (42.3)
Both		15 (5.2)
Comorbidity		
Yes		173 (60.9)
No		111 (39.1)
Biological agents		
Yes		169 (59.5)
No		115 (40.5)
BMI	24.1 ± 4.5	
DAS28	3.5 ± 1.3	
Fatigue	3.3 ± 2.1	
TDQ	15.3 ± 9.1	

BMI: body mass index; DAS28: disease activity score in 28 joints; TDQ: Taiwanese Depression Questionnaire; NTD: New Taiwan dollar; * USD 1 = 32.19 at the study period.

3.2. ASES Subscale Scores

The mean ASES score was 1607.1 (SD = 337.56). Likewise, the subscales of ASES are shown in Table 2 as well. We noted that "physical function subscale" had the highest standardized score, followed by "other symptoms subscale" and "pain subscale", with scores of 89.0, 79.6, and 65.6, respectively.

Table 2. Mean and SD of the three ASES subscale scores (N = 284).

Dimension	Mean	SD	Standardized Score (1)	Rank
Physical function (90–900)	801.4	145.1	89.0	1
Other symptoms (60–600)	477.4	129.4	79.6	2
Pain (50–500)	328.2	126.1	65.6	3
Total score (200–2000)	1607.1	337.6		

SD: standard deviation. (1) Standardized scores: mean ÷ total score × 100%.

3.3. Correlations among Demographic Data, Disease Characteristics, and ASES Scores

Regarding the correlation analysis results, we noted that those engaging in regular exercise had higher self-efficacy (t, −3.45; $p < 0.001$) (Table 3). Most of the measured disease characteristics correlated with the ASES score, with the exception of comorbid conditions and the use of biological agents. For example, disease duration (r, −0.43; $p < 0.001$), swollen joint site (F, 38.34; $p < 0.001$), DAS28 (r, −0.45; $p < 0.001$), fatigue (r, −0.35; $p < 0.001$), and TDQ score (r, −0.42; $p < 0.001$) all correlated negatively with ASES scores (Table 4).

We observed a positive correlation between RA duration and the ASES score, suggesting that those with a longer disease duration since RA onset reported greater self-efficacy. We further analyzed this correlation using disease duration stratified into three time periods: ≤3 years, 4–7 years, and >7 years. The mean ASES scores for the three-time frames were 1260.26 (SD = 358.47), 1512.53 (SD = 412.66), and 1712.53 (SD = 233.79), respectively (test for trend, $p < 0.05$) (Figure 1).

Table 3. Comparison of ASES by participants' baseline characteristics (N = 284).

	ASES Score			
	Mean	**SD**	***p***	**Bonferroni**
Demographic data				
Gender				
Male	1668.25	369.91	0.11 [a]	
Female	1590.53	328.63		
Marital status				
Single	1565.35	343.31	0.31 [a]	
Married	1617.16	337.38		
Educational level				
Low (below junior college)	1584.28	353.08	0.31 [a]	
High (above junior college)	1617.16	319.83		
Monthly income				
≤NTD 30,000	1590.07	349.97	0.20 [a]	
≥NTD 30,001	1646.45	308.66		
Living status				
Living alone	1533.90	297.49	0.17 [a]	
Cohabitating	1617.55	343.39		
Cigarette smoking				
Yes	1639.44	384.16	0.54 [a]	
No	1602.23	332.05		
Regular exercise				
Yes	1673.08	301.72	0.001 [a]	
No	1535.99	361.99		
Age (years)			0.73 [b]	
Disease characteristics				
Disease duration (years)			0.001 [b]	
Swollen joint site				
① Upper limbs	1466.04	348.76		① > ③, ①
② Lower limbs	1785.36	227.34	<0.001 [c]	③ > ①
③ Both	1579.33	327.45		
Comorbidity				
Yes	1587.72	350.61	0.80 [a]	
No	1637.38	318.01		
Biological agents				
Yes	1617.88	307.43	0.88 [a]	
No	1590.21	380.19		
BMI			0.09 [b]	
DAS28			<0.001 [b]	
Fatigue			<0.001 [b]	
TDQ			<0.001 [b]	

ASES: Arthritis Self-Efficacy Scale; SD: standard deviation; BMI: body mass index; DAS28: disease activity score in 28 joints; TDQ: Taiwanese Depression Questionnaire; NTD: New Taiwan dollar. [a] By independent *t* test; [b] by Pearson correlation; [c] by ANOVA test.

Table 4. Multiple stepwise regression analysis predicting ASES scores among RA patients (N = 284).

	Standardized Coefficient *	Unstandardized Coefficient	Adjusted R^2	*p*	VIF	95% Confidence Interval
DAS28 score	−0.23	−55.47	0.20	<0.001	1.14	−79.42–−31.82
Swollen joint site (Upper limbs)	−0.32	−67.97	0.30	<0.001	1.09	−99.71–−43.22
TDQ score	−0.20	−3.51	0.38	<0.001	1.19	−7.27–−0.59
Regular exercise (Yes)	0.14	86.17	0.41	0.004	1.02	32.16–112.19
Fatigue	−0.18	−23.66	0.44	0.004	1.12	−35.66–−16.69
Disease duration	0.20	88.42	0.46	0.003	1.01	67.38–107.46

DAS28: disease activity score in 28 joints; TDQ: Taiwanese Depression Questionnaire; VIF: variance inflation factor. * Positive values indicate a higher level of self-efficacy.

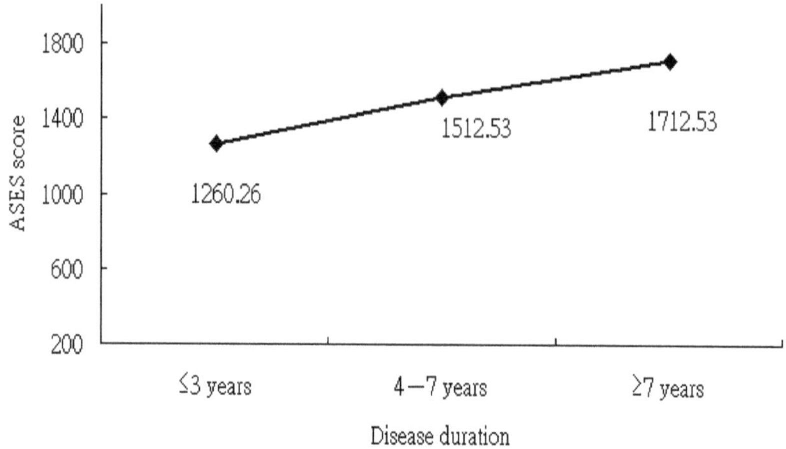

Figure 1. ASES score vs. disease duration of having RA. ASES: Arthritis Self-Efficacy Scale; RA: rheumatoid arthritis.

3.4. Determination of Factors Contributing to Self-Efficacy Using Multiple Linear Stepwise Regression

After fitting multiple linear stepwise regression analysis, we identified six variables that correlated with the ASES score among RA enrollees: DAS28 score, TDQ score, fatigue level, disease duration, swollen joint site, and regular exercise or not, all of which jointly accounted for 46% of the ASES score variance (Table 4). RA patients with higher scores for DAS28, TDQ, and fatigue and those with a shorter disease duration exhibited lower self-efficacy. In addition, those who did not engage in regular exercise and those with swollen upper limbs tended to report a lower level of self-efficacy.

4. Discussion

Robust self-efficacy in patients may improve clinical prognoses for RA persons [12]. It is believed that lower levels of self-efficacy may hamper any advances of modern disease-modifying treatments [15]. Thus, the importance of timely assessment of self-efficacy among RA patients cannot be over-emphasized. To date, only a few studies have explored self-efficacy and its contributing factors among RA patients. A key finding from this study showed that the predictors of RA patients' self-efficacy included those with swollen upper limb joints, higher levels of fatigue, TDQ and DAS28 scores, engaging in limited exercise regimens, and shorter disease duration, all of which explained 46% of ASES variance. These findings can help health professionals learn more about these patients. Additionally, it may serve as a reference for developing individualized strategies to help RA persons cope with the accompanying clinical manifestations.

We observed in this study that RA subjects with swollen upper limbs reported lower self-efficacy. Previous studies have not investigated ASES scores with respect to specific sites of swollen joints, making direct comparison to previous results difficult. Nevertheless, our results corroborate the findings of Walker–Bone, who showed that upper limb impairments were common among those coping with musculoskeletal disorders [30]. We speculate that RA patients with swollen upper limbs were more likely to experience difficulty in carrying out activities of daily living, such as feeding, bathing, dressing, and answering the phone, thereby decreasing their perceived self-efficacy [31]. In addition to conventional anti-arthritic treatments, rehabilitation interventions have shown the potential to restore functional independence to RA patients [32]. For example, hydrotherapy, a *water-based* therapeutic regimen, has been shown to substantially reduce pain and improve wrist range of motion ($p < 0.01$) [33]. Therefore, adding individually tailored rehabilitation regimens to routine care for RA patients should be considered, especially for those who grapple with severe upper limb swelling.

In addition, we noted that symptoms of depression and fatigue also correlated with lower ASES scores. This result appears to echo the concept of metacognitive therapy, which addresses the emergence of interoceptive experience of dishomeostasis throughout the body, also affecting brain functioning through immersion in distressing thoughts and feelings, which consequently act to aggravate disorder-specific negative aspects [34,35], thus abating self-efficacy motivation. Of particular importance is that these negative psychological factors often co-occur with RA [20,36]. Notably, one former study further indicated that depression may mediate the association of self-efficacy with the self-care behaviors among diabetic patients [37]. Accordingly, prior to instituting interventions to improve self-efficacy, it is recommended to have patients referred to the mental health professional for screening of psychological difficulties, including symptoms of depression and fatigue.

Findings from the present study also indicate that individuals who do not exercise regularly may experience lower self-efficacy. A similar association between exercise and self-efficacy level was reported in previous studies of people with and without associated medical conditions [38,39]. We suggest several potential reasons why exercising regularly could be associated with self-efficacy, as observed in our patient cohort. First, accumulating research shows that exercise promotes the release of endorphins, neuropeptides that aid in coping with psychological stress and cognitive function [40], which in turn enhance self-efficacy to some extent. Second, participation in group exercise classes or active hobbies with friends may provide subjects with additional benefits, such as allowing them to socialize and share meaningful moments during the exercise period, thereby encouraging them to seek out further activities that boost self-efficacy.

In our study cohort, we observed that the higher DAS28 scores markedly pertained to the ASES score; this result is in agreement with previous research findings [41,42]. In clinical practice, DAS28 is a widely adopted indicator for disease activity in RA groups, where higher values are indicative of higher disease activity. In this scenario, RA persons with higher DAS28 may experience increased peripheral joint involvement that could hamper their daily activities and, therefore, heighten their doubts about self-capability. Additionally, the duration of RA correlated positively with ASES scores. This finding is consistent with that of a previous study of self-efficacy in patients with other chronic diseases [43]. We infer that RA patients with longer disease duration have gradually learned to accept the consequences and future implications of their disability, and this may have led to higher self-efficacy. Notably, patients in our study whose RA duration was $\leq$3 years reported the lowest level of ASES. For this reason, healthcare providers should pay attention to newly diagnosed RA patients through the establishment of a multidisciplinary care program for evaluating patients' psychophysical status to facilitate early referral for further therapeutic interventions.

While our study is the first to investigate self-efficacy among RA patients, the implications of the results must be considered in light of the following limitations: First, the current analysis was based on a cohort of patients at a single hospital. Although it is not unusual for study conclusions to be drawn from arbitrarily selected cohorts, a potential non-representative cohort might have introduced bias that limits the generalizability of findings to other populations and settings. Similar studies should be conducted with diverse cohorts to determine whether our findings are replicated with different demographic and geographic groups of patients with rheumatologic disorders. Nevertheless, we deliberately determined the appropriate sample size based on the research objectives, the nature of the study, the statistical power required, and relevant factors considered. Second, the cross-sectional nature of this trial might hamper further interpretation regarding the causal directionality of the identified relationships. Third, other potential confounders such as smoking habits, laboratory tests, pain level, personality characteristics and traits, and family-related factors were not assessed and thus not controlled in this study. Further research confronting these issues is warranted. Fourth, the stability of ASES scores over time could be another informative topic of study that was not investigated here.

5. Conclusions

Self-efficacy is an important contributor to the healthy lives of RA persons, which may reinforce their motivation to engage in health promotion behaviors more frequently. Herein, we found a trend toward lower ASES scores among RA patients with higher DAS28 and TDQ scores, fatigue, shorter disease duration, swollen upper limb joints, and a lack of regular exercise regimen. As far as clinical practice is concerned, the healthcare providers may utilize the present results to clarify the groups of patients who potentially report low self-efficacy, especially among those with newly diagnosed RA for less than three years. Not only that, but the healthcare providers would also consider these findings as a reference for designing the program towards self-efficacy improvement for RA subjects. Ensuring that holistic healthcare is available to RA patients may be a critical step to help them better psychologically adapt to their disease and possibly as important as improving the survival rate of patients with this chronic and life-threatening disease.

Author Contributions: I.-Y.H. and W.-J.C. were responsible for data collection and provided comments on the manuscript drafts. M.-C.L., W.-J.C. and H.L. interpreted the data and provided comments on the final draft of the manuscript. T.-Y.T. was responsible for the study conception, design, data analysis, and drafting of the work. All authors have read and agreed to the published version of the manuscript.

Funding: This study was supported by Grant DTCRD112-I-21 from the Buddhist Dalin Tzu Chi Hospital.

Institutional Review Board Statement: This study was approved by the Institutional Ethics Review Board of Dalin Tzu Chi Hospital (No. B11201014). All patients provided written informed consent approved by the participating institutions.

Informed Consent Statement: Not applicable.

Data Availability Statement: Data are available upon reasonable request. The data involved and analyzed during the current work are available from the corresponding authors only on academic research request.

Acknowledgments: All authors thank the participants who responded to our survey. Hsiao I.-Y., Livneh H., and Chen W.-J. equally contributed to this study.

Conflicts of Interest: The authors declare no conflicts of interest.

References

1. Kirkeskov, L.; Bray, K. Employment of patients with rheumatoid arthritis—A systematic review and meta-analysis. *BMC Rheumatol.* **2023**, *7*, 41. [CrossRef]
2. Sokka, T. Work disability in early rheumatoid arthritis. *Clin. Exp. Rheumatol.* **2003**, *21*, S71–S74. [PubMed]
3. Chen, C.I.; Wang, L.; Wei, W.; Yuce, H.; Phillips, K. Burden of rheumatoid arthritis among US medicare population: Co-morbidities, health-care resource utilization and costs. *Rheumatol. Adv. Pract.* **2018**, *2*, I1–I9. [CrossRef] [PubMed]
4. Gabriel, S.; Michaud, K. Epidemiological studies in incidence, prevalence, mortality, and comorbidity of the rheumatic diseases. *Arthritis Res. Ther.* **2009**, *11*, 229. [CrossRef] [PubMed]
5. Innala, L.; Sjöberg, C.; Möller, B.; Ljung, L.; Smedby, T.; Södergren, A.; Magnusson, S.; Rantapää-Dahlqvist, S.; Wållberg-Jonsson, S. Co-morbidity in patients with early rheumatoid arthritis—Inflammation matters. *Arthritis Res. Ther.* **2016**, *18*, 33. [CrossRef]
6. Burska, A.; Boissinot, M.; Ponchel, F. Cytokines as biomarkers in rheumatoid arthritis. *Mediat. Inflamm.* **2014**, *2014*, 545493. [CrossRef]
7. Cook, M.J.; Bellou, E.; Bowes, J.; Sergeant, J.C.; O'Neill, T.W.; Barton, A.; Verstappen, S.M.M. The prevalence of co-morbidities and their impact on physical activity in people with inflammatory rheumatic diseases compared with the general population: Results from the UK Biobank. *Rheumatology* **2018**, *57*, 2172–2182. [CrossRef]
8. Chen, L.; Wu, B.; Mo, L.; Chen, H.; Zhao, Y.; Tan, T.; Chen, L.; Li, Y.; Yao, P.; Tang, Y. Associations between biological ageing and the risk of, genetic susceptibility to, and life expectancy associated with rheumatoid arthritis: A secondary analysis of two observational studies. *Lancet Healthy Longev.* **2024**, *5*, e45–e55. [CrossRef]

9. Ebrahimi Belil, F.; Alhani, F.; Ebadi, A.; Kazemnejad, A. Self-Efficacy of people with chronic conditions: A qualitative directed content analysis. *J. Clin. Med.* **2018**, *7*, 411. [CrossRef]
10. Bandura, A. Self-efficacy: Toward a unifying theory of behavioral change. *Psychol. Rev.* **1977**, *84*, 191–215. [CrossRef]
11. Primdahl, J.; Wagner, L.; Hørslev-Petersen, K. Self-efficacy as an outcome measure and its association with physical disease-related variables in persons with rheumatoid arthritis: A literature review. *Musculoskelet. Care* **2011**, *9*, 125–140. [CrossRef] [PubMed]
12. Garratt, A.M.; Løchting, I.; Smedslund, G.; Hagen, K.B. Measurement properties of instruments assessing self-efficacy in patients with rheumatic diseases. *Rheumatology* **2014**, *53*, 1161–1171. [CrossRef] [PubMed]
13. Degerstedt, Å.; Alinaghizadeh, H.; Thorstensson, C.A.; Olsson, C.B. High self-efficacy—A predictor of reduced pain and higher levels of physical activity among patients with osteoarthritis: An observational study. *BMC Musculoskelet. Disord.* **2020**, *21*, 380. [CrossRef] [PubMed]
14. Brady, T.J. Measures of self-efficacy: Arthritis Self-Efficacy Scale (ASES), Arthritis Self-Efficacy Scale-8 Item (ASES-8), Children's Arthritis Self-Efficacy Scale (CASE), Chronic Disease Self-Efficacy Scale (CDSES), Parent's Arthritis Self-Efficacy Scale (PASE), and Rheumatoid Arthritis Self-Efficacy Scale (RASE). *Arthritis Care Res.* **2011**, *63*, S473–S485. [CrossRef]
15. DiRenzo, D.; Finan, P. Self-Efficacy and the role of non-pharmacologic treatment strategies to improve pain and affect in arthritis. *Curr. Treat. Options Rheumatol.* **2019**, *5*, 168–178. [CrossRef]
16. Nikiphorou, E.; Santos, E.J.F.; Marques, A.; Böhm, P.; Bijlsma, J.W.; Daien, C.I.; Esbensen, B.A.; Ferreira, R.J.O.; Fragoulis, G.E.; Holmes, P.; et al. 2021 EULAR recommendations for the implementation of self-management strategies in patients with inflammatory arthritis. *Ann. Rheum. Dis.* **2021**, *80*, 1278–1285. [CrossRef] [PubMed]
17. Finckh, A.; Gilbert, B.; Hodkinson, B.; Bae, S.C.; Thomas, R.; Deane, K.D.; Alpizar-Rodriguez, D.; Lauper, K. Global epidemiology of rheumatoid arthritis. *Nat. Rev. Rheumatol.* **2022**, *18*, 591–602. [CrossRef]
18. Ye, D.; Mao, Y.; Xu, Y.; Xu, X.; Xie, Z.; Wen, C. Lifestyle factors associated with incidence of rheumatoid arthritis in US adults: Analysis of National Health and Nutrition Examination Survey database and meta-analysis. *BMJ Open* **2021**, *11*, e038137. [CrossRef]
19. Lai, C.; Lai, M.; Lai, K.; Chen, H.-H.; Chiu, Y.-M. Nationwide population-based epidemiologic study of rheumatoid arthritis in Taiwan. *Clin. Exp. Rheumatol.* **2012**, *30*, 358–363.
20. Lu, M.C.; Guo, H.R.; Lin, M.C.; Livneh, H.; Lai, N.S.; Tsai, T.Y. Bidirectional associations between rheumatoid arthritis and depression: A nationwide longitudinal study. *Sci. Rep.* **2016**, *6*, 20647. [CrossRef]
21. Lu, M.C.; Guo, H.R.; Livneh, H.; Lin, M.C.; Lai, N.S.; Tsai, T.Y. The effectiveness of nurse-led case management for patients with rheumatoid arthritis in Taiwan. *Int. J. Clin. Pract.* **2020**, *74*, e13443. [CrossRef] [PubMed]
22. Li, H.H.; Livneh, H.; Chen, W.J.; Fan, W.L.; Lu, M.C.; Guo, H.R.; Tsai, T.Y. Effect of Chinese herbal medicines on hearing loss risk in rheumatoid arthritis patients: Retrospective claims analysis. *Front. Med.* **2021**, *8*, 683211. [CrossRef] [PubMed]
23. Lu, M.C.; Livneh, H.; Yen, C.T.; Huang, H.L.; Lin, M.C.; Yen, S.W.; Lai, N.S.; Tsai, T.Y. Association of use of rehabilitation services with development of dementia among patients with rheumatoid arthritis: Analysis of domestic data in Taiwan. *Front. Med.* **2020**, *7*, 446. [CrossRef]
24. Aletaha, D.; Neogi, T.; Silman, A.J.; Funovits, J.; Felson, D.T.; Bingham, C.O., III; Birnbaum, N.S.; Burmester, G.R.; Bykerk, V.P.; Cohen, M.D.; et al. 2010 Rheumatoid arthritis classification criteria: An American College of Rheumatology/European League Against Rheumatism collaborative initiative. *Arthritis Rheum.* **2010**, *62*, 2569–2581. [CrossRef]
25. Kasturi, S.; Goldstein, B.L.; Malspeis, S.; Karlson, E.W.; Costenbader, K.H. Comparison of the 1987 American College of Rheumatology and the 2010 American College of Rheumatology/European League against Rheumatism criteria for classification of rheumatoid arthritis in the Nurses' Health Study cohorts. *Rheumatol. Int.* **2014**, *34*, 407–411. [CrossRef] [PubMed]
26. Cohen, J. Quantitative methods in psychology: A power primer. *Psychol. Bull.* **1992**, *112*, 155–159. [CrossRef]
27. Lorig, K.; Chastain, R.L.; Ung, E.; Shoor, S.; Holman, H.R. Development and evaluation of a scale to measure perceived self-efficacy in people with arthritis. *Arthritis Rheum.* **1989**, *32*, 37–44. [CrossRef]
28. Tsai, T.Y.; Lu, M.C.; Livneh, H.; Lin, M.C.; Lai, N.S.; Guo, H.R. Psychometric evaluation of the Arthritis Self-Efficacy Scale in Chinese adults with rheumatic diseases: A cross-sectional study. *BMJ Open* **2021**, *11*, e042014. [CrossRef]
29. Peters, M.; Potter, C.M.; Kelly, L.; Fitzpatrick, R. Self-efficacy and health-related quality of life: A cross-sectional study of primary care patients with multi-morbidity. *Health Qual. Life Outcomes* **2019**, *17*, 37. [CrossRef]
30. Walker-Bone, K.; Palmer, K.T.; Reading, I.; Coggon, D.; Cooper, C. Prevalence and impact of musculoskeletal disorders of the upper limb in the general population. *Arthritis Rheum.* **2004**, *51*, 642–651. [CrossRef]
31. Abdullahi, A.; Wong, T.W.L.; Ng, S.S.M. Variation in the rate of recovery in motor function between the upper and lower limbs in patients with stroke: Some proposed hypotheses and their implications for research and practice. *Front. Neurol.* **2023**, *14*, 1225924. [CrossRef] [PubMed]
32. Küçükdeveci, A.A. Nonpharmacological treatment in established rheumatoid arthritis. *Best Pract. Res. Clin. Rheumatol.* **2019**, *33*, 101482. [CrossRef] [PubMed]
33. Aly Yakout, R.; Khlosy, H. Range of motion exercises effect during and after hydrotherapy on patients burned hand function and pain intensity: A comparative study. *Egypt. J. Health Care* **2020**, *11*, 670–687. [CrossRef]
34. Stephan, K.E.; Manjaly, Z.M.; Mathys, C.D.; Weber, L.A.; Paliwal, S.; Gard, T.; Tittgemeyer, M.; Fleming, S.M.; Haker, H.; Seth, A.K.; et al. Allostatic self-efficacy: A metacognitive theory of dyshomeostasis-induced fatigue and depression. *Front. Hum. Neurosci.* **2016**, *10*, 550. [CrossRef]

35. Normann, N.; Morina, N. The efficacy of metacognitive therapy: A systematic review and meta-analysis. *Front. Psychol.* **2018**, *9*, 2211. [CrossRef]
36. Pope, J.E. Management of fatigue in rheumatoid arthritis. *RMD Open* **2020**, *6*, e001084. [CrossRef]
37. Jiang, R.; Ta, X.; Xu, M.; Luo, Z.; Du, Y.; Zhong, X.; Pan, T.; Cao, X. Mediating role of depression between diabetes management self-efficacy and diabetes self-care behavior among elderly type 2 diabetes mellitus patients in China. *Psychol. Res. Behav. Manag.* **2023**, *16*, 1545–1555. [CrossRef]
38. Grasaas, E.; Sandbakk, Ø. Adherence to physical activity recommendations and associations with self-efficacy among Norwegian adolescents: Trends from 2017 to 2021. *Front. Public Health* **2024**, *12*, 1382028. [CrossRef]
39. Martinez-Calderon, J.; Meeus, M.; Struyf, F.; Luque-Suarez, A. The role of self-efficacy in pain intensity, function, psychological factors, health behaviors, and quality of life in people with rheumatoid arthritis: A systematic review. *Physiother. Theory Pract.* **2020**, *36*, 21–37. [CrossRef]
40. Chen, Z.; Lan, W.; Yang, G.; Li, Y.; Ji, X.; Chen, L.; Zhou, Y.; Li, S. Exercise intervention in treatment of neuropsychological diseases: A review. *Front. Psychol.* **2020**, *11*, 569206. [CrossRef]
41. Doumen, M.; De Cock, D.; Pazmino, S.; Bertrand, D.; Joly, J.; Westhovens, R.; Verschueren, P. Treatment response and several patient-reported outcomes are early determinants of future self-efficacy in rheumatoid arthritis. *Arthritis Res. Ther.* **2021**, *23*, 269. [CrossRef] [PubMed]
42. Lee, Y.C.; Cui, J.; Lu, B.; Frits, M.L.; Iannaccone, C.K.; Shadick, N.A.; Weinblatt, M.E.; Solomon, D.H. Pain persists in DAS28 rheumatoid arthritis remission but not in ACR/EULAR remission: A longitudinal observational study. *Arthritis Res. Ther.* **2011**, *13*, R83. [CrossRef] [PubMed]
43. Lu, J.; Sun, S.; Gu, Y.; Li, H.; Fang, L.; Zhu, X.; Xu, H. Health literacy and health outcomes among older patients suffering from chronic diseases: A moderated mediation model. *Front. Public Health* **2022**, *10*, 1069174. [CrossRef] [PubMed]

medicina

MDPI

Review

Anti-SRP Antibodies and Myocarditis in Systemic Sclerosis Overlap Syndrome with Immune-Mediated Necrotizing Myositis (IMNM)

Cristina Alexandru [1,2,†], Anca Donisa [3,†], Florin Bobirca [1,4], Ana Maria Dascalu [1,5,*], Dan Dumitrescu [1,6,*], Ioan Ancuta [1,2], Mihai Bojinca [1,2], Ana Maria Balahura [1,7], Carmen Manea [8], Ionela Belaconi [1,3], Daniela Anghel [1,9], Catalin Dumitrașcu [2], Catalin Alius [1,6], Andreea Cristina Costea [10], Andrei Marin [1,11], Dragos Serban [1,6] and Anca Bobircă [1,2]

1 Faculty of Medicine, "Carol Davila" University of Medicine and Pharmacy, 020021 Bucharest, Romania; ionela.belaconi@umfcd.ro (I.B.); dragos.serban@umfcd.ro (D.S.); anca.bobirca@umfcd.ro (A.B.)
2 Internal Medicine and Rheumatology Department, "Dr. Ion Cantacuzino" Clinical Hospital, 011437 Bucharest, Romania
3 Department of Pneumology, "Marius Nasta" Institute of Pneumology, 010024 Bucharest, Romania
4 Surgery Department, "Dr. Ion Cantacuzino" Clinical Hospital, 011437 Bucharest, Romania
5 Ophthalmology Department, Emergency University Hospital Bucharest, 050098 Bucharest, Romania
6 Fourth General Surgery Department, Emergency University Hospital Bucharest, 050098 Bucharest, Romania
7 Cardiology Department, Clinical Hospital "Prof. Dr. Th. Burghele", 061344 Bucharest, Romania
8 Rheumatology and Internal Medicine Department, "Sfanta Maria" Clinical Hospital Bucharest, 011172 Bucharest, Romania
9 Internal Medicine Department, "Dr. Carol Davila" Central Military Emergency University Hospital, 010242 Bucharest, Romania
10 Department of Nephrology, Diaverum Clinic, 900612 Constanta, Romania
11 Plastic Surgery Department, "Sf. Ioan" Emergency Clinical Hospital, 042122 Bucharest, Romania
* Correspondence: ana.dascalu@umfcd.ro (A.M.D.); dan.dumitrescu@umfcd.ro (D.D.)
† These authors contributed equally to this work.

Abstract: Overlap syndrome of systemic sclerosis and idiopathic inflammatory myopathies is an increasingly frequent entity, but the association with immune-mediated necrotizing myositis has rarely been described. While myositis or myopathy may be features of scleroderma, it is imperative to correctly diagnose an overlap syndrome of these two, since it can be considered a different entity with specific management and a worse prognosis. Anti-signal recognition particle (anti-SRP) antibodies target the striated muscle fiber and inhibit myoblast regeneration, resulting in myofiber atrophy and necrosis. Anti-SRP antibodies are specific in immune-mediated necrotizing myopathy characterized by myonecrosis and minimal inflammatory reaction, with proximal muscle weakness and typical extra-muscular manifestation. There are controversial data on the association of cardiac manifestations and the presence of these antibodies, and recent studies cannot prove a significant correlation between the two. Myocarditis is a complication with an unpredictable, potentially severe outcome from heart failure and dilated cardiomyopathy to fatality. It can be difficult to diagnose, and a myocardial biopsy can be problematic in daily practice; thus, most practitioners rely on cardiac magnetic resonance with suggestive images for the correct diagnosis. This paper seeks to address the challenges associated with the diagnosis and treatment of collagen diseases by evaluating the role of anti-SRP antibodies in the pathogenesis of cardiac involvement.

Keywords: systemic sclerosis; myocarditis; anti-SRP antibodies; necrotizing myositis

1. Introduction

Systemic sclerosis or scleroderma (SSc) is a systemic autoimmune disease, characterized by excessive fibrosis of the skin and internal organs such as the lungs, heart, kidneys, and digestive tract [1]. Idiopathic inflammatory myopathies (IIMs) represent a heterogeneous group of connective tissue diseases characterized by muscular inflammation and extra-muscular damage. The group comprises dermatomyositis, polymyositis, inclusion body myositis, anti-synthetase syndrome, and immune-mediated necrotizing myositis (IMNM) [2]. While myositis or myopathy may be features of scleroderma, it is imperative to correctly diagnose an overlap syndrome of these two, since it can be considered a different entity with specific management and a worse prognosis [3]. Overlap syndrome of scleroderma with idiopathic inflammatory myopathies such as polymyositis or dermatomyositis is more frequent, and usually associated with positive anti-PM/Scl and anti-Ku antibodies [4]. Patients with positive anti-PM/Scl antibodies are more likely to develop myositis, pulmonary interstitial fibrosis, calcinosis, telangiectasia, and dermatomyositis-like skin manifestations.

In contrast, esophageal involvement, pulmonary arterial hypertension, or cardiac involvement are less frequent among these patients [5]. On the other hand, anti-Ku antibodies have been linked to polymyositis–scleroderma overlap since 1981, with patients presenting synovitis, joint contractures, and myositis symptoms but without vascular damage [6]. Patients with SSc are at high risk of developing interstitial lung disease (ILD), a severe complication with great mortality and morbidity; around 30% of cases lead to respiratory failure in the first 5 years after diagnosis [1]. ILD in SSc patients accounts for 17% of SSc-related deaths, with non-specific interstitial pneumonia (NSIP) being the most prevalent subtype on high-resolution computed tomography [HRCT] images [7]. Recent findings have shown that anti-PM/Scl and anti-Ku antibodies are risk factors for severe interstitial lung disease, but relatively modest vascular complications [5]. Another antibody associated with connective tissue diseases is an anti-signal recognition particle (anti-SRP), usually more frequently described in patients with IMNM. Still, these antibodies are also described in several cases of systemic scleroderma or other subtypes of myositis. These antibodies usually come with a specific clinical aspect predominantly proximal muscle pain and dysphagia but chest pain, arthritis, arthralgia, Sicca syndrome, carpal tunnel syndrome, ILD, and skin rash can be present [2,3].

2. Immune-Mediated Necrotizing Myositis (INMN)

INMN is a newly described subtype of idiopathic inflammatory myopathy, frequently presenting with anti-signal recognition particle and anti-3-hydroxy-3-methylglutaryl-coa reductase (anti-HMGCR) antibody positivity [8]. Patients with IMNM have proximal muscle involvement, with a muscle biopsy showing myofiber necrosis with a paucity of lymphocyte infiltrates [9]. Cases of scleroderma overlapping with myopathies with muscle necrosis and damage of small vessels with a "pipe-stern" appearance, with positive anti-SRP antibodies have been described less often [10]. Anti-SRP antibodies are more frequently associated with pain in the proximal muscles and diffuse myonecrosis in the striated muscles, leading to myalgia, dysphagia, and dyspnea with respiratory failure due to fatigue of the respiratory muscles [11]. Recent data support a new theory suggesting that the overlap between scleroderma and myositis represents a distinct disease known as scleromyositis, characterized by specific clinical and immunological features. However, despite a high frequency of IMNM characteristics at muscle biopsy in scleromyositis patients, these patterns are shown to be associated with anti-Ku, anti-PM/SCL, and anti-U1-RNP autoantibodies, rather than with anti-SRP or anti-HMGCR antibodies [12].

Cardiac manifestations in idiopathic inflammatory myopathies and SSc are frequent and can range from subclinical myocardial damage, often identified at cardiac magnetic resonance [CMR], to arrhythmia and heart failure [13]. The cardiac symptoms and their progression are not well defined, and additional studies are needed to establish a specific set of biomarkers in these patients and better characterize the subtypes with a worse outcome. In small studies, anti-SRP antibodies are associated with more frequent myocardial involvement; however, this association was not identified in large studies [14].

3. Cardiac Involvement in Systemic Scleroderma

Cardiac complications in systemic scleroderma are prevalent and frequently underdiagnosed. These complications may arise directly from scleroderma's impact on the myocardium or indirectly from associated conditions such as pulmonary arterial hypertension, interstitial lung disease, or renal crisis. Fibrosis, inflammation, and vascular alterations can affect all cardiac structures, occurring in approximately 80% of systemic scleroderma patients, although they often present without any cardiac symptoms [15]. The direct effects of the myocardium are represented by microvascular coronary artery disease, cardiac fibrosis, myocarditis, systolic or diastolic dysfunctions of the right or left ventricle, conduction, and rhythm anomalies, even with the involvement of the pericardium [16,17]. Cardiac complications, especially arrhythmias and congestive heart failure, represent the second leading cause of death in patients with systemic scleroderma, while in patients with IIM, cardiac complications are responsible for 5% of deaths [18,19]. Additionally, muscle myopathy is associated with a heightened risk of cardiac complications and increased mortality [12]. Microvascular damage and immune dysfunction are the primary pathological mechanisms leading to the accumulation of collagen deposits, which can result in hyperplasia of intramural arteries and intermittent ischemia. Necrotic areas that develop within the myocardium are subsequently replaced by patchy myocardial fibrosis. This fibrotic pattern, regarded as a hallmark of scleroderma of the myocardium, can affect both ventricles and occurs independently of the coronary artery distribution [16]. Cardiac magnetic resonance imaging is the most effective method for detecting cardiac involvement in connective tissue diseases, revealing that heart involvement in patients with SSc is more common than previously recognized [20]. Diastolic dysfunction appears to be common in systemic scleroderma and may affect either ventricle. Impaired ventricular filling is indicative of a fibrotic and rigid ventricle, which can lead to atrial dilatation [20]. Frequent cardiac manifestations are arrhythmias, congestive heart disease, pericarditis, and myocarditis, but primary heart involvement is difficult to establish in patients with SSc [15]. Changes in rhythm, such as supraventricular or ventricular tachycardias can be responsible for sudden death in some patients. Supraventricular arrhythmias are the most frequently observed abnormalities during 24 h Holter monitoring, whereas ventricular arrhythmias, although less common, may present as polymorphic, often characterized by premature contractions [16].

Because of the similarities between the myocardium and skeletal muscles, the heart can also be affected by myositis as part of the same inflammatory process [21]. Although significant cardiac involvement is relatively uncommon, it remains a critical cause of death. This is particularly important in subclinical cases, where proinflammatory cytokines alongside traditional cardiovascular risk factors play a crucial role in diastolic dysfunction [22]. Diastolic dysfunction of the left ventricle is the most common type of cardiac damage in myositis. However, case reports have also documented coronary damage, including angina pectoris, and myocardial infarction [13]. In contrast, subclinical damage appears to be more common. This includes changes such as supraventricular or ventricular arrhythmias, bundle branch blocks, atrioventricular blocks, PR interval prolongations, ventricular premature beats, and abnormal Q waves or ST-T changes, usually detected on the ECG of a patient with myositis [23]. Regarding IIM, the pathogenesis of cardiac changes includes the inflammatory infiltration of the conduction system, with the replacement of cardiomyocytes from it, with fibrosis, and vasculitis of the small vessels that irrigate the myocardium, along with the infiltration of the myocardium itself [24].

The frequency of cardiac involvement in IIM can range from 9.3% to 61%, with arrhythmia being the most common [19,25,26]. Diederichsen et al. showed that cardiac manifestations are more common in newly diagnosed patients naïve to treatment than in controls, proving the negative effect of an inflammatory burden on cardiac function [27].

A recent review which included 29 studies showed the cardiac implications in IIM patients, demonstrating that despite the heterogeneity of IIM, some cardiac patterns can be defined [13]. On the other hand, cardiac changes in patients with myositis can be associated with corticosteroid therapy, making it extremely challenging to distinguish whether these changes are due to the corticosteroids [CSs], or the disease itself. In IIM, corticosteroids are still a reliable therapy in addition to immunosuppressives. CSs are well-known risk factors for hypertension, and increased dosages for a prolonged time are associated with heart failure and decreased ejection fraction [28].

Myocarditis can be difficult to diagnose, being defined as myocardial inflammation on endomyocardial biopsy with specific characteristics [29]. Currently, a myocardial biopsy is rare, and most practitioners rely on cardiac magnetic resonance [CMR] with suggestive images for the correct diagnosis [30]. Myocardial alterations on CMR in IIM patients without any cardiac manifestation are frequent [31]. Myocarditis in IIM can be the first presentation or developed during the follow-up; its prevalence is not well studied, but it can vary around 2.6–3.4%, with a substantial increase at a histopathological examination of 38% of cases [19,32]. The evolution can be severe, from fatality to heart failure or dilated cardiomyopathy. In a study on anti-synthetase syndrome patients with myocarditis, the authors showed a strong correlation between myositis activity and the development of myocarditis, but there was no definition of negative prognostic factors for these patients [32].

Heart involvement is more frequent in overlap syndrome of SSc and myositis [3]. A recent case report by Garcia et al. presented an overlap syndrome of systemic sclerosis and polymyositis with anti-SCL-70 and anti-PL/SCL-100 antibodies with lymphocytic myocarditis responding to cyclophosphamide monthly pulses [33].

4. The Role of Anti-SRP Antibodies

Anti-SRP antibodies are antibodies specific to immune-mediated necrotizing myopathy characterized by myonecrosis and minimal inflammatory reaction. The actual mechanism of anti-SRP pathogenesis has yet to be established. These antibodies target the striated muscle fiber and inhibit myoblast regeneration, resulting in myofiber atrophy and necrosis [8]. Furthermore, in vivo studies revealed that transferring anti-SRP antibodies from patients to mice caused muscular deficit via a complement-related mechanism [34]. There is currently contradictory research about the associations between serum creatine kinase (CK) and anti-SRP antibodies [35,36]. Reversely, antibody serum concentrations in subtypes of IMNM with anti-HMGCR positivity are strongly correlated with CK levels and high antibody titer, suggesting the severity of muscle involvement [37]. Another distinguishing feature of anti-SRP positive is the duration of muscle involvement when compared to other types of myositis. One study found a remission of just 25% after one year and 50% at four years, albeit with a persistently elevated CK level [38].

Anti-SRP IMNM is characterized by proximal muscle weakness, which can be associated with dyspnea and dysphagia. Different studies have defined a distinct extra-muscular phenotype in the presence of anti-SRP antibodies, including chest pain, arthritis, arthralgia, Sicca syndrome, carpal tunnel syndrome, ILD, and skin rash (Figure 1) [11].

Cardiac involvement in the presence of these antibodies is described, with arrhythmias, cardiomyopathy, and gradual evolution toward heart failure. However, data on cardiac involvement come from small cohort studies, clinical cases, or studies conducted on larger cohorts but with a different object, with cardiac involvement only appearing in the description section. Thus, in this paper, we gather all studies on this subject, after a literature search on two medical databases (PubMed/Medline and Google Scholar) using the terms "anti-SRP", "anti-signal recognition particle antibodies", "IMNM", "immune-mediated necrotizing myositis" and "cardiac involvement", "myocardial involvement". The results are structured in Table 1.

In a recent study, following thirty-nine patients with anti-SPR-IMNM, no cardiac involvement was reported in the entire cohort, although the focus of the study was more on muscle strength rather than extra-muscular manifestation [38]. However, a larger study by Suzuki et al. following one hundred patients with anti-SRP IMNM showed that cardiac muscle interest was a rare manifestation, with only two subjects describing it [35].

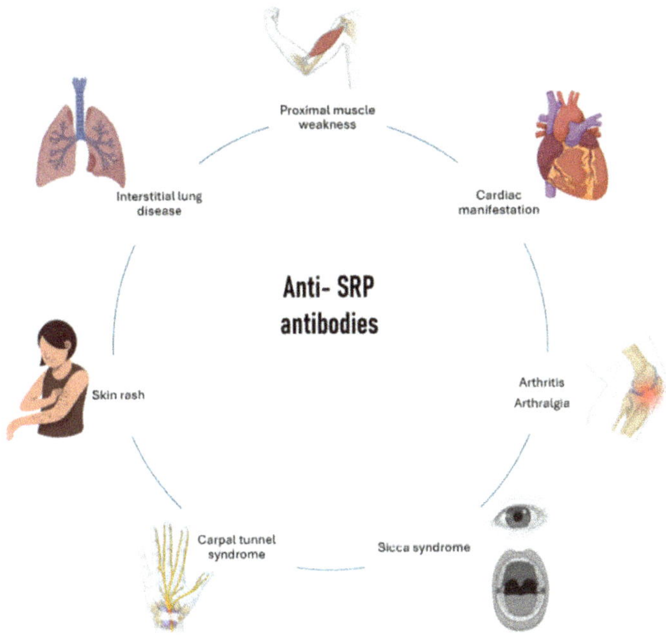

Figure 1. Clinical manifestations associated with anti-signal recognition particle (anti-SRP) antibodies.

Kao et al. followed patients with anti-SRP antibodies and showed that among 790 SSc patients, only 2 had anti-SRP positivity and developed muscle symptoms after a median of 3.5 years. Moreover, among nineteen anti-SRP patients in the cohort (diagnosed with polymyositis, SSc, and anti-synthetase syndrome) cardiac manifestations occurred in 15.8% (three patients), while ILD in 31.57% (six patients) [39]. On the other hand, Hengstman et al. analyzed a large cohort, identifying only five patients diagnosed with polymyositis or dermatomyositis with anti-SRP positivity with severe myalgia and arthritis and resistance to treatment, but none had cardiac manifestations [40]. Later on, they compared a group of anti-SRP patients with polymyositis/dermatomyositis patients with negative anti-SRP, and their results showed no differences in frequency in electrocardiogram abnormalities. Although they reported cardiac anomalies in more than half of patients [clinical symptomatology and electrocardiogram alteration], their results were influenced by cardiovascular factors and concomitant cardiac diseases or ILD [41]. Thus, a well-designed study is needed to clarify the association between anti-SRP antibodies and cardiac manifestations.

One recent study by Bandeira et al. analyzed the cardiac involvement in IIM patients. The results showed that in comparison with patients without cardiac involvement, anti-SRP antibodies are the most commonly identified antibodies (76.9% vs. 31.5%, $p = 0.001$). Moreover, in patients with cardiac manifestation, there was also more frequently reported lung and esophageal involvement, suggesting that patients with systemic manifestations are also more predisposed to cardiac symptomatology and a thorough evaluation is needed [42].

One case report presented severe cardiomyopathy in anti-SRP and anti-MDA-5 IMNM, with progression after immunosuppressive therapy, despite improvement of the clinical myopathy, which needed heart transplantation, supporting the data that this subset of antibodies is a negative prognostic factor [43,44]. Several case reports and case series present a severe course of disease in IMNM patients with anti-SRP positivity presenting with cardiac complications [45–50].

Table 1. Literature search on anti-SRP antibodies and cardiac involvement.

Study	Year	Cohort	Cardiac Involvement
Targoff et al. [49]	1990	12 anti-SRP PM/DM patients	4/12
Hengstman et al. [40]	2002	5 anti-SRP PM/DM patients	0
Miller et al. [50]	2002	7 anti-SRP patients	0
Kao et al. [39]	2004	19 anti-SRP patients (16 PM, 2 SSc, 1 aSS)	3/19
Hengstman et al. [41]	2006	23 anti-SRP patients	6/23
Suzuki et al. [35]	2015	100 anti-SRP patients	2/100
Pinal-Fernandez et al. [38]	2017	37 anti-SRP patients	0
Bandeira et al. [42]	2023	12 anti-SRP patients	3/12

5. Clinical and Paraclinical Presentation

A 74-year-old female, with a history of type 2 diabetes mellitus and arterial hypertension, diagnosed with systemic scleroderma in May 2021, was referred to the rheumatology department in September 2021 to establish the magnitude of organ involvement and to decide the appropriate therapeutic approach. She described Raynaud's phenomenon, arthritis, and mild dyspnea. The physical examination revealed loss of wrinkling, telangiectasias, microstomia, sclerodactyly with puffy fingers achieving a 6/51 Rodnan Score, and velcro bibasilar crackles by lung auscultation (Figure 2).

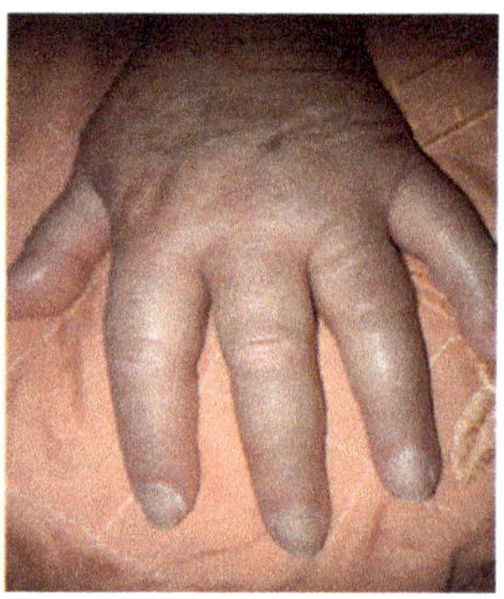

Figure 2. Puffy fingers at the first presentation (September 2021).

Mild anemia (hemoglobin 10.9 g/dL; normal value 11.7–15 g/dL) and high positivity for anti-topoisomerase I antibodies were shown by the blood test evaluation and a late sclerodermic pattern was described at nail video-capillaroscopy. The pulmonary evaluation included chest HRCT [bilateral ground-glass pulmonary infiltrates-NSIP—Figure 3] and spirometry [lung volumes were normal with a slightly decreased DLco (68% of predicted value)], while echocardiography found pulmonary hypertension [43 mmHg] with normal ejection fraction. Throughout the upper endoscopy examination, no indications of esophageal involvement were observed.

Based on the ACR/EULAR criteria [16/28 points] [14], systemic sclerosis with cutaneous, pulmonary, and vascular involvement was diagnosed, and the patient started immunosuppressive treatment. Initially, Mycophenolate mofetil (MMF) was started at 2 g daily, but the patient described intense nausea, abdominal pain and diarrhea. Hence, due to the adverse events associated, MMF was tapered to 1 g daily, together with proton pump inhibitors and calcium channel blockers (CCBs). We decided to switch to intravenous (iv) cyclophosphamide (800 mg monthly for six months) in May 2022 due to the clinical progression (significant progression of the skin fibrosis with a Rodnan score of 14/51) and lung damage with a decrease in DLco (54% of predicted value) and progress of interstitial fibrosis at chest HRCT. It was suggested to start antifibrotic Nintedanib therapy; nevertheless, she did not meet the initiation criteria of the national protocol. The results of the lab tests showed a rising pattern in the levels of inflammatory syndrome (maximum ESR = 59 mm/h; CRP = 33 mg) and creatine kinase [two to three times higher than normal values], and further lung function modification, as indicated by a 50% drop in DLco with stable chest HRCT (Figure 4). A myositis-specific antibody profile was assessed in light of a potential overlapping myositis, and the results indicated that anti-SRP antibodies were present.

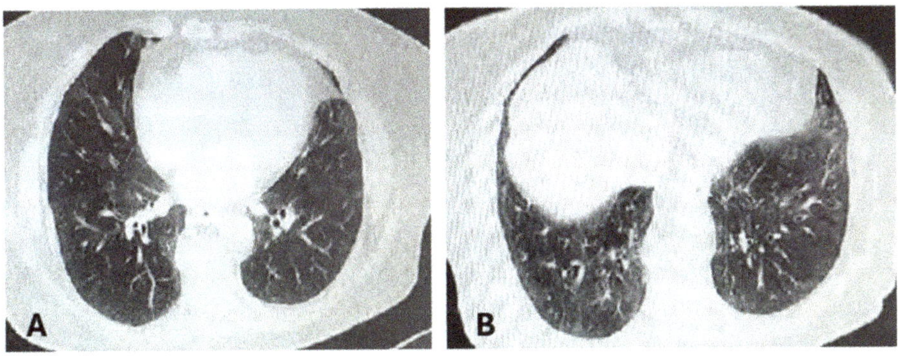

Figure 3. Chest CT September 2021. (**A**) Unsystematized bilateral ground-glass pulmonary infiltrates; (**B**) bilateral basal ground-glass pulmonary infiltrates.

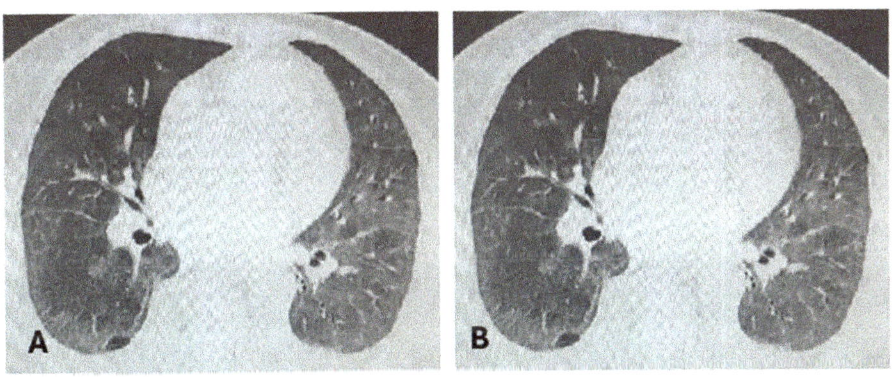

Figure 4. Chest CT September 2022. (**A**) NSIP-like appearance; (**B**) basal aspect of NSIP-like bilateral infiltrates.

The patient experienced a sudden hypertensive spike in November 2022 during the sixth and last cycle of cyclophosphamide. The patient also experienced dyspnea and tachypnea, as well as an 80% desaturation under five liters of oxygen supplementation. The ECG revealed sinus tachycardia and serum troponins were slightly elevated. Importantly, NT-proBNP increased to 35,000 pg/mL. Due to a suspicion of a myocardial infarction other than ST-segment elevation, the patient was referred to the cardiology department. The right ventricle was slightly dilated up to the upper limit of normal values, with normal longitudinal systolic function, mild biatrial dilatation, aortic sclerosis, and possible pulmonary hypertension. Firstly, an echocardiography was performed and it showed a non-dilated left ventricle with moderate global and segmental systolic dysfunction, and hypokinesis of the circumferential apex, inferior wall, and interventricular septum, with intramyocardial hyperechoic areas. Coronary angiography was advised following this incident, but the patient refused. Cardiac magnetic resonance imaging was performed, and the results showed non-dilated ventricles with preserved global systolic function, segmental kinetic disorders, hypokinesis of the left ventricle's lateral wall, indexed myocardial mass within normal limits, replacement myocardial fibrosis with myocarditis pattern, biatrial dilatation, ascending aorta ectasia, and absence of pulmonary artery dilatation (Figure 5).

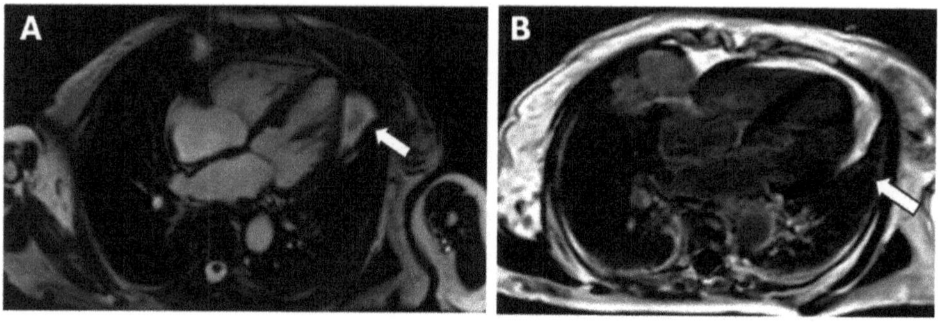

Figure 5. Cardiac MRI. (**A**) Aspect of chronic myocarditis; arrow—the lateral wall of the left ventricle with hypokinesia; no edema; (**B**) LGE PSIR; arrow—Gadolinium accumulation area in the lateral wall of the left ventricle.

No immunosuppressive treatment was administered until January 2023 (Figure 5). A skin and muscle biopsy was performed, after a reasonable disclosure [51] in light of the patient's fatigue, the cardiac episode in November 2022, the elevated CK and CK-MB values in recent months, positive anti-SRP antibodies, muscle atrophy, and the suspicion of immune necrotizing myopathy overlapping systemic sclerosis or maybe a scleromyositis. The histopathological examination indicated a non-specific myopathic appearance with morphological elements consistent with a necrotizing myopathy in the defined clinical-paraclinical context (positive anti-SRP antibodies). There was also a notable variation in the shape of the muscle fibers, with atrophic fibers varying in length and polygonal form, moderate adipose metaplasia, minimal interstitial fibrosis, and rare necrotic fibers. We concluded that the overlapping hypothesis was the most likely to be accurate; therefore, we started the immunosuppressive therapy with Azathioprine 100 mg daily and moderate doses of Prednisone, tapering to a low level.

Although the patient's condition was clinically stable in September 2023, on Azathioprine and 5 mg Prednisone, the DLco decreased by 40% of what was expected, the chest CT scan revealed interstitial changes and slightly altered micronodulations from September 2022 (Figures 6 and 7), and the blood tests continued to reveal a slight anemia and low inflammatory syndrome, so the patient received a single dose of Tocilizumab (400 mg iv administration) with no possibilities to continuing to administrate the biological therapy.

The lung CT scan performed in February 2024 revealed a typical NSIP-like appearance of fibrosis as well as functional deterioration with a DLco of 31% from the predicted one. Thus, the pneumologist decided to start the antifibrotic medication-nintedanib 200 mg/day, and the patient kept taking the specific cardiac drugs, with recurrent interdisciplinary evaluation and favorable cardiac evolution.

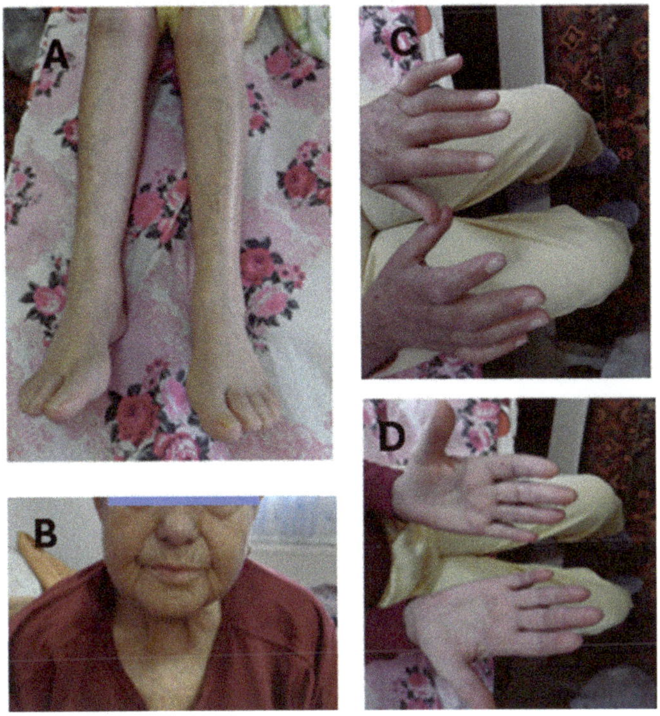

Figure 6. Clinical aspect of the patient in January 2023: (**A**) patient's legs with no edema and hair loss; (**B**) patient's hands- sclerodactyly; (**C**) patient's face showing microstomia; (**D**) patient's hand-telangiectasias.

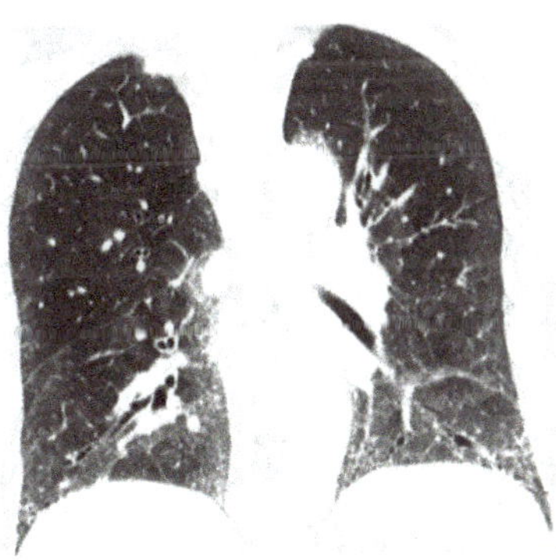

Figure 7. Chest CT September 2023. Bilateral infiltrates slightly changed compared to September 2022; reconstruction in coronal plane.

6. Discussion

The anti-SRP antibodies are very uncommon among SSc patients, with a prevalence of around 0.7%, and even lower in overlap syndrome [52]. IMNM is a less prevalent subtype of IIM, accounting for 18–39% of cases, with an average age of onset of 40–50 years, contrary to our case with an elderly disease onset [8].

There are several studies describing cardiac complications in SSc and IMNM, and although in the past there was a strong correlation between anti-SRP antibodies and cardiac manifestations, our research has not proved this correlation (Table 1). This theory needs to be validated in large, well-controlled studies, but a major concern still remains, and supplementary cardiac investigations are recommended in these patients. Such cases are difficult to diagnose and there is no general protocol on the management in these cases. In Figure 8, we try to summarize the diagnosis and treatment steps.

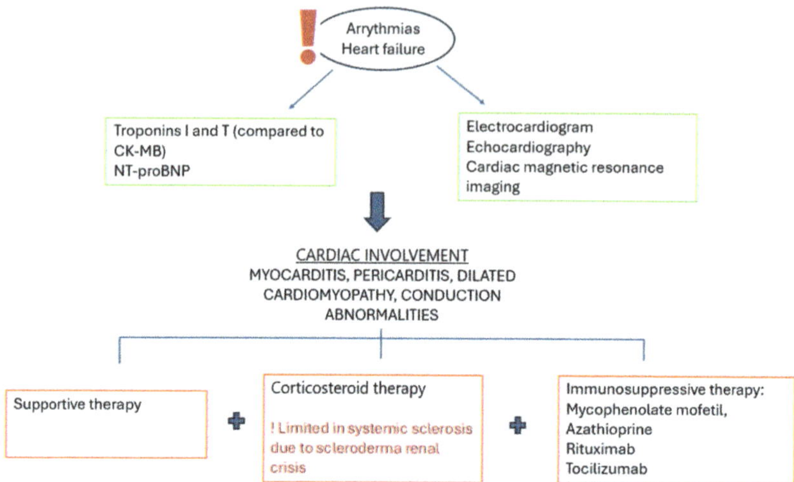

Figure 8. General management steps of cardiac involvement in anti-SRP patients.

Other antibodies that are more frequently associated with cardiac manifestation in IIM patients are anti Jo1 anti bodies (33.3%) and anti SSA/SSB antibodies (33.3%), but heart involvement in connective tissue diseases is still an undervalued field and in great need of further studies [42].

The most frequent cardiac manifestation in SSc and in IIM are arrhythmias, and our patients develop tachycardia as a symptom of the underlying myocarditis [15,26]. In terms of age interfering with the disease characteristics, younger age is associated with a more difficult-to-treat form of IMNM in anti-SRP-positive patients, in contrast with other subtypes of IIM [35,38]. In our case, although the muscle injury was minor by the literature, cardiac complications such as myocarditis provided diagnostic and therapeutic challenges. A similar pattern was described by Ma et al., showing progressive cardiac involvement, regardless of the good clinical response under immunotherapy [43]. The early identification of cardiac involvement can be achieved by measuring troponins I and T, which rapidly detect myocardial injury, especially troponin I in acute coronary damage, with troponin T also influenced by skeletal muscle damage; both are more specific compared to CK-MB measurement. Another relevant tool in the case of these individuals is NTproBNP, which can identify hemodynamic and structural abnormalities in their preclinical period [2]. Nailfold video-capillaroscopy is an essential diagnostic tool in SSc patients with Raynaud's phenomenon, with a specific pattern, and it can have a prognostic factor too. In IIM, although alteration is identified, there is no specificity for myositis, nor for other autoimmune diseases [53,54].

We experienced challenges in establishing our patient's accurate diagnosis; although initially SSc was a facile diagnosis, when the patient later developed muscle involvement, asthenia, muscle atrophy, muscle cytolysis, and cardiac involvement equivalent to myocarditis, with anti-SRP positivity, a series of theories appeared: to integrate cardiac and muscle involvement in the context of SSc, to reconsider the diagnosis as scleromyositis (a new diagnostic entity in rheumatology that is under-explored or neglected), or to conclude that we were faced with an overlapping syndrome of SSc and IMNM. We could argue that the following subpoints support the confirmation of scleromyositis in our patient: elevated muscle enzymes, more frequent cardiac involvement [myocarditis], muscular manifestations, and rapid progression of pulmonary involvement. The classical hallmarks of muscle biopsy, which include vasculopathy and fibrotic lesions without necrosis and inflammation, and the absence of anti-Pm/Scl antibodies work against the diagnosis [12]. But we concluded that the overlapping syndrome of SS and IMNM is the appropriate diagnosis sustained by the muscular biopsy findings—a necrotizing myopathy in the context of anti-SRP positivity and the severity of organ involvement, such as cardiac pulmonary hypertension and myocarditis, ILD [55].

Regarding the acute onset of cardiac manifestation, we took into account the possible adverse effects of Cyclophosphamide (CYC), although Cyclophosphamide has been for years the standard of treatment for systemic sclerosis, particularly in cases of heart involvement [myocarditis] [56]. Administered intravenously or orally in SSc, CYC has some potential risks including hemorrhagic cystitis, alopecia, vomiting, diarrhea, and skin and bladder cancer, as well as possibly irreversible infertility; cardiac side effects are not as prevalent [57,58]. CyC is a strong alkylating medication used in oncology. Many cardiac adverse events associated with its metabolites have been reported in the literature. They are divided into two categories: irreversible, which is heart failure caused by the death of cardiomyocytes as a result of oxidative stress or the platelets' reactivity-arachidonic pathway, and reversible, which is cardiac remodeling due to the impairment of cardiomyocytes' function as a result of proinflammatory cytokines [59]. Such side effects are not typically reported in SSc, as a consequence of the lowest dosages used for ILD, but when autologous stem cell transplantation (ASCT) was used more often for SS patients, the dosage of CYC had to be increased, which resulted in the automatic onset of secondary cardiac dysfunction. It is important to discuss the case of a patient with SSc with ILD who had no prior cardiac involvement and no cardiac risk, and was treated with CYC 12g IV over four days for ASCT. At twelve hours after ASCT, the patient developed acute heart failure (BNP of 7136 ng/L and widespread hypokinesia with an LVEFo10%). The patient passed away on day nine following ASCT despite receiving intense supportive care. A necropsy revealed significant pericarditis, intracavitary thrombus, and myonecrosis without any signs of inflammation, fibrosis, or hypertrophy, leading the examiners to conclude that the cause of death was acute cardiotoxicity caused by CYC [60]. Although acute CYC cardiotoxicity is potentially lethal, it currently appears to be quite rare, mostly due to pre-existing cardiovascular involvement not being given proper consideration. Consequently, extensive pre-transplant disease-specific screening is essential to prevent underlying undiagnosed SSc-related cardiopathy because this kind of therapeutic approach will be the future medicine for our SSc patients with severe organ involvement [61].

Considering our patient's pre-existing cardiovascular risk factors and cardiac damage in the context of scleroderma, the concept of cumulative cardiac toxicity of CYC could be brought into consideration (possible pulmonary hypertension). Evaluation using a CMR of the acute event revealed alterations suggesting myocarditis that are more likely due to collagen disease but could also be induced by CYC [4.5 g cumulative dosage over 6 months].

There is no formal recommendation for the treatment of cardiac involvement either in scleroderma or in myositis. Usually, the treatment is supportive, depending on the type of cardiac damage. In some studies, a slight amelioration of cardiac output was observed during immunosuppressive treatment, especially in combination with corticosteroids, but with high precaution due to the high risk of scleroderma renal crisis [62]. There have been cases of patients with dermatomyositis and Raynaud's with ECG changes such as multifocal atrial tachycardia, ventricular premature beats, or blocks, changes that resolved after treatment with Rituximab and corticosteroids [63]. Other patients with myocardial hypokinesia showed normalization in 6 months after treatment with CS and immunosuppressants [64]. Some patients with myositis may present Prinzmetal vasospastic angina, especially in those with Raynaud's syndrome, which has been successfully treated with high-dose BCC [65]. Due to a lack of cases, treatment in anti-SRP IMNM is not systematically studied, and the efficacy of immunosuppressive treatment is coming from case reports and small cohort studies. A small study showed a favorable response to Rituximab in 76% of cases (13/17), but the duration of the good response is yet to be established [38]. Rituximab has shown promise in the treatment of cardiac and pulmonary complications associated with collagen diseases; nevertheless, there is also evidence of the involvement of tocilizumab [TCZ] in these manifestations. Several Asian studies describe the beneficial effects of TCZ in managing cardiac involvement among patients with SS who have previously received other immunosuppressive treatments, including Rituximab. Following TCZ treatment, the patients' MRI and ECG showed improvement, probably as a result of IL6 inhibition blocking the inflammatory and fibrotic process, which involves myocardial remodeling [66,67]. Starting from the data indicating the use of TCZ in COVID-19 myocardial disease, we also considered that, in the instance of our patient, a single intravenous dosage of 8 mg/kg may have additional benefits for long-term cardiac outcomes [68].

ILD is a common manifestation in SSc, especially in cases with diffuse fibrosis and anti-Scl 70 antibodies. On the other hand, ILD is associated with anti-SRP IMNM in about 20% of cases [11]. Despite treatment with cyclophosphamide 6 pulses, followed by maintenance therapy with azathioprine, pulmonary fibrosis progressed and nintedanib was initiated.

This paper has several limitations. Firstly, this analysis is based on a single clinical case, and conducting studies on larger cohorts would be advantageous for deriving more definitive conclusions regarding cardiac involvement and the presence of anti-SRP antibodies. Another limitation is the scarcity of data available in the literature, as most insights are derived from case reports and small case series. Additionally, studies involving larger patient populations do not primarily focus on evaluating cardiac manifestations in these patients, which introduces a potential bias due to the study design.

7. Conclusions

In conclusion, this is a case that brings several challenges for both diagnosis and treatment, which could be used as a guide for possible warning outcomes related to antibody seropositivity. Cardiac involvement in connective tissue diseases presents a significant diagnostic challenge, particularly in cases of acute heart failure, which necessitates rapid diagnosis and prompt therapeutic intervention due to its association with high mortality rates in these patients. The current literature lacks sufficient evidence to definitively establish the relationship between anti-SRP antibodies and cardiac dysfunction, highlighting the need for large-scale, rigorously designed studies. While the use of immunosuppressive therapies has shown increasing efficacy in managing pulmonary complications in systemic sclerosis and idiopathic inflammatory myopathies (IIMs), treatment strategies for cardiac involvement remain underdeveloped. This area is complicated by the need to account for both traditional cardiovascular risk factors, which may limit immunosuppressant options, and the potential adverse effects of these therapies [5,35].

Author Contributions: Conceptualization, C.A. (Cristina Alexandru), A.D., F.B. and A.M.D.; methodology, D.D., I.A. and M.B.; software, A.M.B.; validation, C.M., I.B., D.A. and C.D.; formal analysis, C.A. (Catalin Alius), A.C.C. and A.M.; investigation, D.S.; resources, A.M.D.; data curation, A.B.; writing—original draft preparation, C.A. (Cristina Alexandru), A.D., F.B., A.M.D., D.D., I.A., M.B., A.M.B. and C.M.; writing—review and editing, I.B., D.A., C.D., C.A. (Catalin Alius), A.C.C., A.M., D.S. and A.B.; visualization, C.A. (Cristina Alexandru); supervision, A.B.; project administration, A.D.; funding acquisition, A.M.D. All authors have read and agreed to the published version of the manuscript.

Funding: This research received no external funding.

Institutional Review Board Statement: Not applicable.

Informed Consent Statement: Written informed consent has been obtained from the patient to publish this paper.

Data Availability Statement: No new data were created.

Conflicts of Interest: The authors declare no conflicts of interest.

References

1. Kuwana, M.; Gil-Vila, A.; Selva-O'Callaghan, A. Role of autoantibodies in the diagnosis and prognosis of interstitial lung disease in autoimmune rheumatic disorders. *Ther. Adv. Musculoskelet. Dis.* **2021**, *13*, 1759720X211032457. [CrossRef] [PubMed]
2. Chen, F.; Peng, Y.; Chen, M. Diagnostic approach to cardiac involvement in idiopathic inflammatory myopathies: A strategy combining cardiac troponin I but not T assay with other methods. *Int. Heart J. Int. Heart J. Assoc.* **2018**, *59*, 256–262. [CrossRef]
3. Ranque, B.; Bérezné, A.; Le-Guern, V.; Pagnoux, C.; Allanore, Y.; Launay, D.; Hachulla, E.; Authier, F.J.; Gherardi, R.; Kahan, A.; et al. Myopathies related to systemic sclerosis: A case-control study of associated clinical and immunological features. *Scand. J. Rheumatol.* **2010**, *39*, 498–505. [CrossRef] [PubMed]
4. Mahler, M.; Raijmakers, R. Novel aspects of autoantibodies to the PM/Scl complex: Clinical, genetic and diagnostic insights. *Autoimmun. Rev.* **2007**, *6*, 432–437. [CrossRef]
5. Cavazzana, I.; Vojinovic, T.; Airo, P.; Fredi, M.; Ceribelli, A.; Pedretti, E.; Lazzaroni, M.G.; Garrafa, E.; Franceschini, F. Systemic Sclerosis-Specific Antibodies: Novel and Classical Biomarkers. *Clin. Rev. Allergy Immunol.* **2022**, *64*, 412–430. [CrossRef] [PubMed]
6. Mimori, T.; Akizuki, M.; Yamagata, H.; Inada, S.; Yoshida, S.; Homma, M. Characterization of a high molecular weight acidic nuclear protein recognized by autoantibodies in sera from patients with polymyositis-scleroderma overlap. *J. Clin. Investig.* **1981**, *68*, 611–620. [CrossRef] [PubMed]
7. Elhai, M.; Meune, C.; Boubaya, M.; Avouac, J.; Hachulla, E.; Balbir-Gurman, A.; Riemekasten, G.; Airò, P.; Joven, B.; Vettori, S.; et al. Mapping and predicting mortality from systemic sclerosis. *Ann. Rheum. Dis.* **2017**, *76*, 1897–1905. [CrossRef]
8. Watanabe, Y.; Uruha, A.; Suzuki, S.; Nakahara, J.; Hamanaka, K.; Takayama, K.; Suzuki, N.; Nishino, I. Clinical features and prognosis in anti-SRP and anti-HMGCR necrotizing myopathy. *J. Neurol. Neurosurg. Psychiatry* **2016**, *87*, 1038–1044. [CrossRef]
9. Anquetil, C.; Boyer, O.; Wesner, N.; Benveniste, O.; Allenbach, Y. Myositis-specific autoantibodies, a cornerstone in immune-mediated necrotizing myopathy. *Autoimmun. Rev.* **2019**, *18*, 223–230. [CrossRef]
10. Pope, J.E. Scleroderma overlap syndromes. *Curr. Opin. Rheumatol.* **2002**, *14*, 704–710. [CrossRef]
11. Ma, X.; Bu, B.T. Anti-SRP immune-mediated necrotizing myopathy: A critical review of current concepts. *Front. Immunol.* **2022**, *13*, 1019972. [CrossRef] [PubMed]
12. Giannini, M.; Ellezam, B.; Leclair, V.; Lefebvre, F.; Troyanov, Y.; Hudson, M.; Senécal, J.L.; Geny, B.; Landon-Cardinal, O.; Meyer, A. Scleromyositis: A distinct novel entity within the systemic sclerosis and autoimmune myositis spectrum. Implications for care and pathogenesis. *Front. Immunol.* **2023**, *13*, 974078. [CrossRef] [PubMed]
13. Fairley, J.L.; Wicks, I.; Peters, S.; Day, J. Defining cardiac involvement in idiopathic inflammatory myopathies: A systematic review. *Rheumatology* **2021**, *61*, 103–120. [CrossRef] [PubMed]
14. Allenbach, Y.; Benveniste, O. Peculiar clinicopathological features of immune-mediated necrotizing myopathies. *Curr. Opin. Rheumatol.* **2018**, *30*, 655–663. [CrossRef]
15. Bruni, C.; Ross, L. Cardiac involvement in systemic sclerosis: Getting to the heart of the matter. *Best Pract. Res. Clin. Rheumatol.* **2021**, *35*, 101668. [CrossRef]
16. Ross, L.; Costello, B.; Brown, Z.; Hansen, D.; Lindqvist, A.; Stevens, W.; Burns, A.; Prior, D.; Nikpour, M.; La Gerche, A.; et al. Myocardial fibrosis and arrhythmic burden in systemic sclerosis. *Rheumatology* **2022**, *61*, 4497–4502. [CrossRef]
17. Glynn, P.; Hale, S.; Hussain, T.; Freed, B.H. Cardiovascular Imaging for Systemic Sclerosis Monitoring and Management. *Front. Cardiovasc. Med.* **2022**, *9*, 846213. [CrossRef]
18. Bairkdar, M.; Dong, Z.; Andell, P.; Hesselstrand, R.; Holmqvist, M. Arrhythmia in patients with systemic sclerosis: Incidence, risk factors and impact on mortality in a Swedish register-based study. *RMD Open* **2024**, *10*, e004532. [CrossRef] [PubMed]
19. Gupta, R.; Wayangankar, S.A.; Targoff, I.N.; Hennebry, T.A. Clinical cardiac involvement in idiopathic inflammatory myopathies: A systematic review. *Int. J. Cardiol.* **2011**, *148*, 261–270. [CrossRef]
20. Giucă, A.; Gegenava, T.; Mihai, C.M.; Jurcuţ, C.; Săftoiu, A.; Gîrniţă, D.M.; Popescu, B.A.; Ajmone Marsan, N.; Jurcuț, R. Sclerodermic Cardiomyopathy-A State-of-the-Art Review. *Diagnostics* **2022**, *12*, 669. [CrossRef]
21. Myhr, K.A.; Pecini, R. Management of Myocarditis in Myositis: Diagnosis and Treatment. *Curr. Rheumatol. Rep.* **2020**, *22*, 49. [CrossRef] [PubMed]
22. Schwartz, T.; Diederichsen, L.P.; Lundberg, I.E.; Sjaastad, I.; Sanner, H. Cardiac involvement in adult and juvenile idiopathic inflammatory myopathies. *RMD Open* **2016**, *2*, e000291. [CrossRef] [PubMed]
23. Lundberg, I.E. The heart in dermatomyositis and polymyositis. *Rheumatology* **2006**, *45* (Suppl. S4), iv18–iv21. [CrossRef]
24. Leone, O.; Veinot, J.P.; Angelini, A.; Baandrup, U.T.; Basso, C.; Berry, G.; Bruneval, P.; Burke, M.; Butany, J.; Calabrese, F.; et al. 2011 Consensus statement on endomyocardial biopsy from the Association for European Cardiovascular Pathology and the Society for Cardiovascular Pathology. *Cardiovasc. Pathol.* **2012**, *21*, 245–274. [CrossRef]
25. Dankó, K.; Ponyi, A.; Constantin, T.; Borgulya, G.; Szegedi, G. Long-Term Survival of Patients With Idiopathic Inflammatory Myopathies According to Clinical Features. *Medicine* **2004**, *83*, 35–42. [CrossRef]
26. Kassardjian, C.D.; Lennon, V.A.; Alfugham, N.B.; Mahler, M.; Milone, M. Clinical Features and Treatment Outcomes of Necrotizing Autoimmune Myopathy. *JAMA Neurol.* **2015**, *72*, 996. [CrossRef]

27. Diederichsen, L.P.; Simonsen, J.A.; Diederichsen, A.C.P.; Kim, W.Y.; Hvidsten, S.; Hougaard, M.; Junker, P.; Lundberg, I.E.; Petersen, H.; Hansen, E.S.; et al. Cardiac abnormalities assessed by non-invasive techniques in patients with newly diagnosed idiopathic inflammatory myopathies. *Clin. Exp. Rheumatol.* **2015**, *33*, 706–714. [PubMed]
28. Adamczak, D.M.; Oduah, M.T.; Kiebalo, T.; Nartowicz, S.; Bęben, M.; Pochylski, M.; Ciepłucha, A.; Gwizdała, A.; Lesiak, M.; Straburzyńska-Migaj, E.; et al. Heart Failure with Preserved Ejection Fraction—A Concise Review. *Curr. Cardiol. Rep.* **2020**, *22*, 82. [CrossRef] [PubMed]
29. Al-Akchar, M.; Shams, P.; Kiel, J. *Acute Myocarditis*; StatPearls Publishing: Treasure Island, FL, USA, 2017.
30. Bernhard, B.; Schnyder, A.; Garachemani, D.; Fischer, K.; Tanner, G.; Safarkhanlo, Y.; Stark, A.W.; Schütze, J.; Pavlicek-Bahlo, M.; Greulich, S.; et al. Prognostic Value of Right Ventricular Function in Patients with Suspected Myocarditis Undergoing Cardiac Magnetic Resonance. *JACC Cardiovasc. Imaging* **2023**, *16*, 28–41. [CrossRef]
31. Khoo, T.; Stokes, M.B.; Teo, K.; Proudman, S.; Basnayake, S.; Sanders, P.; Limaye, V. Cardiac involvement in idiopathic inflammatory myopathies detected by cardiac magnetic resonance imaging. *Clin. Rheumatol.* **2019**, *38*, 3471–3476. [CrossRef]
32. Dieval, C.; Deligny, C.; Meyer, A.; Cluzel, P.; Champtiaux, N.; Lefevre, G.; Saadoun, D.; Sibilia, J.; Pellegrin, J.L.; Hachulla, E.; et al. Myocarditis in Patients with Antisynthetase Syndrome. *Medicine* **2015**, *94*, e798. [CrossRef] [PubMed]
33. Garcia, S.; Martins, F.R.; Oliveira, D.; Samões, B.; Martins, A.; Terroso, G.; Costa, L. Lymphocytic myocarditis in an overlap syndrome of systemic sclerosis and polymyositis. *Clin. Rheumatol.* **2022**, *41*, 581–582. [CrossRef] [PubMed]
34. Bergua, C.; Chiavelli, H.; Allenbach, Y.; Arouche-Delaperche, L.; Arnoult, C.; Bourdenet, G.; Jean, L.; Zoubairi, R.; Guerout, N.; Mahler, M.; et al. In vivo pathogenicity of IgG from patients with anti-SRP or anti-HMGCR autoantibodies in immune-mediated necrotising myopathy. *Ann. Rheum. Dis.* **2019**, *78*, 131–139. [CrossRef] [PubMed]
35. Suzuki, S.; Nishikawa, A.; Kuwana, M.; Nishimura, H.; Watanabe, Y.; Nakahara, J.; Hayashi, Y.K.; Suzuki, N.; Nishino, I. Inflammatory myopathy with anti-signal recognition particle antibodies: Case series of 100 patients. *Orphanet J. Rare Dis.* **2015**, *10*, 61. [CrossRef]
36. Benveniste, O.; Drouot, L.; Jouen, F.; Charuel, J.L.; Bloch-Queyrat, C.; Behin, A.; Amoura, Z.; Marie, I.; Guiguet, M.; Eymard, B.; et al. Correlation of anti-signal recognition particle autoantibody levels with creatine kinase activity in patients with necrotizing myopathy. *Arthritis Rheum.* **2011**, *63*, 1961–1971. [CrossRef]
37. Werner, J.L.; Christopher-Stine, L.; Ghazarian, S.R.; Pak, K.S.; Kus, J.E.; Daya, N.R.; Lloyd, T.E.; Mammen, A.L. Antibody levels correlate with creatine kinase levels and strength in anti–3-hydroxy-3-methylglutaryl-coenzyme A reductase–associated autoimmune myopathy. *Arthritis Rheum.* **2012**, *64*, 4087–4093. [CrossRef]
38. Pinal-Fernandez, I.; Parks, C.; Werner, J.L.; Albayda, J.; Paik, J.J.; Danoff, S.K.; Casciola-Rosen, L.; Christopher-Stine, L.; Mammen, A.L. Longitudinal Course of Disease in a Large Cohort of Myositis Patients with Autoantibodies Recognizing the Signal Recognition Particle. *Arthritis Care Res.* **2017**, *69*, 263–270. [CrossRef]
39. Kao, A.H.; Lacomis, D.; Lucas, M.; Fertig, N.; Oddis, C.V. Anti–signal recognition particle autoantibody in patients with and patients without idiopathic inflammatory myopathy. *Arthritis Rheum.* **2004**, *50*, 209–215. [CrossRef]
40. Hengstman, G.J.D.; Brouwer, R.; Vree Egberts, W.T.M.; Seelig, H.P.; Jongen, P.J.H.; van Venrooij, W.J.; van Engelen, B.G. Clinical and serological characteristics of 125 Dutch myositis patients. *J. Neurol.* **2002**, *249*, 69–75. [CrossRef]
41. Hengstman, G.J.D.; ter Laak, H.J.; Vree Egberts, W.T.M.; Lundberg, I.E.; Moutsopoulos, H.M.; Vencovsky, J.; Doria, A.; Mosca, M.; van Venrooij, W.J.; van Engelen, B.G. Anti-signal recognition particle autoantibodies: Marker of a necrotising myopathy. *Ann. Rheum. Dis.* **2006**, *65*, 1635–1638. [CrossRef]
42. Bandeira, M.; Dourado, E.; Melo, A.T.; Martins, P.; Fraga, V.; Ferraro, J.L.; Saraiva, A.; Sousa, M.; Parente, H.; Soares, C.; et al. Predictors of cardiac involvement in idiopathic inflammatory myopathies. *Front. Immunol.* **2023**, *14*, 1146817. [CrossRef] [PubMed]
43. Ma, X.; Xu, L.; Li, Y.; Bu, B. Immunotherapy reversed myopathy but not cardiomyopathy in a necrotizing autoimmune myopathy patient with positive anti-SRP and MDA-5 autoantibodies. *BMC Cardiovasc. Disord.* **2021**, *21*, 88. [CrossRef]
44. Bobirca, A.; Alexandru, C.; Musetescu, A.E.; Bobirca, F.; Florescu, A.T.; Constantin, M.; Tebeica, T.; Florescu, A.; Isac, S.; Bojinca, M.; et al. Anti-MDA5 Amyopathic Dermatomyositis—A Diagnostic and Therapeutic Challenge. *Life* **2022**, *12*, 1108. [CrossRef]
45. Thiébaut, M.; Terrier, B.; Menacer, S.; Berezne, A.; Bussone, G.; Goulvestre, C.; Bellance, R.; Guillevin, L.; Vignaux, O.; Mouthon, L. Antisignal Recognition Particle Antibodies–Related Cardiomyopathy. *Circulation* **2013**, *127*, e434–e436. [CrossRef] [PubMed]
46. Takeguchi-Kikuchi, S.; Hayasaka, T.; Katayama, T.; Kano, K.; Takahashi, K.; Saito, T.; Sawada, J.; Minoshima, A.; Sakamoto, N.; Akasaka, K.; et al. Anti-signal Recognition Particle Antibody-positive Necrotizing Myopathy with Secondary Cardiomyopathy: The First Myocardial Biopsy- and Multimodal Imaging-proven Case. *Intern. Med.* **2019**, *58*, 3189–3194. [CrossRef] [PubMed]
47. Tanaka, M.; Gamou, N.; Shizukawa, H.; Tsuda, E.; Shimohama, S. Myopericarditis in a case of anti-signal recognition particle [anti-SRP] antibody-positive myopathy. *Rinsho Shinkeigaku* **2016**, *56*, 862–865. [CrossRef] [PubMed]
48. Vargas-Hitos, J.A.; Sáez-Urán, L.M.; Rosales-Castillo, A.; Jiménez-Alonso, J. Constitutional syndrome and chest pain as clinical onset feature of necrotizing myopathy with myocardial involvement. *Int. J. Rheum. Dis.* **2017**, *20*, 1767–1769. [CrossRef]
49. Targoff, I.N.; Johnson, A.E.; Miller, F.W. Antibody to signal recognition particle in polymyositis. *Arthritis Rheum.* **1990**, *33*, 1361–1370. [CrossRef]
50. Miller, T. Myopathy with antibodies to the signal recognition particle: Clinical and pathological features. *J. Neurol. Neurosurg. Psychiatry* **2002**, *73*, 420–428. [CrossRef]

51. Serban, D.; Spataru, R.I.; Vancea, G.; Balasescu, S.A.; Socea, B.; Tudor, C.; Dascalu, A.M. Informed consent in all surgical specialties: From legal obligation to patient satisfaction. *Rom. J. Leg. Med.* **2020**, *28*, 317–321. [CrossRef]
52. Leurs, A.; Dubucquoi, S.; Machuron, F.; Balden, M.; Renaud, F.; Rogeau, S. Extended myositis-specific and -associated antibodies profile in systemic sclerosis: A cross-sectional study. *Jt. Bone Spine* **2021**, *88*, 105048. [CrossRef] [PubMed]
53. Anghel, D.; Sîrbu, C.A.; Petrache, O.G.; Opriș-Belinski, D.; Negru, M.M.; Bojincă, V.C.; Pleșa, C.F.; Ioniță Radu, F. Nailfold Videocapillaroscopy in Patients with Rheumatoid Arthritis and Psoriatic Arthropathy on ANTI-TNF-ALPHA Therapy. *Diagnostics* **2023**, *13*, 2079. [CrossRef]
54. Sambataro, D.; Sambataro, G.; Libra, A.; Vignigni, G.; Pino, F.; Fagone, E.; Fruciano, M.; Gili, E.; Pignataro, F.; Del Papa, N.; et al. Nailfold Videocapillaroscopy Is a Useful Tool to Recognize Definite Forms of Systemic Sclerosis and Idiopathic Inflammatory Myositis in Interstitial Lung Disease Patients. *Diagnostics* **2020**, *10*, 253. [CrossRef]
55. Bhansing, K.J.; Lammens, M.; Knaapen, H.K.; van Riel, P.L.; van Engelen, B.G.; Vonk, M.C. Scleroderma-polymyositis overlap syndrome versus idiopathic polymyositis and systemic sclerosis: A descriptive study on clinical features and myopathology. *Arthritis Res. Ther.* **2014**, *16*, R111. [CrossRef] [PubMed]
56. Vonk, M.C. Is there still a role for cyclophosphamide in the treatment of systemic sclerosis? *J. Scleroderma Relat. Disord.* **2021**, *6*, 117–122. [CrossRef]
57. Kowal-Bielecka, O.; Fransen, J.; Avouac, J.; Becker, M.; Kulak, A.; Allanore, Y.; Distler, O.; Clements, P.; Cutolo, M.; Czirjak, L.; et al. Update of EULAR recommendations for the treatment of systemic sclerosis. *Ann. Rheum. Dis.* **2017**, *76*, 1327–1339. [CrossRef] [PubMed]
58. Serban, D.; Smarandache, A.M.; Cristian, D.; Tudor, C.; Duta, L.; Dascalu, A.M. Medical errors and patient safety culture—Shifting the healthcare paradigm in Romanian hospitals. *Rom. J. Leg. Med.* **2020**, *28*, 195–201. [CrossRef]
59. Morelli, M.B.; Bongiovanni, C.; Da Pra, S.; Miano, C.; Sacchi, F.; Lauriola, M.; D'Uva, G. Cardiotoxicity of Anticancer Drugs: Molecular Mechanisms and Strategies for Cardioprotection. *Front. Cardiovasc. Med.* **2022**, *9*, 847012. [CrossRef]
60. Martin, M.; Fornecker, L.M.; Marcellin, L.; Mousseaux, E.; Hij, A.; Snowden, J.A.; Farge, D.; Martin, T. Acute and fatal cardiotoxicity following high-dose cyclophosphamide in a patient undergoing autologous stem cell transplantation for systemic sclerosis despite satisfactory cardiopulmonary screening. *Bone Marrow Transpl.* **2017**, *52*, 1674–1677. [CrossRef]
61. Burt, R.K.; Oliveira, M.C.; Shah, S.J.; Moraes, D.A.; Simoes, B.; Gheorghiade, M.; Schroeder, J.; Ruderman, E.; Farge, D.; Chai, Z.J.; et al. Cardiac involvement and treatment-related mortality after non-myeloablative haemopoietic stem-cell transplantation with unselected autologous peripheral blood for patients with systemic sclerosis: A retrospective analysis. *Lancet* **2013**, *381*, 1116–1124. [CrossRef]
62. Opinc, A.H.; Makowski, M.A.; Łukasik, Z.M.; Makowska, J.S. Cardiovascular complications in patients with idiopathic inflammatory myopathies: Does heart matter in idiopathic inflammatory myopathies? *Heart Fail. Rev.* **2021**, *26*, 111–125. [CrossRef] [PubMed]
63. Touma, Z.; Arayssi, T.; Kibbi, L.; Masri, A.F. Successful treatment of cardiac involvement in dermatomyositis with rituximab. *Jt. Bone Spine* **2008**, *75*, 334–337. [CrossRef] [PubMed]
64. Allanore, Y. Effects of corticosteroids and immunosuppressors on idiopathic inflammatory myopathy related myocarditis evaluated by magnetic resonance imaging. *Ann. Rheum. Dis.* **2006**, *65*, 249–252. [CrossRef] [PubMed]
65. Riemekasten, G.; Opitz, C.; Audring, H.; Barthelmes, H.; Meyer, R.; Hiepe, F.; Burmester, G.R. Beware of the heart: The multiple picture of cardiac involvement in myositis. *Rheumatology* **1999**, *38*, 1153–1157. [CrossRef]
66. Lee, Z.C.; Noviani, M.; Yap, J.; Chin, C.W.L.; Ng, S.A.; Low, A.H.L. Tocilizumab for systemic sclerosis with cardiac involvement: A case report. *Clin. Exp. Rheumatol.* **2022**, *40*, 2006–2007. [CrossRef] [PubMed]
67. Ishizaki, Y.; Ooka, S.; Doi, S.; Kawasaki, T.; Sakurai, K.; Mizushima, M.; Kiyokawa, T.; Takakuwa, Y.; Tonooka, K.; Kawahata, K. Treatment of myocardial fibrosis in systemic sclerosis with tocilizumab. *Rheumatology* **2021**, *60*, e205–e206. [CrossRef]
68. Schreiber, A.; Elango, K.; Sossou, C.; Fakhra, S.; Asad, S.; Ahsan, C. COVID-19 Induced Cardiomyopathy Successfully Treated with Tocilizumab. *Case Rep. Cardiol.* **2022**, *2022*, 9943937. [CrossRef]

medicina

MDPI

Review

The Challenges of Local Intra-Articular Therapy

Gailute Kirdaite [1,*], Jaroslav Denkovskij [2], Diana Mieliauskaite [1], Jolita Pachaleva [2] and Eiva Bernotiene [2,3]

1 Department of Personalised Medicine, State Research Institute Centre for Innovative Medicine, LT-08406 Vilnius, Lithuania

2 Department of Regenerative Medicine, State Research Institute Centre for Innovative Medicine, LT-08406 Vilnius, Lithuania; eiva.bernotiene@imcentras.lt (E.B.)

3 Faculty of Fundamental Sciences, Vilnius Gediminas Technical University, VilniusTech, Sauletekio al. 11, LT-10223 Vilnius, Lithuania

* Correspondence: gailute.kirdaite@imcentras.lt

Abstract: Fibroblast-like synoviocytes (FLSs) are among the main disease-driving players in most cases of monoarthritis (MonoA), oligoarthritis, and polyarthritis. In this review, we look at the characteristics and therapeutic challenges at the onset of arthritis and during follow-up management. In some cases, these forms of arthritis develop into autoimmune polyarthritis, such as rheumatoid arthritis (RA), whereas local eradication of the RA synovium could still be combined with systemic treatment using immunosuppressive agents. Currently, the outcomes of local synovectomies are well studied; however, there is still a lack of a comprehensive analysis of current local intra-articular treatments highlighting their advantages and disadvantages. Therefore, the aim of this study is to review local intra-articular therapy strategies. According to publications from the last decade on clinical studies focused on intra-articular treatment with anti-inflammatory molecules, a range of novel slow-acting forms of steroidal drugs for the local treatment of synovitis have been investigated. As pain is an essential symptom, caused by both inflammation and cartilage damage, various molecules acting on pain receptors are being investigated in clinical trials as potential targets for local intra-articular treatment. We also overview the new targets for local treatment, including surface markers and intracellular proteins, non-coding ribonucleic acids (RNAs), etc.

Keywords: monoarthritis; inflammation; synovectomy; local treatment; fibroblast like synoviocytes; non-coding ribonucleic acids (RNAs)

1. Introduction

The European League Against Rheumatism (EULAR) has launched a Europe-wide campaign, "Don't delay, connect today", to raise awareness of the major public health concerns of rheumatic and musculoskeletal diseases (RMDs). Guidelines from the Osteoarthritis Research Society International (OARSI) and the Food and Drug Administration (FDA), as well as recommendations from the EULAR, emphasize the importance of early anti-inflammatory therapy (EIT) and the treat-to-target strategy (T2T) [1–3]. According to EULAR recommendations, a rheumatologist should see the patient within 6 weeks of the onset of arthritis and decide on a treatment strategy. The "window of opportunity" is usually up to three months, which is a crucial timeframe to choose an effective treatment strategy to stop the progression of the disease in its early stages [4,5].

Therefore, the management of inflammatory arthritis, especially monoarthritis (MonoA), before it develops into oligoarthritis and polyarthritis remains a challenge. The duration of acute MonoA is two to four weeks. Making an accurate diagnosis in such a short period is only sometimes possible. In most cases, acute MonoA is caused by a variety of causes ranging from benign to life-threatening. Thus, the onset of inflammatory arthritis (IA) may be MonoA, which needs to be carefully differentiated from diseases with different pathogenesis, such as gout (urine-type crystals), traumatic arthritis (trauma), infectious arthritis (virus or bacteria), paraneoplastic arthritis (cancer), and others [6–8]. It should be noted that several cases of MonoA have also been described since the beginning of 2021 after COVID-19 [9].

The PubMed scientific literature data on this topic could be more coherent, so we decided to review these issues. Thus, it remains to resolve and understand the main problem of MonoA as a choice of intervention strategy for synovial local inflammation. According to the literature, about 50% of MonoA cases resolve spontaneously; the rest develop into oligo- or polyarticular disease, but a significant proportion remains as persistent inflammatory MonoA. We attempt to analyze the data based on a basic pathogenetic message that FLSs are the key players in the majority of MonoA cases. As FLSs are key targets for local therapy, we focused on new targets related to surface markers and intracellular proteins, non-coding ribonucleic acids (RNAs), signaling, etc. Therefore, there is an urgent need to suppress or eradicate local inflammation, from which aggressive fibroblast-like synoviocytes (FLSs) are activated to induce cartilage degradation and may trigger a systemic autoimmune response [10,11], including rheumatoid arthritis (RA). Synovial inflammation has recently been suggested as a target for the treatment of osteoarthritis (OA) as well [12,13]. Thus, the synovitis-related phenotype or endotype of OA is an important factor in designing more effective disease-modifying interventions in these cases [14]. There is very little knowledge on the incidence and prevalence of early IA in primary care settings. Therefore, in most studies, the prevalence of early undifferentiated arthritis is around 30% [15–17].

Today, the scientific data on local synovectomy are well studied, one by one, but it is necessary to summarize the comparative data on this treatment modality. These challenges concern the scientific, medical, and pharmaceutical communities as they seek to establish a strong link between new intra-articular (i.a.) treatments. Thus, we analyzed local treatments from the US National Library of Medicine (clinicaltrials.gov, accessed on 1 January 2023) database with the following criteria: 2013–2023 years completed trials with results publications, adult population, and intra-articular arthritis treatment (in particular anti-inflammatory effects on synovium).

Therefore, in this paper, we will analyze the long-term monitoring results of MonoA and explore the local treatment strategies available today.

2. Materials and Methods

We tried to analyze the data based on the pathogenesis basic knowledge that FLSs are key players in most cases of arthritis (see graphical abstract). In the 1st step, the PubMed database was searched for the keyword 'monoarthritis' only. Monoarthritis was represented by 353 case reports, but these cases were not included in the pooled data.

Therefore, in the 2nd step, we had to solve and understand the main problem of the choice of the intervention strategy for local inflammation of the synovium, so we used different combinations of terms for local treatment approaches in the PubMed database search: 'monoarthritis', 'local treatment', 'intra-articular treatment', 'synovectomy', and 'synovitis treatment'. On the basis of our analysis of these clinically evaluated synovectomies, we concluded that there is still a lack of data on selective local treatment.

In the 3rd step, we analyzed 53 contemporary local treatments from the US National Library of Medicine (clinicaltrials.gov) database according to the following criteria: completed trials with results, 10-year follow-up period, adult population, and intra-articular arthritis treatment. In the clinical studies, we searched for new intra-articular approaches, especially for OA patients with inflammatory phenotype where FLSs are less aggressive.

In the 4th step, we asked about new advances in the inhibition of aggressive FLS suppression, using an RA example. As FLSs are key targets for local therapy, we focused on new targets related to surface markers and intracellular proteins, non-coding ribonucleic acids (RNAs), signaling, etc.

3. Local Treatment of Arthritis

3.1. Monoarthritis: Treatment Challenges

The experience with MonoA shows that local treatment of joint synovitis is feasible, especially when large joints are affected (Figure 1).

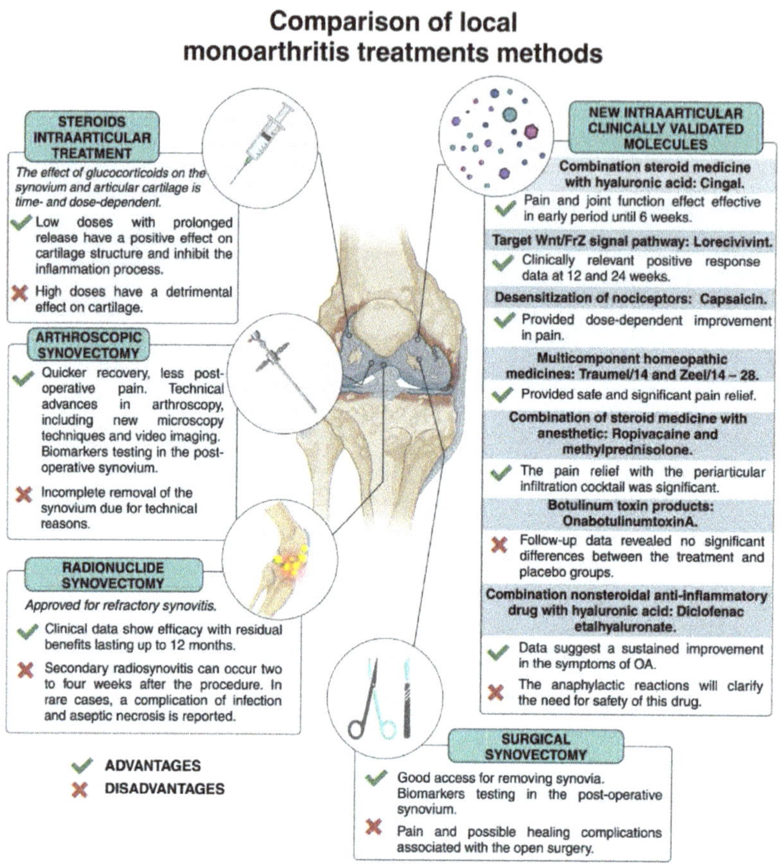

Figure 1. Advantages and disadvantages of local monoarthritis treatments. Created with BioRender.com (accessed on 4 July 2024).

In general, each of the local procedures used in clinical practice has its own advantages and disadvantages, and open and arthroscopic surgical interventions remove inflamed tissue while providing the opportunity to study biomarkers [18–20]. Currently, needle ultrasound and arthroscopy biopsy are used to assess synovitis [21,22], but new contrast-enhanced magnetic resonance imaging (MRI) techniques are better able as a reference method to characterize the synovium and cartilage [23]. A decrease in orthopedic joints is linked to the development of more conventional new systemic biologics, medications, etc. [24,25].

The EULAR recommendations on intra-articular therapy for different inflammatory arthritis should be considered [26]. The effect of corticosteroids on articular cartilage is time- and dose-dependent: a low dose has a beneficial effect, whereas a high dose has a detrimental effect on cartilage degradation [27]. There is a diverse scientific debate on the predictive factors of response to intra-articular steroid injections in knee osteoarthritis: degree of synovitis, site of discharge, and cartilage protection [28]. Intra-articular injections of glucocorticoids are probably the most common and widely used for local inhibition of synovial inflammation. This EULAR Guideline describes the basic principles for the use of i.a. steroid injections for knee pain relief in combination with release or for RA in cases where there is a need to adjust the disease-modifying antirheumatic drugs DMARDs therapy in one or more remaining active joints [26]. As previously described, in the MonoA, steroid therapy is the first choice for suppressing local inflammation; this treatment modality is good at suppressing synovitis and symptoms. In cases where steroids are injected close to the synovium (e.g., into the fat pad of the knee joint), the anti-inflammatory efficacy may be very similar to the same precise needle placement into the synovial cavity due to the distribution of the steroid through the tissues surrounding the joint [29]. Synovial inflammation has recently been proposed as an essential target for the treatment of OA [12]. Today, the FDA has approved low-dose, slow-release drugs for the treatment of OA local synovitis [30].

3.2. *Recent Developments of Intra-Articular Medication*

We analyzed and summarized 10 years of clinical studies in Table 1. Thus, novel molecules have been described as clinically validated i.a. therapies for synovitis treatment strategies. Joint damage due to synovial inflammation and cartilage breakdown are two of the factors that cause pain. Therefore, analgetic treatment is also very essential for local treatment. Brief comments on the solutions to these problems are given below.

Table 1. New clinically tested treatment options for local synovial inflammation.

Clinical Studies Showing Positive Local Intra-Articular Anti-Inflammatory and Analgesic Effects		
	STEROIDS	
	1. Triamcinolone acetonide extended-release. Product name and description: FX006 (Zilreta), a microsphere-based extended-release triamcinolone acetonide.	
Phase	Design (*n* = patients), tested medication doses, follow-up duration.	Outcomes
Phase 2	Double-blind, multicenter study (228 patients); Dose FX006 (containing 10, 40, or 60 mg of triamcinolone acetonide) or 40 mg of immediate-release triamcinolone acetonide (TA). Follow-up 12 weeks.	FX006 40 mg dose provided pain relief from 2 to 12 weeks. This medication was significantly superior to TA at five to ten weeks. Adverse events were mild and similar in the treatment groups [31].
Phase 2b	306 participants were randomized (1:1:1) to receive single i.a. injections of FX006 32 mg (*n* = 104) or 16 mg (n = 102) or saline placebo (*n* – 100). Follow-up 12 weeks.	FX006 32 mg versus 16 mg produced a dose-dependent analgesic response, the treatment was well tolerated, and the safety profile was similar to that of saline placebo [32].
Phase 3b	Single-arm, open-label study, participants (*n* = 208). All patients received the first (day 1) intra-articular triamcinolone acetonide extended-release (TA-ER) injection. The second-injection patients received a flexible (at either week 12, 16, 20, or 24) schedule, which depends on the first-injection response duration. Patients who received two injections were evaluated for 52 weeks.	TA-ER administration with a flexible dosing schedule repeated twice according to patient response was well tolerated, with no radiographic evidence of knee joint cartilage effects [33].
Phase 2	Randomized, multicenter, open-label, single-dose study, 30 patients with hip OA were randomly assigned 1:1 to receive single i.a. injections in the hip joint of TA-ER 32 mg or triamcinolone acetonide TA crystalline suspension (TAcs) 40 mg. Pharmacokinetic (PK) analysis of this medication concentration was performed up to day 85.	The systemic plasma concentration exposure was substantially lower for TA-ER versus TAcs during follow-up. Thus, TA-ER was generally well tolerated, with a safety profile comparable to that of Tacs [34].
Phase 2	Randomized, open-label, single-dose study 25 patients randomly received a single ultrasound-guided i.a. injection in the shoulder joint of TA-ER 32 mg or TAcs 40 mg. PK analysis of these medication concentration was performed up to day 85.	The pharmacokinetic results showed that TA-ER was well tolerated with the systemic safe profile compared to TAcs crystalline suspension [35].
Phase 2	Open-label study sequentially enrolled 81 patients. After SF aspiration, the i.a. injection of 32 mg FX006 or 40 mg TAcs was given to each patient at baseline and during follow-up visits (FX006: weeks 1–6–12–16–20; TAcs: week 6).	After injection of FX006 microspheres, the SF and plasma PK observations are consistent with slow release of TA relative to TAcs in patients with knee OA. The slow release of FX006 microspheres reduced systemic TA exposure relative to TAcs [36].

Table 1. *Cont.*

Clinical Studies Showing Positive Local Intra-Articular Anti-Inflammatory and Analgesic Effects		
2. Liposome formulation of dexamethasone sodium phosphate. Product name and description: TLC599 is a water-soluble corticosteroid, dexamethasone sodium phosphate (DSP), produced using new BioSeizer® technology, which encapsulates therapeutically active molecules in multilayer lipid membranes to ensure an extremely long drug release time.		
Phase 2a	Randomized, placebo-controlled, dose-finding study, n = 75 patients. Two single injections of TLC599 (12 mg and 18 mg DSP) and placebo (normal saline) were given, and pain relief was observed in clinical data up to week 24.	The 12 mg dose level of TLC599 showed effective pain relief and improvement in physical function. Treatment was safe and without side effects [37].
3. Combination steroid medicine with hyaluronic acid (HA). Product name and description: Triamcinolone hexacetonide with a commercial cross-linked HA viscosupplement (Cingal).		
	Multicenter, double-blind, saline-controlled clinical trial randomized 368 subjects. A single injection of Cingal (4 mL, 88 mg HA plus 18 mg triamcinolone hexacetonide (TH)), Monovisc (4 mL, 88 mg HA), or saline solution (4 mL, 0.9%). The pain score monitoring was assessed at 12 weeks and 26 weeks.	The pain and function were significantly better in Cingal group compared to saline groups. Cingal had a better effect in the early period, but after 6 weeks and beyond, the effect was similar compared to Monovisc alone [38].
WNT INHIBITORS		
4. Target Wnt/FrZ signal pathway. Product name and description: SM04690 (Lorecivivint (LOR)), which acts as an inhibitor of the Wnt signaling pathway, is thought to play an important role in cartilage degeneration by affecting the differentiation of chondrocytes, osteoblasts, and synovial cells.		
Phase 2b	Multicenter, randomized, double-blind, placebo-controlled trial, n = 695 patients. This study's objective was to identify effective LOR doses: 0.03, 0.07, 0.15, or 0.23 mg. Follow-up 24 weeks.	The optimal dose was identified as 0.07 mg LOR [39].
	Post hoc analysis of this clinical trial identified the proportions of LOR responders.	Patient-reported outcomes (PROs) provide clinically relevant positive response data on measures of pain, function, and patient global assessment compared with placebo, with benefits that persisted at 24 weeks [40].
	Post hoc analysis of this clinical trial identified the proportions of LOR responders.	The PRO comparison of control groups, dry needle sham, and saline-based placebo injections for the treatment of knee OA showed equivalent patient-reported outcomes at all time points up to week 24, with no physiological impact [41].
Summary: The results of the clinical study suggested that the optimal dose for future studies was 0.07 mg LOR [39]. A post hoc analysis yielded clinically relevant positive response data at 12 and 24 weeks in participants with moderate and severe knee OA [40,41].		
PAIN MANAGEMENT		
5. Molecule induces desensitization of nociceptors. Product name and description: The Capsaicin (CNTX-4975) molecule is involved in the long-term desensitization of nociceptors associated with calcium influx into nociceptive nerve endings.		
Phase 2	Multicenter double-blind study, n = 172 patients. Randomization: placebo group, CNTX-4975 0.5 mg and 1.0 mg groups. Follow-up 24 weeks.	CNTX-4975 1.0 mg at 24 weeks significantly reduced OA knee pain; CNTX-4975 0.5 mg significantly reduced pain at 12 weeks, but no effect on pain effect was evident at 24 weeks. Adverse events were mild and similar in the treatment groups [42].
6. Multicomponent homeopathic medicines. Product name and description: Traumel/14 and Zeel/14–28 ingredients are of vegetable, mineral, and other organic origin, diluted to so-called "low strength" because they contain measurable molecular concentrations of potential active substances with anti-inflammatory, antioxidant, and chondroprotective properties.		
	The double-blind, multicenter, randomized, saline-controlled trial, n = 232 patients. The investigational medicinal product is 4.2 mL (2.0 mL for Zeel/14 and 2.2 mL for Traumel/14 on days 1, 8, and 15 of treatment). Follow-up 29, 71, 85 days.	In this study, intra-articular Traumel14/Zeel14 provided safe and significant pain relief [43].

Table 1. *Cont.*

Clinical Studies Showing Positive Local Intra-Articular Anti-Inflammatory and Analgesic Effects		
7. Combination of steroid medicine with anesthetic. Product name and description: Ropivacaine and methylprednisolone were infiltrated with the periarticular infiltration of this cocktail for the reduction in pain.		
	The prospective non-randomized pilot 9-month period study, $n = 50$ patients. After total knee arthroplasty (TKA), the solution contained a cocktail of ropivacaine, clonidine, epinephrine, and ketorolac with 1 mL of methylprednisolone (40 mg), which was infiltrated in the periarticular tissues, control group was second knee with the infiltration the same solutions mixture except for methylprednisolone. Patients' follow-ups for pain evaluation were the first three days after surgery.	The reduction in pain with the periarticular infiltration ropivacaine and methylprednisolone cocktail was significant [44].
8. Botulinum toxin products. Product name and description: OnabotulinumtoxinA—the regulation of response to nociception in various diseases.		
	The multicenter, double-blind, randomized, placebo-controlled study enrolled 176 patients, and 158 completed the study. Randomization: i.a. onabotulinumtoxinA 400 U or 200 U and placebo (saline), followed up for 24 weeks.	Follow-up data revealed no significant differences between the treatment and placebo groups in the reduction in WOMAC mean pain score. Treatment was safe and without serious effects [45].
9. Combination nonsteroidal anti-inflammatory drug with HA. Product name and description: Diclofenac etalhyaluronate (DF) molecule covalently bonded to HA has a long-lasting anti-inflammatory effect.		
Phase 3	The multicenter, open-label, noncomparative study, $n = 166$ patients. Treatment regimen was i.a. 30 mg DF-HA every 4 weeks for 1 year (13 times in total). Follow-up 52 weeks.	The results showed that DF-HA was well tolerated and the data suggest a sustained improvement in the symptoms of OA [46].
Phase 3	Multicenter, randomized, double-blind, placebo-controlled trial, $n = 440$ patients. DF-HA 30 mg or placebo once every 4 weeks for 20 weeks (a total of 6 injections). Follow-up for 24 weeks.	The significant improvement in the WOMAC pain subscale score compared to placebo was over 12 weeks. The observed anaphylactic reactions will clarify the need for the safety of this drug [47].

Summary: Thus, today, new steroid formats are approved for the local treatment of OA knees, hips, and shoulder joints with a slow-acting drug that has no detrimental effect on the cartilage or other aspects of the joint structure; the pain relief is dose-dependent. The 3b clinical study with a flexible dosing schedule repeated twice according to patient response was well tolerated and effective until 52 weeks [33]. Other studies in which steroids were administered slowly showed encouraging results in terms of pain relief and improvement in physical function at around 24 weeks [30–32,34–37]. Another important aspect is the combination of steroids with HA, which has been evaluated and found to have a beneficial anti-inflammatory effect in combination with viscosupplementation [38]; this combination is effective against pain in the early phase of the disease for up to 6 weeks. WNT inhibitors are being investigated and this drug has a positive effect on cartilage degeneration by affecting chondrocyte differentiation and inhibition of osteoblasts and synovial cells [39,40]. Meanwhile, molecules, involved in the long-term desensitization of nociceptors associated with calcium influx into nociceptive nerve endings show a beneficial pain inhibitory effect [42]. The regulation of the nociceptive response with botulinum toxin has not shown a beneficial effect on synovium pain [45]. Various combinations (steroids with anesthetics or NSAIDs with HA) are currently being clinically validated, and these agents have shown pain suppression [44,46,47]. Attention must be paid to nonsteroidal anti-inflammatory drugs in combination with HA regarding anaphylactic reactions [47]. Consequently, multicomponent homeopathic medicines are also used in the clinical practice for pain relief [43]. The effects of all of these drugs are dose-dependent, with duration ranging from 12 weeks to 52 weeks. The summarized data are represented in Figure S1. Local treatment of early synovitis with targeted intra-articular suppression is essential, but at the same time, the per os treatment must be chosen to select an effective treatment strategy and to halt disease progression in the early stages [4,5]. MonoA data for local treatment, especially intra-articular treatment, have revealed that key target molecules are involved in OA. In the clinical studies described above, we analyzed novel molecules approved for intra-articular therapy, particularly targeting OA patients with an inflammatory phenotype where FLSs are less aggressive. Another approach is the investigation of new targets in inflammatory tissues after synovectomy in pre-clinical studies. As fibroblast-like synoviocytes are one of the targets of local treatment, we focused on these synovitis-promoting players. The behavior of FLS in RA is an excellent example for exploring new targets related to surface markers and intracellular proteins of these cells, non-coding RNAs, signal transduction, etc.

3.3. Fibroblast-like Synoviocytes as Potential Targets for Early Local Therapy

In RA, fibroblast-like synoviocytes have intrinsic pathogenic properties and actively contribute to the disease process. They proliferate and promote joint destruction by stimulating inflammation. However, the reasons why they turn from beneficial to harmful in RA remain to be fully understood. Studies have shown that persistent inflammation can induce molecular changes in FLSs that transform them from passive responders to inflammation to active aggressors [48,49]. RA FLSs have specific characteristics that distinguish them from healthy FLSs. These characteristics remain unchanged even when RA FLSs are isolated from an environment rich in inflammatory cytokines [11,49]. Potential therapeutic strategies could target FLS surfaces and intracellular proteins, FLS metabolism, and signaling pathways that increase FLS invasive and migratory potential, non-coding ribonucleic acid, oxidative stress molecules, etc. Current therapeutic approaches focus on modifying the immune response, specifically by targeting pro-inflammatory cytokines, B cells, or T cells [50]. Some of these drugs may also influence the invasive behavior of FLSs, especially those that inhibit cytokines or signal transduction pathways [51,52]. Although these drugs can reduce the level of FLS activity in RA, they may not always be effective, which is why patients still suffer from this disease. In such cases, the use of a combination of alternative or complementary therapies may be useful to manage the disease effectively. Potential therapeutic targets related to FLS are described in Figure 2 and the following sections.

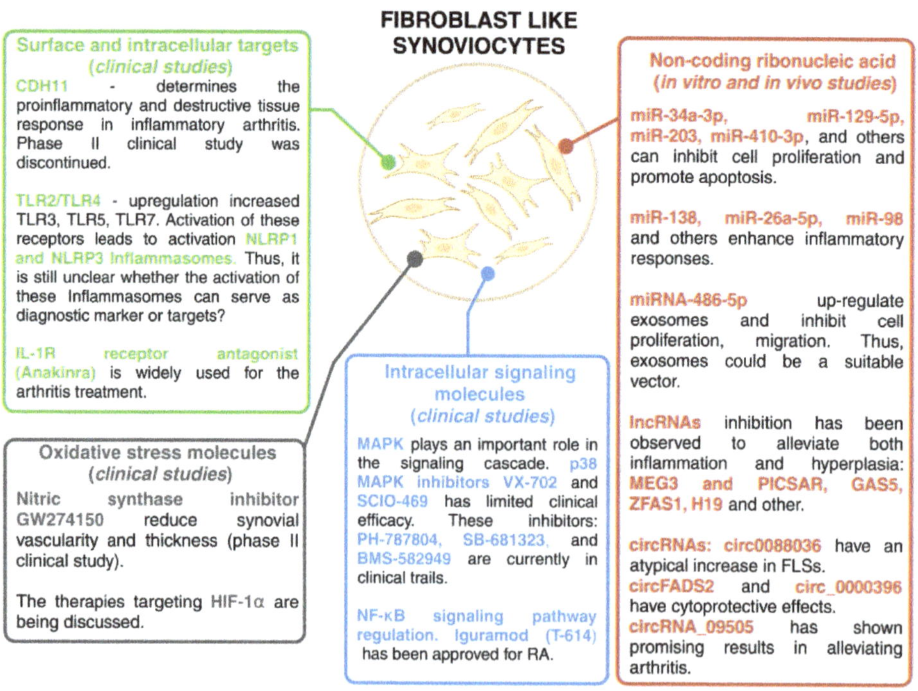

Figure 2. Potential therapeutic targets related to FLSs. Created with BioRender.com.

3.3.1. Cell Surface Targets

The discovery of different FLS phenotypes that contribute to synovitis leads to the possibility of targeting cells based on their surface phenotype. This implies the identification of pathogenic cell-specific surface proteins and the development of innovative treatment strategies targeting specific RA FLS phenotypes. RA FLSs lineages are characterized by the expression of specific markers such as CD10, CD34, CD55, CD90, CD248, and podoplanin (PDPN) [53–56]. These surface markers characterize RA FLS subgroups with significant functional differences. For example, previous studies have shown that cadherin 11 (CDH11) significantly contributes to homotypic FLS aggregation in in vitro and in vivo models [57,58]. CDH11 has attracted considerable attention as a potential marker of RA and has been widely regarded as a promising target. Nevertheless, a clinical trial investigating the efficacy of a monoclonal antibody directed against CDH11 in a phase II study was discontinued due to low efficacy.

Other potential markers and targets of RA include Toll-like receptors (TLRs) and inflammasomes. Pattern recognition receptors (PRRs) such as TLRs recognize pathogen-associated molecular patterns (PAMPs) or damage-associated molecular patterns (DAMPs). If regulatory mechanisms fail, TLR activation can trigger local inflammation and contribute to inflammatory or autoimmune diseases. Necrotic cells in inflamed joints may be a source of endogenous ligands for these receptors. Heat shock proteins and low molecular weight hyaluronan were originally thought to activate TLR2/TLR4 heterodimers directly, but pure ligands do not effectively activate these receptors [59]. However, citrullination of endogenous ligands such as fibrinogen and histones can stimulate the TLR4-mediated pathway [60,61]. The involvement of the TLR4-mediated pathway in the development of RA is suggested by the significant inhibition of monocyte activation observed in these patients with ACPA when treated with anti-TLR4 antibodies [62]. TLR4 can increase the production of pro-inflammatory cytokines and chemokines, such as IL-6 and IL-17, by binding to exogenous ligands, such as peptidoglycan, in the FLS of RA patients and in peripheral blood mononuclear cells (PBMCs), leading to inflammation and degeneration of cartilage [63]. In addition to the up-regulation of TLR2 and TLR4, an increased expression of TLR3, TLR5, and TLR7 has been observed in FLSs from RA patients compared to individuals with OA or without inflammatory diseases [64–67]. Activation of these receptors leads to enhanced local inflammatory responses, including the formation of nucleotide-binding oligomerization domain (NOD)-like receptor family pyrin domain-rich receptor 1 (NLRP1) and NLRP3 inflammasomes [68].

Inflammasomes are multicellular protein complexes that activate the release of pro-inflammatory cytokines such as interleukin-1β (IL-1β) in response to cellular stress or infection. Activation of the NLRP3 inflammasome contributes to the development of autoimmune diseases such as ankylosing spondylitis, systemic sclerosis, systemic lupus erythematosus, and RA [69,70]. Two signals are required to activate the NLRP3 inflammasome. The first signal is transduced via membrane receptors such as TLRs. Meanwhile, the second signal is linked to stimuli such as changes in ATP, K^+ and Ca^{2+} levels, lysosomal destabilization, mitochondrial dysfunction, reactive oxygen species, and uric acid crystals [71–73]. Targeting TLRs and inflammasomes is promising for modulating the immune response and possibly treating inflammatory disorders. However, it is still unclear whether the activation of these inflammasomes can serve as diagnostic markers to differentiate undifferentiated early inflammatory arthritis into specific diseases such as RA.

The question is whether these different populations are definitive subsets with a consistent phenotype or whether the FLS phenotype is flexible and microenvironment-dependent, leading to differences in the relative prevalence of the various putative phenotypes.

3.3.2. Intracellular Signaling Molecules

Various cell signaling molecules have been investigated as potential biomarkers of RA, which can help diagnose, monitor, and predict the disease's progression.

There are several strategies to combat FLSs, including inhibition of components of the mitogen-activated protein kinase (MAPK) cascade, inhibition of kinases that activate c-Jun N-terminal kinase (JNK), and blocking the nuclear factor-κB (NFκB) pathway [74].

MAPK regulates the production of pro-inflammatory cytokines and plays an important role in the signaling cascade downstream of interleukin (IL)-1, IL-17, and tumor necrosis factor (TNF)-α receptors [75,76]. Activation of MAPK family members occurs primarily in synovial tissues. Their activation is important for the production of pro-inflammatory cytokines such as TNF, IL-6, and IL-1. p38 kinase is a potential target for the treatment of RA, but clinical trials have yet to identify effective inhibitors. The results show that the p38 MAPK inhibitor VX-702 has limited clinical efficacy and is accompanied by transient inhibition of inflammatory biomarkers [77]. However, it may not offer a significant and permanent inhibitory impact on the chronic inflammation observed in RA. For instance, the clinical trial, including SCIO-469, an orally administered inhibitor of p38-α MAPK, did not show greater efficacy than a placebo in individuals diagnosed with rheumatoid arthritis [78]. PH-797804, SB-681323, and BMS-582949 are p38 inhibitors currently in clinical trials [74]. As an alternative approach, higher members of the MAPK cascade, such as MKK3, MKK6, and MAP3K5, have been investigated as potential targets in pre-clinical models [79].

Targeting JNK in this pathway has shown encouraging results in alleviating the clinical symptoms of RA. JNK1 plays a crucial role in maintaining and promoting inflammation in the synovium [80]. It is expressed in FLS and macrophage-like synoviocytes (MLS), and targeting JNK1 with blocking agents can reduce its endogenous expression in both synovial cell types [81,82]. For example, the use of the JNK inhibitor SP600125 has decreased c-Jun transcription and enhanced the accumulation of phospho-Jun, thereby attenuating the inflammatory response. In addition, the JNK inhibitor AS601245 can relieve symptoms of collagen-induced arthritis rat model (CIA) rats [83].

Current pharmacological drugs used for treatment therapy specifically target or interact with the NF-κB signaling pathway. The NF-κB signaling pathway regulates a variety of cellular processes, including inflammation, immune response, and cell survival [74,84]. These drugs act by modulating NF-κB activity, inhibiting its activation or blocking downstream signaling events. For example, methotrexate (MTX) is an effective drug for the treatment of RA and affects TNF-α levels in early RA patients via the NF-κB pathway [85]. Prednisolone, a synthetic glucocorticoid, inhibits the transcription of inflammatory genes via the NF-κB signaling pathway and is clinically used to reduce RA inflammation [86].

In addition, new drugs are currently being investigated and developed to reduce the activity of aggressive FLS by modulating the NF-κB signaling pathway. Iguramod (T-614) is a new disease-modifying anti-rheumatic drug that inhibits NF-κB activation and is approved for the treatment of RA in Japan and China [87]. Denosumab inhibits NF-κB ligand–receptor activator and can partially restore bone erosions in RA patients. The combination of Denosumab with DMARDs may be considered in RA patients with progressive bone erosions. Previous studies have demonstrated the efficacy of an antagonist targeting cysteinyl leukotriene receptor 1 (CysLT1) in inhibiting NF-kB pathway activation as well as interleukin-6 (IL-6) and interleukin-8 (IL-8) secretion in FLS [88]. The results of this study suggest that modulation of CysLT1 and leukotriene B4 (LTB4) receptors may be an effective therapeutic strategy to reduce inflammation and slow the progression of RA patients [89]. However, further studies are needed to confirm their efficacy and to investigate their clinical application. The integration of multiple biomarkers and the use of advanced technologies may increase their diagnostic and prognostic value in the future [10,90,91].

3.3.3. Non-Coding Ribonucleic Acids

Non-coding ribonucleic acids (ncRNAs) have emerged as potential biomarkers for rheumatoid arthritis (RA). ncRNAs are RNA molecules that do not encode proteins but play important regulatory roles in gene expression and cellular processes, including signaling pathways. ncRNAs comprise a diverse group of molecules, including microRNAs (miRNAs), long non-coding RNAs (lncRNAs), and circular RNAs (circRNAs).

The level of miRNAs can influence the secretion of inflammatory cytokines or metalloproteinases (MMPs), which in turn can impact the progression of RA [92]. Certain miRNAs have been found to inhibit cell proliferation and promote apoptosis [93], while others have been shown to contribute to the inflammatory environment, possibly leading to tissue damage [94,95]. Animal and cell culture experiments have shown promising results when certain miRNAs alleviate or enhance RA symptoms. For example, when overexpressed, miR-34a-3p [96], miR-129-5p [97], miR-203 [98], miR-410-3p [99], and others can inhibit cell proliferation and promote apoptosis by targeting different proteins. On the other hand, miR-138 [100], miR-26a-5p [94], miR-98 [101], and similar miRNAs enhance inflammatory responses. In addition, miRNA-486-5p up-regulation in exosomes has been found to inhibit cell proliferation and migration, suggesting that exosomes could be a suitable vector for the therapeutic delivery of miRNA-486-5p [102]. Long non-coding RNAs (lncRNAs) over 200 nucleotides in length are widely expressed in many human tissues and can be a diagnostic tool for RA [103]. However, like miRNAs, they may have dual effects. Some lncRNAs have anti-inflammatory properties, while others can enhance inflammatory reactions. For example, inhibition of specific long non-coding RNAs (lncRNAs) has been observed to alleviate both inflammation and hyperplasia. The involvement of non-coding RNAs (ncRNA) FER1L4 and MEG3 in RA has been demonstrated in [104,105]. MEG3 upregulation has an inflammation-suppressive effect by modulating the AKT/mTOR signaling cascade [106]. PICSAR, an additional (ncRNA), influences several cellular processes, including cell proliferation, migration, invasion, and the synthesis of IL-6, IL-8, and MMP-3. It exerts this influence by interacting with miR-4701-5p [107]. The role of the miR-222-3p/Sirt1 axis is central to the action of GAS5 in mitigating RA FSL proliferation, inflammation, and apoptosis [108]. Silencing of the lncRNA ZFAS1 may mitigate inflammation and hyperplasia by competitively binding to miR-296-5p and regulating MMP-15 expression in the context of an experimental arthritis model. Inhibition of ZFAS1 has been observed to alleviate both inflammation and hyperplasia. This effect is achieved by binding ZFAS1 to miR-296-5p, which subsequently regulates MMP-15 expression [109]. Furthermore, IncRNAs expressing lncRNA-H19 injected into the ankles of collagen-induced arthritis (CIA) mice ameliorate the progression by competing with miR-124a, which directly acts on CDK2 and MCP-1 [110].

Circular RNAs (circRNAs) are a recently discovered class of endogenous ncRNA molecules whose importance in regulating gene expression is increasingly recognized. CircRNAs have been found to be abnormally elevated in RA and to contribute to disease progression. These circRNAs have been identified as abnormally increased in RA and contribute to the advancement of the disease. These ncRNAs have great potential and promising targets for the treatment of RA. They have several functional properties, including RNA polymerase II elongation, regulation of RNA maturation, and protein localization [111]. Several studies have started to investigate the involvement of circRNAs in the pathogenesis of RA. As an example, the molecule circ0088036 has been observed to have an atypical increase in FLSs. This abnormality contributes to the progression of RA by acting as a molecular sponge for miR-140-3p, thereby augmenting the production of SIRT 1 [112]. Other circRNAs, circFADS2 and circ_0000396, have been shown to have cytoprotective effects against apoptosis and suppress cell proliferation [113]. Furthermore, it has been observed that circRNA_09505 plays a significant role in promoting the expression of AKT1 by regulating the IkBa/NF-kB signaling pathway in macrophages. Notably, the knockdown of circRNA_09505 has shown promising results in alleviating arthritis and inflammation in mice with collagen-induced arthritis (CIA) [114]. RNA plays a crucial role in the pathophysiology of rheumatoid arthritis (RA) and has great potential for diagnostic and therapeutic target treatment. Despite challenges related to identification and characterization, tissue specificity, standardization and reproducibility, functional characterization, validation, and clinical utility, ncRNA are promising potential biomarkers of RA due to their stability, detectability in various body fluids, and involvement in regulatory processes [115–117]. However, further studies are needed to fully understand the complex mechanisms underlying these different forms of RNA.

3.3.4. Oxidative Stress Molecules

Oxidative stress is defined as a harmful condition characterized by an imbalance of oxidative molecules, such as reactive oxygen species (ROS), leading to an excess of prooxidants [118]. This imbalance can lead to disruption of redox signaling and molecular damage. Under physiological conditions, ROS are required to maintain the cellular redox status and play an important role in cell signaling pathways, differentiation, proliferation, growth, apoptosis, regulation of the cytoskeleton, and phagocytosis. However, when ROS levels exceed physiological levels, they can have detrimental effects on many cellular components, such as cell membranes, lipids, proteins, and nucleic acids [119,120]. In RA patients and animal models, there is a significant association between blood ROS levels and RA severity. Several studies have shown alteration in the expression of nitric oxide (NO) and inducible nitric oxide synthase (iNOS), which lead to impaired infiltration of T- and B-cells into the joints by interfering with their chemotaxis and adhesion [121,122]. Furthermore, promising results have been observed with NOS and iNOS inhibitors L-NAME and iNOS inhibitor GW274150 in reducing the inflammatory response and synovial thickness, offering the potential for targeted treatments [123,124]. In addition, patients with active RA are characterized by increased ROS levels and reduced antioxidant capacity, leading to increased levels of lipid peroxidation, which can be observed in synovial fluid and blood samples [125–128]. Based on previous studies, a positive correlation between lipid peroxidation biomarker malondialdehyde (MDA) and proinflammatory cytokines has been observed in the serum of individuals with RA [129]. Furthermore, studies have shown that reactive oxygen metabolites (ROM) are increased in blood samples from RA patients and positively correlate with disease activity [130]. In line with these findings, it has been observed that RA patients have reduced levels of antioxidants in serum and synovial fluid [131,132].

A link between oxidative damage to synovial tissue, mitochondrial dysfunction, and hypoxic status in arthritic joints has also been demonstrated. For example, inflammatory mediators and hypoxic conditions can impair the mitochondrial state of synovial cells, leading to metabolic shifts and increased mutation rates. Furthermore, oxidative stress can alter energy metabolism, increase ROS production, and raise mitochondrial mutagenesis, thereby contributing to inflammatory processes and impaired angiogenesis in RA patients. The metabolic disparity between healthy synovial tissue and RA-affected synovial tissue particularly highlights the alterations in cellular metabolism known as the Warburg effect or aerobic glycolysis [133]. This phenomenon describes the overexpression of glycolytic enzymes in RA synovial tissue and its potential impact on inflammatory cytokines, cell proliferation, and disease activity [134,135]. In the context of RA, studies have shown that hypoxia-inducible factor (HIF)-1α is important in maintaining oxygen balance and regulating the expression of genes involved in angiogenesis and inflammation in the synovium. Various factors, including hypoxia, ROS, cytokines, hormones, and mechanical stress, influence HIF-1α activation. In terms of clinical relevance, the potential of therapies targeting HIF-1α or angiogenic factors as an alternative approach to the treatment of RA has been suggested [136,137]. Furthermore, studies on the Notch signaling pathway in the context of RA have revealed its role in regulating cellular processes and promoting inflammation. It has also been suggested that the Notch signaling pathway could be used as a pharmacological treatment for RA [138].

In general, local treatment of early synovitis with conventional glucocorticoids and synovectomy involves targeted suppression or eradication of aggressive fibroblast-like synoviocytes. In advanced RA, combining immunosuppressants with local FLS-targeted therapy can more effectively control disease activity.

4. Conclusions and Future Directions

In the course of MonoA, local synovitis treatment involves targeted inhibition or destruction of fibroblast-like synoviocytes. Today, several new intra-articular therapies have been approved in clinical studies, especially for osteoarthritis patients with an inflammatory endotype where FLSs are less aggressive. Currently, various slow-acting steroidal drugs for the local treatment of synovitis, which do not have a detrimental effect on cartilage, are gradually being marketed in clinics. Various combination therapies (steroids with HA, steroids with anesthetic, nonsteroidal anti-inflammatory drugs with HA, etc.) are currently approved in clinical practice and have proven to be effective in pain relief. Thus, personalized medicine initiatives involve the choice and decision of medicines based on the unique clinical characteristics or risk factors and biomarker expression of each patient [130]. A local approach to the elimination of synovial tissue inflammation will lead to the discovery of new local targets related to surface markers and intracellular proteins, non-coding RNAs, signaling molecules, and improvement in the treatment techniques and protocols.

Supplementary Materials: The following supporting information can be downloaded at: https://www.mdpi.com/article/10.3390/medicina60111819/s1, Table S1: Local treatments: advantages and disadvantages.

Author Contributions: Writing—original draft, G.K. and J.D.; writing—review and editing, G.K., J.D., D.M., J.P. and E.B.; conceptualization, G.K. and E.B. All authors have read and agreed to the published version of the manuscript.

Funding: We wish to acknowledge financial support from the European Research Executive Agency according to the project "Twinning for Promoting Excellence, Ability and Knowledge to develop novel approaches for targeting inflammatory and degenerative age-related joint diseases (TWINFLAG)". GRANT_NUMBER: 101079489.

Institutional Review Board Statement: Not applicable.

Informed Consent Statement: Not applicable.

Data Availability Statement: Publicly available datasets were analyzed in this study and are referred to in the list of references.

Conflicts of Interest: The authors declare no conflicts of interest.

References

1. Lane, N.E.; Brandt, K.; Hawker, G.; Peeva, E.; Schreyer, E.; Tsuji, W.; Hochberg, M.C. OARSI-FDA Initiative: Defining the Disease State of Osteoarthritis. *Osteoarthr. Cartil.* **2011**, *19*, 478–482. [CrossRef] [PubMed]
2. Smolen, J.S.; Breedveld, F.C.; Burmester, G.R.; Bykerk, V.; Dougados, M.; Emery, P.; Kvien, T.K.; Navarro-Compán, M.V.; Oliver, S.; Schoels, M.; et al. Treating Rheumatoid Arthritis to Target: 2014 Update of the Recommendations of an International Task Force. *Ann. Rheum. Dis.* **2016**, *75*, 3–15. [CrossRef] [PubMed]
3. Stoffer, M.A.; Schoels, M.M.; Smolen, J.S.; Aletaha, D.; Breedveld, F.C.; Burmester, G.; Bykerk, V.; Dougados, M.; Emery, P.; Haraoui, B.; et al. Evidence for Treating Rheumatoid Arthritis to Target: Results of a Systematic Literature Search Update. *Ann. Rheum. Dis.* **2016**, *75*, 16–22. [CrossRef]
4. Combe, B.; Landewe, R.; Lukas, C.; Bolosiu, H.D.; Breedveld, F.; Dougados, M.; Emery, P.; Ferraccioli, G.; Hazes, J.M.W.; Klareskog, L.; et al. EULAR Recommendations for the Management of Early Arthritis: Report of a Task Force of the European Standing Committee for International Clinical Studies Including Therapeutics (ESCISIT). *Ann. Rheum. Dis.* **2007**, *66*, 34–45. [CrossRef]
5. Combe, B.; Landewe, R.; Daien, C.I.; Hua, C.; Aletaha, D.; Álvaro-Gracia, J.M.; Bakkers, M.; Brodin, N.; Burmester, G.R.; Codreanu, C.; et al. 2016 Update of the EULAR Recommendations for the Management of Early Arthritis. *Ann. Rheum. Dis.* **2017**, *76*, 948–959. [CrossRef]
6. Ellis, J.M. Acute Monoarthritis. *JAAPA Off. J. Am. Acad. Physician Assist.* **2019**, *32*, 25–31. [CrossRef]
7. Siva, C.; Velazquez, C.; Mody, A.; Brasington, R. Diagnosing Acute Monoarthritis in Adults: A Practical Approach for the Family Physician. *Am. Fam. Physician* **2003**, *68*, 83–90. [PubMed]
8. Becker, J.A.; Daily, J.P.; Pohlgeers, K.M. Acute Monoarthritis: Diagnosis in Adults. *Am. Fam. Physician* **2016**, *94*, 810–816.
9. Cincinelli, G.; Di Taranto, R.; Orsini, F.; Rindone, A.; Murgo, A.; Caporali, R. A Case Report of Monoarthritis in a COVID-19 Patient and Literature Review: Simple Actions for Complex Times. *Medicine* **2021**, *100*, e26089. [CrossRef]

10. Ding, Q.; Hu, W.; Wang, R.; Yang, Q.; Zhu, M.; Li, M.; Cai, J.; Rose, P.; Mao, J.; Zhu, Y.Z. Signaling Pathways in Rheumatoid Arthritis: Implications for Targeted Therapy. *Signal Transduct. Target. Ther.* **2023**, *8*, 68. [CrossRef]
11. Nygaard, G.; Firestein, G.S. Restoring Synovial Homeostasis in Rheumatoid Arthritis by Targeting Fibroblast-like Synoviocytes. *Nat. Rev. Rheumatol.* **2020**, *16*, 316–333. [CrossRef] [PubMed]
12. Mathiessen, A.; Conaghan, P.G. Synovitis in Osteoarthritis: Current Understanding with Therapeutic Implications. *Arthritis Res. Ther.* **2017**, *19*, 18. [CrossRef] [PubMed]
13. Han, D.; Fang, Y.; Tan, X.; Jiang, H.; Gong, X.; Wang, X.; Hong, W.; Tu, J.; Wei, W. The Emerging Role of Fibroblast-like Synoviocytes-Mediated Synovitis in Osteoarthritis: An Update. *J. Cell. Mol. Med.* **2020**, *24*, 9518–9532. [CrossRef] [PubMed]
14. Van Spil, W.E.; Kubassova, O.; Boesen, M.; Bay-Jensen, A.-C.; Mobasheri, A. Osteoarthritis Phenotypes and Novel Therapeutic Targets. *Biochem. Pharmacol.* **2019**, *165*, 41–48. [CrossRef]
15. de Rooy, D.P.C.; van der Linden, M.P.M.; Knevel, R.; Huizinga, T.W.J.; van der Helm-van Mil, A.H.M. Predicting Arthritis Outcomes—What Can Be Learned from the Leiden Early Arthritis Clinic? *Rheumatol. Oxf. Engl.* **2011**, *50*, 93–100. [CrossRef]
16. Combe, B.; Benessiano, J.; Berenbaum, F.; Cantagrel, A.; Daurès, J.-P.; Dougados, M.; Fardellone, P.; Fautrel, B.; Flipo, R.-M.; Goupille, P.; et al. The ESPOIR Cohort: A Ten-Year Follow-up of Early Arthritis in France: Methodology and Baseline Characteristics of the 813 Included Patients. *Joint Bone Spine* **2007**, *74*, 440–445. [CrossRef]
17. Quinn, M.A.; Green, M.J.; Marzo-Ortega, H.; Proudman, S.; Karim, Z.; Wakefield, R.J.; Conaghan, P.G.; Emery, P. Prognostic Factors in a Large Cohort of Patients with Early Undifferentiated Inflammatory Arthritis after Application of a Structured Management Protocol. *Arthritis Rheum.* **2003**, *48*, 3039–3045. [CrossRef]
18. Orr, C.; Vieira-Sousa, E.; Boyle, D.L.; Buch, M.H.; Buckley, C.D.; Cañete, J.D.; Catrina, A.I.; Choy, E.H.S.; Emery, P.; Fearon, U.; et al. Synovial Tissue Research: A State-of-the-Art Review. *Nat. Rev. Rheumatol.* **2017**, *13*, 463–475. [CrossRef]
19. de Hair, M.J.H.; Harty, L.C.; Gerlag, D.M.; Pitzalis, C.; Veale, D.J.; Tak, P.P. Synovial Tissue Analysis for the Discovery of Diagnostic and Prognostic Biomarkers in Patients with Early Arthritis. *J. Rheumatol.* **2011**, *38*, 2068–2072. [CrossRef]
20. Soroosh, S.G.; Ghatfan, A.; Farbod, A.; Meftah, E. Synovial Biopsy for Establishing a Definite Diagnosis in Undifferentiated Chronic Knee Monoarthritis. *BMC Musculoskelet. Disord.* **2023**, *24*, 23. [CrossRef]
21. Ike, R.W.; Kalunian, K.C. Will Rheumatologists Ever Pick up the Arthroscope Again? *Int. J. Rheum. Dis.* **2021**, *24*, 1235–1246. [CrossRef]
22. Andreozzi, V.; Monaco, E.; Garufi, C.; Spinelli, F.R.; Rossi, G.; Dagget, M.; Conti, F.; Ferretti, A. In-Office Needle Arthroscopic Synovial Biopsy Is an Effective Diagnostic Tool in Patients With Inflammatory Arthritis. *Arthrosc. Sports Med. Rehabil.* **2022**, *4*, e2099–e2106. [CrossRef]
23. Bernotiene, E.; Bagdonas, E.; Kirdaite, G.; Bernotas, P.; Kalvaityte, U.; Uzieliene, I.; Thudium, C.S.; Hannula, H.; Lorite, G.S.; Dvir-Ginzberg, M.; et al. Emerging Technologies and Platforms for the Immunodetection of Multiple Biochemical Markers in Osteoarthritis Research and Therapy. *Front. Med.* **2020**, *7*, 572977. [CrossRef]
24. Momohara, S.; Tanaka, S.; Nakamura, H.; Mibe, J.; Iwamoto, T.; Ikari, K.; Nishino, J.; Kadono, Y.; Yasui, T.; Takahashi, K.; et al. Recent Trends in Orthopedic Surgery Performed in Japan for Rheumatoid Arthritis. *Mod. Rheumatol.* **2011**, *21*, 337–342. [CrossRef] [PubMed]
25. Jämsen, E.; Virta, L.J.; Hakala, M.; Kauppi, M.J.; Malmivaara, A.; Lehto, M.U.K. The Decline in Joint Replacement Surgery in Rheumatoid Arthritis Is Associated with a Concomitant Increase in the Intensity of Anti-Rheumatic Therapy: A Nationwide Register-Based Study from 1995 through 2010. *Acta Orthop.* **2013**, *84*, 331–337. [CrossRef] [PubMed]
26. Uson, J.; Rodriguez-García, S.C.; Castellanos-Moreira, R.; O'Neill, T.W.; Doherty, M.; Boesen, M.; Pandit, H.; Möller Parera, I.; Vardanyan, V.; Terslev, L.; et al. EULAR Recommendations for Intra-Articular Therapies. *Ann. Rheum. Dis.* **2021**, *80*, 1299–1305. [CrossRef] [PubMed]
27. Wernecke, C.; Braun, H.J.; Dragoo, J.L. The Effect of Intra-Articular Corticosteroids on Articular Cartilage: A Systematic Review. *Orthop. J. Sports Med.* **2015**, *3*, 2325967115581163. [CrossRef]
28. Maricar, N.; Callaghan, M.J.; Felson, D.T.; O'Neill, T.W. Predictors of Response to Intra-Articular Steroid Injections in Knee Osteoarthritis—A Systematic Review. *Rheumatol. Oxf. Engl.* **2013**, *52*, 1022–1032. [CrossRef]
29. Hirsch, G.; O'Neill, T.W.; Kitas, G.; Sinha, A.; Klocke, R. Accuracy of Injection and Short-Term Pain Relief Following Intra-Articular Corticosteroid Injection in Knee Osteoarthritis - an Observational Study. *BMC Musculoskelet. Disord.* **2017**, *18*, 44. [CrossRef]
30. Paik, J.; Duggan, S.T.; Keam, S.J. Triamcinolone Acetonide Extended-Release: A Review in Osteoarthritis Pain of the Knee. *Drugs* **2019**, *79*, 455–462. [CrossRef]
31. Bodick, N.; Lufkin, J.; Willwerth, C.; Kumar, A.; Bolognese, J.; Schoonmaker, C.; Ballal, R.; Hunter, D.; Clayman, M. An Intra-Articular, Extended-Release Formulation of Triamcinolone Acetonide Prolongs and Amplifies Analgesic Effect in Patients with Osteoarthritis of the Knee: A Randomized Clinical Trial. *J. Bone Jt. Surg.* **2015**, *97*, 877–888. [CrossRef] [PubMed]
32. Conaghan, P.G.; Cohen, S.B.; Berenbaum, F.; Lufkin, J.; Johnson, J.R.; Bodick, N. Brief Report: A Phase IIb Trial of a Novel Extended-Release Microsphere Formulation of Triamcinolone Acetonide for Intraarticular Injection in Knee Osteoarthritis. *Arthritis Rheumatol.* **2018**, *70*, 204–211. [CrossRef] [PubMed]
33. Spitzer, A.I.; Richmond, J.C.; Kraus, V.B.; Gomoll, A.; Jones, D.G.; Huffman, K.M.; Peterfy, C.; Cinar, A.; Lufkin, J.; Kelley, S.D. Safety and Efficacy of Repeat Administration of Triamcinolone Acetonide Extended-Release in Osteoarthritis of the Knee: A Phase 3b, Open-Label Study. *Rheumatol. Ther.* **2019**, *6*, 109–124. [CrossRef]

34. Kivitz, A.; Mehra, P.; Hanson, P.; Kwong, L.; Cinar, A.; Lufkin, J.; Kelley, S. A Randomized, Open-Label, Single-Dose Study to Assess Safety and Systemic Exposure of Triamcinolone Acetonide Extended-Release in Patients With Hip Osteoarthritis. *Rheumatol. Ther.* **2022**, *9*, 679–691. [CrossRef] [PubMed]
35. Hanson, P.; Kivitz, A.; Mehra, P.; Kwong, L.; Cinar, A.; Lufkin, J.; Kelley, S.D. Safety and Systemic Exposure of Triamcinolone Acetonide Following Ultrasound-Guided Intra-Articular Injection of Triamcinolone Extended-Release or Standard Triamcinolone Acetonide in Patients with Shoulder Osteoarthritis: An Open-Label, Randomized Study. *Drugs RD* **2021**, *21*, 285–293. [CrossRef]
36. Kraus, V.B.; Conaghan, P.G.; Aazami, H.A.; Mehra, P.; Kivitz, A.J.; Lufkin, J.; Hauben, J.; Johnson, J.R.; Bodick, N. Synovial and Systemic Pharmacokinetics (PK) of Triamcinolone Acetonide (TA) Following Intra-Articular (IA) Injection of an Extended-Release Microsphere-Based Formulation (FX006) or Standard Crystalline Suspension in Patients with Knee Osteoarthritis (OA). *Osteoarthr. Cartil.* **2018**, *26*, 34–42. [CrossRef]
37. Hunter, D.J.; Chang, C.-C.; Wei, J.C.-C.; Lin, H.-Y.; Brown, C.; Tai, T.-T.; Wu, C.-F.; Chuang, W.C.-M.; Shih, S.-F. TLC599 in Patients with Osteoarthritis of the Knee: A Phase IIa, Randomized, Placebo-Controlled, Dose-Finding Study. *Arthritis Res. Ther.* **2022**, *24*, 52. [CrossRef]
38. Hangody, L.; Szody, R.; Lukasik, P.; Zgadzaj, W.; Lénárt, E.; Dokoupilova, E.; Bichovsk, D.; Berta, A.; Vasarhelyi, G.; Ficzere, A.; et al. Intraarticular Injection of a Cross-Linked Sodium Hyaluronate Combined with Triamcinolone Hexacetonide (Cingal) to Provide Symptomatic Relief of Osteoarthritis of the Knee: A Randomized, Double-Blind, Placebo-Controlled Multicenter Clinical Trial. *Cartilage* **2018**, *9*, 276–283. [CrossRef]
39. Yazici, Y.; McAlindon, T.E.; Gibofsky, A.; Lane, N.E.; Lattermann, C.; Skrepnik, N.; Swearingen, C.J.; Simsek, I.; Ghandehari, H.; DiFrancesco, A.; et al. A Phase 2b Randomized Trial of Lorecivivint, a Novel Intra-Articular CLK2/DYRK1A Inhibitor and Wnt Pathway Modulator for Knee Osteoarthritis. *Osteoarthr. Cartil.* **2021**, *29*, 654–666. [CrossRef]
40. Tambiah, J.R.S.; Kennedy, S.; Swearingen, C.J.; Simsek, I.; Yazici, Y.; Farr, J.; Conaghan, P.G. Individual Participant Symptom Responses to Intra-Articular Lorecivivint in Knee Osteoarthritis: Post Hoc Analysis of a Phase 2B Trial. *Rheumatol. Ther.* **2021**, *8*, 973–985. [CrossRef]
41. Tambiah, J.R.S.; Simsek, I.; Swearingen, C.J.; Kennedy, S.; Cole, B.J.; McAlindon, T.E.; Yazici, Y. Comparing Patient-Reported Outcomes From Sham and Saline-Based Placebo Injections for Knee Osteoarthritis: Data From a Randomized Clinical Trial of Lorecivivint. *Am. J. Sports Med.* **2022**, *50*, 630–636. [CrossRef] [PubMed]
42. Stevens, R.M.; Ervin, J.; Nezzer, J.; Nieves, Y.; Guedes, K.; Burges, R.; Hanson, P.D.; Campbell, J.N. Randomized, Double-Blind, Placebo-Controlled Trial of Intraarticular Trans-Capsaicin for Pain Associated With Osteoarthritis of the Knee. *Arthritis Rheumatol.* **2019**, *71*, 1524–1533. [CrossRef] [PubMed]
43. Lozada, C.J.; Del Rio, E.; Reitberg, D.P.; Smith, R.A.; Kahn, C.B.; Moskowitz, R.W. A Double-Blind, Randomized, Saline-Controlled Study of the Efficacy and Safety of Co-Administered Intra-Articular Injections of Tr14 and Ze14 for Treatment of Painful Osteoarthritis of the Knee: The MOZArT Trial. *Eur. J. Integr. Med.* **2017**, *13*, 54–63. [CrossRef]
44. Kulkarni, M.; Mallesh, M.; Wakankar, H.; Prajapati, R.; Pandit, H. Effect of Methylprednisolone in Periarticular Infiltration for Primary Total Knee Arthroplasty on Pain and Rehabilitation. *J. Arthroplast.* **2019**, *34*, 1646–1649. [CrossRef]
45. McAlindon, T.E.; Schmidt, U.; Bugarin, D.; Abrams, S.; Geib, T.; DeGryse, R.E.; Kim, K.; Schnitzer, T.J. Efficacy and Safety of Single-Dose onabotulinumtoxinA in the Treatment of Symptoms of Osteoarthritis of the Knee: Results of a Placebo-Controlled, Double-Blind Study. *Osteoarthritis Cartilage* **2018**, *26*, 1291–1299. [CrossRef]
46. Nishida, Y.; Kano, K.; Osato, T.; Seo, T. Open-Label Phase 3 Study of Diclofenac Conjugated to Hyaluronate (Diclofenac Etalhyaluronate: ONO-5704/SI-613) for Treatment of Osteoarthritis: 1-Year Follow-Up. *BMC Musculoskelet. Disord.* **2021**, *22*, 233. [CrossRef]
47. Nishida, Y.; Kano, K.; Nobuoka, Y.; Seo, T. Efficacy and Safety of Diclofenac-Hyaluronate Conjugate (Diclofenac Etalhyaluronate) for Knee Osteoarthritis: A Randomized Phase III Trial in Japan. *Arthritis Rheumatol.* **2021**, *73*, 1646–1655. [CrossRef] [PubMed]
48. Müller-Ladner, U.; Kriegsmann, J.; Franklin, B.N.; Matsumoto, S.; Geiler, T.; Gay, R.E.; Gay, S. Synovial Fibroblasts of Patients with Rheumatoid Arthritis Attach to and Invade Normal Human Cartilage When Engrafted into SCID Mice. *Am. J. Pathol.* **1996**, *149*, 1607–1615.
49. Bottini, N.; Firestein, G.S. Duality of Fibroblast-like Synoviocytes in RA: Passive Responders and Imprinted Aggressors. *Nat. Rev. Rheumatol.* **2013**, *9*, 24–33. [CrossRef]
50. Choy, E.H.; Kavanaugh, A.F.; Jones, S.A. The Problem of Choice: Current Biologic Agents and Future Prospects in RA. *Nat. Rev. Rheumatol.* **2013**, *9*, 154–163. [CrossRef]
51. McGarry, T.; Orr, C.; Wade, S.; Biniecka, M.; Wade, S.; Gallagher, L.; Low, C.; Veale, D.J.; Fearon, U. JAK/STAT Blockade Alters Synovial Bioenergetics, Mitochondrial Function, and Proinflammatory Mediators in Rheumatoid Arthritis. *Arthritis Rheumatol.* **2018**, *70*, 1959–1970. [CrossRef] [PubMed]
52. Sanchez-Lopez, E.; Cheng, A.; Guma, M. Can Metabolic Pathways Be Therapeutic Targets in Rheumatoid Arthritis? *J. Clin. Med.* **2019**, *8*, 753. [CrossRef] [PubMed]
53. Croft, A.P.; Naylor, A.J.; Marshall, J.L.; Hardie, D.L.; Zimmermann, B.; Turner, J.; Desanti, G.; Adams, H.; Yemm, A.I.; Müller-Ladner, U.; et al. Rheumatoid Synovial Fibroblasts Differentiate into Distinct Subsets in the Presence of Cytokines and Cartilage. *Arthritis Res. Ther.* **2016**, *18*, 270. [CrossRef]
54. Denkovskij, J.; Rudys, R.; Bernotiene, E.; Minderis, M.; Bagdonas, S.; Kirdaite, G. Cell Surface Markers and Exogenously Induced PpIX in Synovial Mesenchymal Stem Cells. *Cytom. Part J. Int. Soc. Anal. Cytol.* **2015**, *87*, 1001–1011. [CrossRef]

55. Mizoguchi, F.; Slowikowski, K.; Wei, K.; Marshall, J.L.; Rao, D.A.; Chang, S.K.; Nguyen, H.N.; Noss, E.H.; Turner, J.D.; Earp, B.E.; et al. Functionally Distinct Disease-Associated Fibroblast Subsets in Rheumatoid Arthritis. *Nat. Commun.* **2018**, *9*, 789. [CrossRef]
56. Stephenson, W.; Donlin, L.T.; Butler, A.; Rozo, C.; Bracken, B.; Rashidfarrokhi, A.; Goodman, S.M.; Ivashkiv, L.B.; Bykerk, V.P.; Orange, D.E.; et al. Single-Cell RNA-Seq of Rheumatoid Arthritis Synovial Tissue Using Low-Cost Microfluidic Instrumentation. *Nat. Commun.* **2018**, *9*, 791. [CrossRef]
57. Chang, S.K.; Gu, Z.; Brenner, M.B. Fibroblast-like Synoviocytes in Inflammatory Arthritis Pathology: The Emerging Role of Cadherin-11. *Immunol. Rev.* **2010**, *233*, 256–266. [CrossRef]
58. Lee, D.M.; Kiener, H.P.; Agarwal, S.K.; Noss, E.H.; Watts, G.F.M.; Chisaka, O.; Takeichi, M.; Brenner, M.B. Cadherin-11 in Synovial Lining Formation and Pathology in Arthritis. *Science* **2007**, *315*, 1006–1010. [CrossRef] [PubMed]
59. Ebid, R.; Lichtnekert, J.; Anders, H.-J. Hyaluronan Is Not a Ligand but a Regulator of Toll-like Receptor Signaling in Mesangial Cells: Role of Extracellular Matrix in Innate Immunity. *ISRN Nephrol.* **2014**, *2014*, 714081. [CrossRef]
60. Sohn, D.H.; Rhodes, C.; Onuma, K.; Zhao, X.; Sharpe, O.; Gazitt, T.; Shiao, R.; Fert-Bober, J.; Cheng, D.; Lahey, L.J.; et al. Local Joint Inflammation and Histone Citrullination in a Murine Model of the Transition from Preclinical Autoimmunity to Inflammatory Arthritis. *Arthritis Rheumatol.* **2015**, *67*, 2877–2887. [CrossRef]
61. Sanchez-Pernaute, O.; Filkova, M.; Gabucio, A.; Klein, M.; Maciejewska-Rodrigues, H.; Ospelt, C.; Brentano, F.; Michel, B.A.; Gay, R.E.; Herrero-Beaumont, G.; et al. Citrullination Enhances the Pro-Inflammatory Response to Fibrin in Rheumatoid Arthritis Synovial Fibroblasts. *Ann. Rheum. Dis.* **2013**, *72*, 1400–1406. [CrossRef] [PubMed]
62. Hatterer, E.; Shang, L.; Simonet, P.; Herren, S.; Daubeuf, B.; Teixeira, S.; Reilly, J.; Elson, G.; Nelson, R.; Gabay, C.; et al. A Specific Anti-Citrullinated Protein Antibody Profile Identifies a Group of Rheumatoid Arthritis Patients with a Toll-like Receptor 4-Mediated Disease. *Arthritis Res. Ther.* **2016**, *18*, 224. [CrossRef] [PubMed]
63. Farrugia, M.; Baron, B. The Role of Toll-Like Receptors in Autoimmune Diseases through Failure of the Self-Recognition Mechanism. *Int. J. Inflamm.* **2017**, *2017*, 8391230. [CrossRef] [PubMed]
64. Chamberlain, N.D.; Vila, O.M.; Volin, M.V.; Volkov, S.; Pope, R.M.; Swedler, W.; Mandelin, A.M.; Shahrara, S. TLR5, a Novel and Unidentified Inflammatory Mediator in Rheumatoid Arthritis That Correlates with Disease Activity Score and Joint TNF-α Levels. *J. Immunol.* **2012**, *189*, 475–483. [CrossRef]
65. Huang, Q.; Ma, Y.; Adebayo, A.; Pope, R.M. Increased Macrophage Activation Mediated through Toll-like Receptors in Rheumatoid Arthritis. *Arthritis Rheum.* **2007**, *56*, 2192–2201. [CrossRef]
66. Kim, K.-W.; Cho, M.-L.; Lee, S.-H.; Oh, H.-J.; Kang, C.-M.; Ju, J.H.; Min, S.-Y.; Cho, Y.-G.; Park, S.-H.; Kim, H.-Y. Human Rheumatoid Synovial Fibroblasts Promote Osteoclastogenic Activity by Activating RANKL via TLR-2 and TLR-4 Activation. *Immunol. Lett.* **2007**, *110*, 54–64. [CrossRef] [PubMed]
67. Brentano, F.; Schorr, O.; Gay, R.E.; Gay, S.; Kyburz, D. RNA Released from Necrotic Synovial Fluid Cells Activates Rheumatoid Arthritis Synovial Fibroblasts via Toll-like Receptor 3. *Arthritis Rheum.* **2005**, *52*, 2656–2665. [CrossRef]
68. Tsuchiya, K.; Hosojima, S.; Hara, H.; Kushiyama, H.; Mahib, M.R.; Kinoshita, T.; Suda, T. Gasdermin D Mediates the Maturation and Release of IL-1α Downstream of Inflammasomes. *Cell Rep.* **2021**, *34*, 108887. [CrossRef]
69. Li, Z.; Guo, J.; Bi, L. Role of the NLRP3 Inflammasome in Autoimmune Diseases. *Biomed. Pharmacother.* **2020**, *130*, 110542. [CrossRef]
70. Sakalyte, R.; Denkovskij, J.; Bernotiene, E.; Stropuviene, S.; Mikulenaite, S.O.; Kvederas, G.; Porvaneckas, N.; Tutkus, V.; Venalis, A.; Butrimiene, I. The Expression of Inflammasomes NLRP1 and NLRP3, Toll-Like Receptors, and Vitamin D Receptor in Synovial Fibroblasts From Patients With Different Types of Knee Arthritis. *Front. Immunol.* **2021**, *12*, 767512. [CrossRef]
71. Pazár, B.; Ea, H.-K.; Narayan, S.; Kolly, L.; Bagnoud, N.; Chobaz, V.; Roger, T.; Lioté, F.; So, A.; Busso, N. Basic Calcium Phosphate Crystals Induce Monocyte/Macrophage IL-1β Secretion through the NLRP3 Inflammasome in Vitro. *J. Immunol.* **2011**, *186*, 2495–2502. [CrossRef] [PubMed]
72. Yi, Y.-S. Role of Inflammasomes in Inflammatory Autoimmune Rheumatic Diseases. *Korean J. Physiol. Pharmacol. Off. J. Korean Physiol. Soc. Korean Soc. Pharmacol.* **2018**, *22*, 1–15. [CrossRef]
73. Jin, C.; Frayssinet, P.; Pelker, R.; Cwirka, D.; Hu, B.; Vignery, A.; Eisenbarth, S.C.; Flavell, R.A. NLRP3 Inflammasome Plays a Critical Role in the Pathogenesis of Hydroxyapatite-Associated Arthropathy. *Proc. Natl. Acad. Sci. USA* **2011**, *108*, 14867–14872. [CrossRef] [PubMed]
74. Liu, S.; Ma, H.; Zhang, H.; Deng, C.; Xin, P. Recent Advances on Signaling Pathways and Their Inhibitors in Rheumatoid Arthritis. *Clin. Immunol.* **2021**, *230*, 108793. [CrossRef] [PubMed]
75. Lu, N.; Malemud, C.J. Extracellular Signal-Regulated Kinase: A Regulator of Cell Growth, Inflammation, Chondrocyte and Bone Cell Receptor-Mediated Gene Expression. *Int. J. Mol. Sci.* **2019**, *20*, 3792. [CrossRef]
76. McGeachy, M.J.; Cua, D.J.; Gaffen, S.L. The IL-17 Family of Cytokines in Health and Disease. *Immunity* **2019**, *50*, 892–906. [CrossRef]
77. Damjanov, N.; Kauffman, R.S.; Spencer-Green, G.T. Efficacy, Pharmacodynamics, and Safety of VX-702, a Novel P38 MAPK Inhibitor, in Rheumatoid Arthritis: Results of Two Randomized, Double-Blind, Placebo-Controlled Clinical Studies. *Arthritis Rheum.* **2009**, *60*, 1232–1241. [CrossRef] [PubMed]
78. Genovese, M.C.; Cohen, S.B.; Wofsy, D.; Weinblatt, M.E.; Firestein, G.S.; Brahn, E.; Strand, V.; Baker, D.G.; Tong, S.E. A 24-Week, Randomized, Double-Blind, Placebo-Controlled, Parallel Group Study of the Efficacy of Oral SCIO-469, a P38 Mitogen-Activated Protein Kinase Inhibitor, in Patients with Active Rheumatoid Arthritis. *J. Rheumatol.* **2011**, *38*, 846–854. [CrossRef]

79. Yoshizawa, T.; Hammaker, D.; Boyle, D.L.; Corr, M.; Flavell, R.; Davis, R.; Schett, G.; Firestein, G.S. Role of MAPK Kinase 6 in Arthritis: Distinct Mechanism of Action in Inflammation and Cytokine Expression. *J. Immunol.* **2009**, *183*, 1360–1367. [CrossRef]
80. Han, Z.; Boyle, D.L.; Chang, L.; Bennett, B.; Karin, M.; Yang, L.; Manning, A.M.; Firestein, G.S. C-Jun N-Terminal Kinase Is Required for Metalloproteinase Expression and Joint Destruction in Inflammatory Arthritis. *J. Clin. Investig.* **2001**, *108*, 73–81. [CrossRef]
81. Guma, M.; Ronacher, L.M.; Firestein, G.S.; Karin, M.; Corr, M. JNK-1 Deficiency Limits Macrophage-Mediated Antigen-Induced Arthritis. *Arthritis Rheum.* **2011**, *63*, 1603–1612. [CrossRef] [PubMed]
82. Vickers, N.J. Animal Communication: When I'm Calling You, Will You Answer Too? *Curr. Biol.* **2017**, *27*, R713–R715. [CrossRef] [PubMed]
83. Gaillard, P.; Jeanclaude-Etter, I.; Ardissone, V.; Arkinstall, S.; Cambet, Y.; Camps, M.; Chabert, C.; Church, D.; Cirillo, R.; Gretener, D.; et al. Design and Synthesis of the First Generation of Novel Potent, Selective, and in Vivo Active (Benzothiazol-2-Yl)Acetonitrile Inhibitors of the c-Jun N-Terminal Kinase. *J. Med. Chem.* **2005**, *48*, 4596–4607. [CrossRef]
84. Sun, S.-C. The Non-Canonical NF-κB Pathway in Immunity and Inflammation. *Nat. Rev. Immunol.* **2017**, *17*, 545–558. [CrossRef]
85. Yu, J.; Zhou, P. The Advances of Methotrexate Resistance in Rheumatoid Arthritis. *Inflammopharmacology* **2020**, *28*, 1183–1193. [CrossRef]
86. Ferreira, J.F.; Ahmed Mohamed, A.A.; Emery, P. Glucocorticoids and Rheumatoid Arthritis. *Rheum. Dis. Clin. N. Am.* **2016**, *42*, 33–46, vii. [CrossRef]
87. Xie, S.; Li, S.; Tian, J.; Li, F. Iguratimod as a New Drug for Rheumatoid Arthritis: Current Landscape. *Front. Pharmacol.* **2020**, *11*, 73. [CrossRef] [PubMed]
88. Dong, H.; Liu, F.; Ma, F.; Xu, L.; Pang, L.; Li, X.; Liu, B.; Wang, L. Montelukast Inhibits Inflammatory Response in Rheumatoid Arthritis Fibroblast-like Synoviocytes. *Int. Immunopharmacol.* **2018**, *61*, 215–221. [CrossRef]
89. Venugopal, N.; Acharya, P.; Zarei, M.; Talahalli, R.R. Cysteinyl Leukotriene Receptor Antagonism: A Promising Pharmacological Strategy for Lowering the Severity of Arthritis. *Inflammopharmacology* **2019**, *27*, 923–931. [CrossRef]
90. Imas, J.J.; Ruiz Zamarreño, C.; Zubiate, P.; Sanchez-Martín, L.; Campión, J.; Matías, I.R. Optical Biosensors for the Detection of Rheumatoid Arthritis (RA) Biomarkers: A Comprehensive Review. *Sensors* **2020**, *20*, 6289. [CrossRef]
91. Zhao, S.S.; Moots, R.J. Biomarkers for Treatment Response in Rheumatoid Arthritis: Where Are They? *Rheumatol. Immunol. Res.* **2020**, *1*, 1–3. [CrossRef] [PubMed]
92. Huang, J.; Fu, X.; Chen, X.; Li, Z.; Huang, Y.; Liang, C. Promising Therapeutic Targets for Treatment of Rheumatoid Arthritis. *Front. Immunol.* **2021**, *12*, 686155. [CrossRef] [PubMed]
93. Zhang, C.; Fang, L.; Liu, X.; Nie, T.; Li, R.; Cui, L.; Wang, J.; Ji, Y. miR-22 Inhibits Synovial Fibroblasts Proliferation and Proinflammatory Cytokine Production in RASF via Targeting SIRT1. *Gene* **2020**, *724*, 144144. [CrossRef] [PubMed]
94. Huang, Z.; Xing, S.; Liu, M.; Deng, W.; Wang, Y.; Huang, Z.; Huang, Y.; Huang, X.; Wu, C.; Guo, X.; et al. MiR-26a-5p Enhances Cells Proliferation, Invasion, and Apoptosis Resistance of Fibroblast-like Synoviocytes in Rheumatoid Arthritis by Regulating PTEN/PI3K/AKT Pathway. *Biosci. Rep.* **2019**, *39*, BSR20182192. [CrossRef] [PubMed]
95. Wang, Y.; Hou, L.; Yuan, X.; Xu, N.; Zhao, S.; Yang, L.; Zhang, N. miR-483-3p Promotes Cell Proliferation and Suppresses Apoptosis in Rheumatoid Arthritis Fibroblast-like Synoviocytes by Targeting IGF-1. *Biomed. Pharmacother.* **2020**, *130*, 110519. [CrossRef]
96. Hou, C.; Wang, D.; Zhang, L. MicroRNA-34a-3p Inhibits Proliferation of Rheumatoid Arthritis Fibroblast-like Synoviocytes. *Mol. Med. Rep.* **2019**, *20*, 2563–2570. [CrossRef]
97. Zhang, Y.; Yan, N.; Wang, X.; Chang, Y.; Wang, Y. MiR-129-5p Regulates Cell Proliferation and Apoptosis via IGF-1R/Src/ERK/Egr-1 Pathway in RA-Fibroblast-like Synoviocytes. *Biosci. Rep.* **2019**, *39*, BSR20192009. [CrossRef]
98. Stanczyk, J.; Ospelt, C.; Karouzakis, E.; Filer, A.; Raza, K.; Kolling, C.; Gay, R.; Buckley, C.D.; Tak, P.P.; Gay, S.; et al. Altered Expression of microRNA-203 in Rheumatoid Arthritis Synovial Fibroblasts and Its Role in Fibroblast Activation. *Arthritis Rheum.* **2011**, *63*, 373–381. [CrossRef]
99. Wang, Y.; Xu, N.; Zhao, S.; Jiao, T.; Fu, W.; Yang, L.; Zhang, N. miR-410-3p Suppresses Cytokine Release from Fibroblast-Like Synoviocytes by Regulating NF-κB Signaling in Rheumatoid Arthritis. *Inflammation* **2019**, *42*, 331–341. [CrossRef]
100. Shao, L.; Hou, C. miR-138 Activates NF-κB Signaling and PGRN to Promote Rheumatoid Arthritis via Regulating HDAC4. *Biochem. Biophys. Res. Commun.* **2019**, *519*, 166–171. [CrossRef]
101. Li, Z.; Chen, H.; Wang, F.; Wang, Z.; Zhao, Q.; Liu, S.; Huang, B.; Lou, S.; Zuo, J. Down-Regulation of microRNA-98 Promoted Apoptosis of TNF-α Stimulated Human Fibroblast-like Synoviocytes via up-Regulating IL-10. *Gene* **2019**, *706*, 124–130. [CrossRef] [PubMed]
102. Chen, J.; Liu, M.; Luo, X.; Peng, L.; Zhao, Z.; He, C.; He, Y. Exosomal miRNA-486-5p Derived from Rheumatoid Arthritis Fibroblast-like Synoviocytes Induces Osteoblast Differentiation through the Tob1/BMP/Smad Pathway. *Biomater. Sci.* **2020**, *8*, 3430–3442. [CrossRef] [PubMed]
103. Sun, L.; Tu, J.; Liu, C.; Pan, A.; Xia, X.; Chen, X. Analysis of lncRNA Expression Profiles by Sequencing Reveals That Lnc-AL928768.3 and Lnc-AC091493.1 Are Novel Biomarkers for Disease Risk and Activity of Rheumatoid Arthritis. *Inflammopharmacology* **2020**, *28*, 437–450. [CrossRef]
104. Liu, Y.-R.; Yang, L.; Xu, Q.-Q.; Lu, X.-Y.; Ma, T.-T.; Huang, C.; Li, J. Long Noncoding RNA MEG3 Regulates Rheumatoid Arthritis by Targeting NLRC5. *J. Cell. Physiol.* **2019**, *234*, 14270–14284. [CrossRef]

105. Yu, H.; Ding, C.; Dai, S.; Sun, J.; Wang, S.; Zhang, Z. Long Noncoding RNA FER1L4 Regulates Rheumatoid Arthritis via Targeting NLRC5. *Clin. Exp. Rheumatol.* **2020**, *38*, 713–723. [PubMed]
106. Li, G.; Liu, Y.; Meng, F.; Xia, Z.; Wu, X.; Fang, Y.; Zhang, C.; Zhang, Y.; Liu, D. LncRNA MEG3 Inhibits Rheumatoid Arthritis through miR-141 and Inactivation of AKT/mTOR Signalling Pathway. *J. Cell. Mol. Med.* **2019**, *23*, 7116–7120. [CrossRef]
107. Bi, X.; Guo, X.H.; Mo, B.Y.; Wang, M.L.; Luo, X.Q.; Chen, Y.X.; Liu, F.; Olsen, N.; Pan, Y.F.; Zheng, S.G. LncRNA PICSAR Promotes Cell Proliferation, Migration and Invasion of Fibroblast-like Synoviocytes by Sponging miRNA-4701-5p in Rheumatoid Arthritis. *EBioMedicine* **2019**, *50*, 408–420. [CrossRef]
108. Yang, Z.; Lin, S.-D.; Zhan, F.; Liu, Y.; Zhan, Y.-W. LncRNA GAS5 Alleviates Rheumatoid Arthritis through Regulating miR-222-3p/Sirt1 Signalling Axis. *Autoimmunity* **2021**, *54*, 13–22. [CrossRef]
109. Zheng, J.; Zeng, P.; Zhang, H.; Zhou, Y.; Liao, J.; Zhu, W.; Jia, N.; Lin, L. Long Noncoding RNA ZFAS1 Silencing Alleviates Rheumatoid Arthritis via Blocking miR-296-5p-Mediated down-Regulation of MMP-15. *Int. Immunopharmacol.* **2021**, *90*, 107061. [CrossRef]
110. Fu, X.; Song, G.; Ni, R.; Liu, H.; Xu, Z.; Zhang, D.; He, F.; Huang, G. LncRNA-H19 Silencing Suppresses Synoviocytes Proliferation and Attenuates Collagen-Induced Arthritis Progression by Modulating miR-124a. *Rheumatol. Oxf. Engl.* **2021**, *60*, 430–440. [CrossRef]
111. Xia, X.; Tang, X.; Wang, S. Roles of CircRNAs in Autoimmune Diseases. *Front. Immunol.* **2019**, *10*, 639. [CrossRef] [PubMed]
112. Zhong, S.; Ouyang, Q.; Zhu, D.; Huang, Q.; Zhao, J.; Fan, M.; Cai, Y.; Yang, M. Hsa_circ_0088036 Promotes the Proliferation and Migration of Fibroblast-like Synoviocytes by Sponging miR-140-3p and Upregulating SIRT 1 Expression in Rheumatoid Arthritis. *Mol. Immunol.* **2020**, *125*, 131–139. [CrossRef] [PubMed]
113. Li, G.; Tan, W.; Fang, Y.; Wu, X.; Zhou, W.; Zhang, C.; Zhang, Y.; Liu, Y.; Jiu, G.; Liu, D. circFADS2 Protects LPS-Treated Chondrocytes from Apoptosis Acting as an Interceptor of miR-498/mTOR Cross-Talking. *Aging* **2019**, *11*, 3348–3361. [CrossRef]
114. Yang, J.; Cheng, M.; Gu, B.; Wang, J.; Yan, S.; Xu, D. CircRNA_09505 Aggravates Inflammation and Joint Damage in Collagen-Induced Arthritis Mice via miR-6089/AKT1/NF-κB Axis. *Cell Death Dis.* **2020**, *11*, 833. [CrossRef] [PubMed]
115. Winkle, M.; El-Daly, S.M.; Fabbri, M.; Calin, G.A. Noncoding RNA Therapeutics - Challenges and Potential Solutions. *Nat. Rev. Drug Discov.* **2021**, *20*, 629–651. [CrossRef]
116. Hueso, M.; Mallén, A.; Suñé-Pou, M.; Aran, J.M.; Suñé-Negre, J.M.; Navarro, E. ncRNAs in Therapeutics: Challenges and Limitations in Nucleic Acid-Based Drug Delivery. *Int. J. Mol. Sci.* **2021**, *22*, 11596. [CrossRef]
117. Rocca, R.; Grillone, K.; Citriniti, E.L.; Gualtieri, G.; Artese, A.; Tagliaferri, P.; Tassone, P.; Alcaro, S. Targeting Non-Coding RNAs: Perspectives and Challenges of in-Silico Approaches. *Eur. J. Med. Chem.* **2023**, *261*, 115850. [CrossRef]
118. Smallwood, M.J.; Nissim, A.; Knight, A.R.; Whiteman, M.; Haigh, R.; Winyard, P.G. Oxidative Stress in Autoimmune Rheumatic Diseases. *Free Radic. Biol. Med.* **2018**, *125*, 3–14. [CrossRef]
119. Filippin, L.I.; Vercelino, R.; Marroni, N.P.; Xavier, R.M. Redox Signalling and the Inflammatory Response in Rheumatoid Arthritis. *Clin. Exp. Immunol.* **2008**, *152*, 415–422. [CrossRef]
120. Quiñonez-Flores, C.M.; González-Chávez, S.A.; Del Río Nájera, D.; Pacheco-Tena, C. Oxidative Stress Relevance in the Pathogenesis of the Rheumatoid Arthritis: A Systematic Review. *BioMed Res. Int.* **2016**, *2016*, 6097417. [CrossRef]
121. Takatani, Y.; Ono, K.; Suzuki, H.; Inaba, M.; Sawada, M.; Matsuda, N. Inducible Nitric Oxide Synthase during the Late Phase of Sepsis Is Associated with Hypothermia and Immune Cell Migration. *Lab. Investig. J. Tech. Methods Pathol.* **2018**, *98*, 629–639. [CrossRef] [PubMed]
122. Liu, Y.; Wei, W.; Hong, C.; Wang, Y.; Sun, X.; Ma, J.; Zheng, F. Calreticulin Induced Endothelial ICAM-1 up-Regulation Associated with Tristetraprolin Expression Alteration through PI3K/Akt/eNOS/P38 MAPK Signaling Pathway in Rheumatoid Arthritis. *Mol. Immunol.* **2019**, *107*, 10–20. [CrossRef] [PubMed]
123. Dey, S.; Bishayi, B. Effect of iNOS Inhibitor LNMMA along with Antibiotics Chloramphenicol or Ofloxacin in Murine Peritoneal Macrophages Regulates S.Aureus Infection as Well as Inflammation: An in Vitro Study. *Microb. Pathog.* **2017**, *105*, 307–320. [CrossRef]
124. Seymour, M.; Pétavy, F.; Chiesa, F.; Perry, H.; Lukey, P.T.; Binks, M.; Donatien, P.D.; Freidin, A.J.; Eckersley, R.J.; McClinton, C.; et al. Ultrasonographic Measures of Synovitis in an Early Phase Clinical Trial: A Double-Blind, Randomised, Placebo and Comparator Controlled Phase IIa Trial of GW274150 (a Selective Inducible Nitric Oxide Synthase Inhibitor) in Rheumatoid Arthritis. *Clin. Exp. Rheumatol.* **2012**, *30*, 254–261. [PubMed]
125. Attia, A.M.M.; Ibrahim, F.A.A.; Abd El-Latif, N.A.; Aziz, S.W.; Elwan, A.M.; Abdel Aziz, A.A.A.; Elgendy, A.; Elgengehy, F.T. Therapeutic Antioxidant and Anti-Inflammatory Effects of Laser Acupuncture on Patients with Rheumatoid Arthritis. *Lasers Surg. Med.* **2016**, *48*, 490–497. [CrossRef]
126. Mateen, S.; Moin, S.; Khan, A.Q.; Zafar, A.; Fatima, N. Increased Reactive Oxygen Species Formation and Oxidative Stress in Rheumatoid Arthritis. *PloS ONE* **2016**, *11*, e0152925. [CrossRef]
127. Phull, A.-R.; Nasir, B.; Haq, I.U.; Kim, S.J. Oxidative Stress, Consequences and ROS Mediated Cellular Signaling in Rheumatoid Arthritis. *Chem. Biol. Interact.* **2018**, *281*, 121–136. [CrossRef]
128. Helli, B.; Mowla, K.; Mohammadshahi, M.; Jalali, M.T. Effect of Sesamin Supplementation on Cardiovascular Risk Factors in Women with Rheumatoid Arthritis. *J. Am. Coll. Nutr.* **2016**, *35*, 300–307. [CrossRef]

129. Vaghef-Mehrabany, E.; Homayouni-Rad, A.; Alipour, B.; Sharif, S.-K.; Vaghef-Mehrabany, L.; Alipour-Ajiry, S. Effects of Probiotic Supplementation on Oxidative Stress Indices in Women with Rheumatoid Arthritis: A Randomized Double-Blind Clinical Trial. *J. Am. Coll. Nutr.* **2016**, *35*, 291–299. [CrossRef]
130. Nakajima, A.; Aoki, Y.; Shibata, Y.; Sonobe, M.; Terajima, F.; Takahashi, H.; Saito, M.; Taniguchi, S.; Yamada, M.; Nakagawa, K. Identification of Clinical Parameters Associated with Serum Oxidative Stress in Patients with Rheumatoid Arthritis. *Mod. Rheumatol.* **2014**, *24*, 926–930. [CrossRef]
131. da Fonseca, L.J.S.; Nunes-Souza, V.; Goulart, M.O.F.; Rabelo, L.A. Oxidative Stress in Rheumatoid Arthritis: What the Future Might Hold Regarding Novel Biomarkers and Add-On Therapies. *Oxid. Med. Cell. Longev.* **2019**, *2019*, 7536805. [CrossRef]
132. Abdollahzad, H.; Aghdashi, M.A.; Asghari Jafarabadi, M.; Alipour, B. Effects of Coenzyme Q10 Supplementation on Inflammatory Cytokines (TNF-α, IL-6) and Oxidative Stress in Rheumatoid Arthritis Patients: A Randomized Controlled Trial. *Arch. Med. Res.* **2015**, *46*, 527–533. [CrossRef] [PubMed]
133. DeBerardinis, R.J.; Chandel, N.S. We Need to Talk about the Warburg Effect. *Nat. Metab.* **2020**, *2*, 127–129. [CrossRef] [PubMed]
134. López-Armada, M.J.; Fernández-Rodríguez, J.A.; Blanco, F.J. Mitochondrial Dysfunction and Oxidative Stress in Rheumatoid Arthritis. *Antioxidants* **2022**, *11*, 1151. [CrossRef] [PubMed]
135. Zuo, J.; Tang, J.; Lu, M.; Zhou, Z.; Li, Y.; Tian, H.; Liu, E.; Gao, B.; Liu, T.; Shao, P. Glycolysis Rate-Limiting Enzymes: Novel Potential Regulators of Rheumatoid Arthritis Pathogenesis. *Front. Immunol.* **2021**, *12*, 779787. [CrossRef]
136. Westra, J.; Molema, G.; Kallenberg, C.G.M. Hypoxia-Inducible Factor-1 as Regulator of Angiogenesis in Rheumatoid Arthritis-Therapeutic Implications. *Curr. Med. Chem.* **2010**, *17*, 254–263. [CrossRef]
137. Szekanecz, Z.; Koch, A.E. Targeting Angiogenesis in Rheumatoid Arthritis. *Curr. Rheumatol. Rev.* **2008**, *4*, 298–303. [CrossRef]
138. Chen, J.; Cheng, W.; Li, J.; Wang, Y.; Chen, J.; Shen, X.; Su, A.; Gan, D.; Ke, L.; Liu, G.; et al. Notch-1 and Notch-3 Mediate Hypoxia-Induced Activation of Synovial Fibroblasts in Rheumatoid Arthritis. *Arthritis Rheumatol.* **2021**, *73*, 1810–1819. [CrossRef]

medicina

MDPI

Review

Sjögren's Disease and Gastroesophageal Reflux Disease: What Is Their Evidence-Based Link?

Diana Mieliauskaitė * and Vilius Kontenis

Department of Personalised Medicine, State Research Institute Center for Innovative Medicine, Santariskiu st. 5, LT-08405 Vilnius, Lithuania; vilius.kontenis@imcentras.lt

* Correspondence: diana.mieliauskaite@imcentras.lt

Abstract: Sjögren's disease (SjD), or primary Sjögren's syndrome (pSS), is a heterogeneous chronic autoimmune disorder with multiple clinical manifestations that can develop into non-Hodgkin's lymphoma in mucosa-associated lymphoid tissue. SjD is one of the autoimmune diseases with the maximum delayed diagnosis due to its insidious onset, heterogeneous clinical features and varied course. It is increasingly recognized that extraglandular manifestations represent a clinical challenge for patients with SjD. The European League Against Rheumatism (EULAR) Sjögren's Syndrome (SS) Disease Activity Index (ESSDAI) is a systemic disease activity index designed to measure disease activity in patients with primary Sjogren's syndrome. It consists of 12 domains: cutaneous, pulmonary, renal, articular, muscular, peripheral nervous system, central nervous system, hematological, glandular, constitutional, lymphadenopathy and lymphoma, biological. More than a quarter of patients with pSS may have systemic features that are not included in the ESSDAI classification, i.e., various cardiovascular, ophthalmic, ENT, and other systemic or organ involvement that increase the magnitude of the systemic phenotype in the disease. The ESSDAI also excludes the gastrointestinal (GI) tract, and unfortunately, GI manifestations are not routinely assessed. Gastroesophageal reflux disease (GERD) is one of the most prevalent gastrointestinal disorders, impairing quality of life and consuming a large volume of medical resources. Recently carried out the Mendelian randomized trial confirmed the causal link between SjD and gastroesophageal reflux disease (GERD) and showed that GERD is a risk factor for SjD. This review aims to provide an overview of the research describing evidenced based links between Sjögren's disease and gastroesophageal reflux disease, with the intention of ensuring that any systemic pathology in Sjögren's disease is properly assessed and that management of the disease is directed towards the patient. A comprehensive literature search was carried out on PubMed, Web of Science, Scopus and the Cochrane Library databases. Two researchers searched for published studies indexed from inception to 1 September 2024 using the keywords 'Sjögren's syndrome' OR 'Sjögren's disease' AND 'gastroesophageal reflux disease' AND 'microbiota' OR microbiota dysbiosis'. We limited our search for scientific articles to human studies, and only included articles in English. Overall, there is a lack of evidence-based studies assessing the association between GERD and Sjögren's disease and the changes in the microbiota associated with GERD in a multidisciplinary setting. Such studies are needed for the future, as this will improve the early diagnosis of Sjögren's disease and the personalized management of the disease.

Keywords: Sjögren's disease; gastroesophageal reflux disease; extraglandular manifestations; microbiota; Mendelian randomized study

1. Introduction

Sjögren's disease (SjD), or primary Sjögren's syndrome (pSS), is a heterogeneous chronic autoimmune disorder with multiple clinical manifestations that can develop into non-Hodgkin's lymphoma in mucosa-associated lymphoid tissue [1]. An analysis of the results from 62 studies provided an up-to-date summary of the available evidence on the incidence, prevalence, age of symptom onset and age of diagnosis of SjD globally, based on the 2016 ACR/EULAR diagnostic criteria. This summary identified a prevalence ranging from 12.4 to 13.1 per 100,000 person-years or 22.0 to 770.0 per 100,000 persons (once metrics were scaled to100,000 persons) [2]. SjD is one of the autoimmune diseases with the most delayed diagnoses due to its insidious onset, heterogeneous clinical features and varied course [3].

It is increasingly recognized that extraglandular manifestations represent a clinical challenge for patients with SjD, as the clinical features of the disease vary [4]. The European League Against Rheumatism (EULAR) Sjögren's Syndrome (SS) Disease Activity Index (ESSDAI) is a systemic disease activity index designed to measure disease activity in patients with primary Sjogren's syndrome. The ESSDAI is used as the gold standard for assessing disease activity in clinical trials. It consists of 12 domains (cutaneous, pulmonary, renal, articular, muscular, peripheral nervous system (PNS), central nervous system (CNS), hematological, glandular, constitutional, lymphadenopathy and lymphoma, biological) [5].

EULAR Sjogren's Syndrome Patient Reported Index (ESSPRI), and other patient-reported outcomes (PROs), such as the visual analog scale (VAS) for symptoms and EULAR sicca score (ESS), are used to assess the disease activity of primary Sjögren's syndrome (pSS) [6]. More than a quarter of patients with pSS may have systemic features that are not included in the ESSDAI classification, i.e., various cardiovascular, ophthalmic, ENT and other systemic or organ involvement that increase the magnitude of the systemic phenotype in the disease. The ESSDAI also excludes the gastrointestinal tract [7]. Although the ESSDAI, ESSPRI and PROs do not include the gastrointestinal tract, the main gastrointestinal manifestations of Sjogren's disease can occur in the esophagus, stomach, pancreas, liver and small intestine, and unfortunately are not routinely assessed [8,9] (Figure 1).

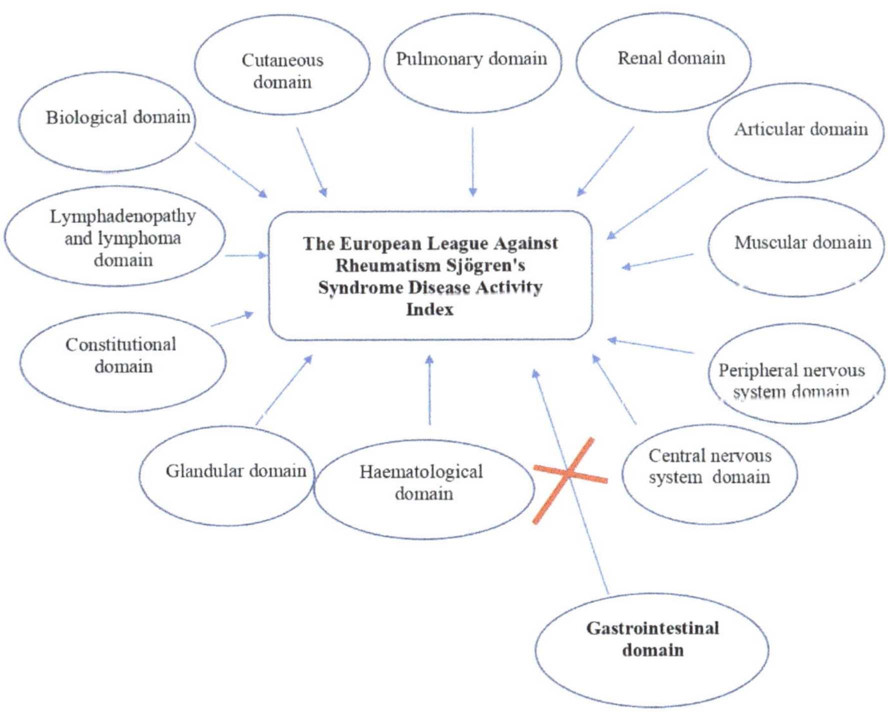

Figure 1. The European League Against Rheumatism (EULAR) Sjögren's Syndrome (SS) Disease Activity Index (ESSDAI)—a systemic disease activity index designed to measure disease activity in patients with primary Sjogren's syndrome.

Gastroesophageal reflux disease (GERD) is one of the most prevalent gastrointestinal disorders, impairing quality of life and consuming a large volume of medical resources. Epidemiological studies show that the prevalence of GERD is steadily increasing worldwide. The prevalence of GERD ranges from 2.5% to 51.2%, depending on the population studied and the clinical features assessed, but the pooled prevalence of those studies that evaluated the criteria of weekly heartburn or regurgitation frequency was 13.3% (95% CI 12.0–14.6%) [10].

Notably, the just-published Mendelian randomized trial confirmed that there is a causal link between Sjögren's disease and gastroesophageal reflux disease, and that GERD is a risk factor for SjD, while Sjögren's disease itself has no effect on gastroesophageal reflux disease [11].

This review aims to provide an overview of the research describing evidenced based links between Sjögren's disease and gastroesophageal reflux disease, with the intention of ensuring that any systemic pathology in Sjögren's disease is properly assessed and that management of the disease is directed towards the patient.

2. Materials and Methods

A comprehensive literature search was carried out on the PubMed, Web of Science, Scopus and the Cochrane Library databases. Two researchers searched for published studies indexed from inception to 1 September 2024 using the keywords 'Sjögren's syndrome' OR 'Sjögren's disease' AND 'gastroesophageal reflux disease' AND 'gastrointestinal manifestations' AND 'microbiota' OR microbiota dysbiosis'. We limited our search for scientific articles to human studies, and only included articles in English.

3. Sjogren's Disease and Clinical Heterogeneity

The pathogenesis of SjD is multifactorial, resulting from the interaction between genetic factors and exogenous and endogenous factors, leading to an abnormal autoimmune response involving T and B lymphocytes. Inflammation maintains, perpetuates and enhances tissue damage, leading to progressive functional impairment of the affected organs [1,12]. SjD is a systemic disease that can affect almost all organs and systems. This clinical presentation is due to a variety of mechanisms: secondary exocrinopathy, autoimmune epithelitis with periepithelial lymphocytic infiltration of target organs, and organ autoimmunity with specific autoantibodies, and a systemic presentation involving immune complexes or cryoglobulinaemia and clonal lymphocyte expansion [12].

Patients with Sjögren's disease are heterogeneous in terms of their clinical symptoms, systemic manifestations and risks. A recent study identified different groups of patients with Sjögren's disease based on subjective symptoms, objective test results and biological parameters. The results of this study underline the fact that, even in patients with predominantly systemic symptoms, the symptom burden is high and should not be ignored. These results reinforce the need for appropriate assessment of patient complaints in all subgroups of Sjögren's disease, irrespective of systemic activity [13].

3.1. Gastrointestinal Manifestations in Sjogren's Disease

Since 2015, the annual reviews of *Clinical and Experimental Rheumatology* have summarized the innovations in Sjögren's disease research from that year. These annual reviews highlight the heterogeneity of the disease and the importance of the early detection of both glandular and extraglandular manifestations. Also, a recent systematic review highlighted the importance of early diagnosis of pSS, with recommendations for early recognition of the disease, particularly focusing on the recognition of organ-specific "hidden" signs of systemic disease. Although the annual *Clinical and Experimental Rheumatology* reviews aim to emphasize the importance of an early diagnosis of pSS, focusing on the recognition of organ-specific "hidden" signs of systemic disease, there are very few reviews of studies on the gastrointestinal manifestations of Sjogren's disease, and no mention of GERD [14–24]. The 2018 review presents the results of a study showing that elevated levels of fecal calprotectin, a good marker of gastrointestinal inflammation, were found in a subgroup of patients with pSS and were associated with gastrointestinal tract comorbidities. Also, a study was reviewed in which severe intestinal dysbiosis was associated with clinical and laboratory signs of systemic disease activity, as well as with laboratory signs of gastrointestinal tract damage [18].

In a retrospective analysis of the Spanish Sjögrenser cohort, gastrointestinal involvement occurred in approximately 16% of patients, particularly as an autoimmune disorder, and in half of the patients, gastrointestinal involvement occurred at the same time as or after the diagnosis. Chronic atrophic gastritis was the most common form reported in approximately 30% of patients, followed by primary biliary cholangitis and autoimmune hepatitis. Pancreatic involvement was reported in 10% of patients and 7% had coeliac disease. Patients with gastrointestinal involvement were significantly older at the time of diagnosis of SS, were more likely to be female, and had a higher prevalence of autoimmune hypothyroidism and C3 hypo-complementemia [19].

In recent years, convincing evidence has suggested that patients with systemic rheumatic diseases, in particular pSS, may have an increased risk of coeliac disease (CD). A recent multicenter, case–control, Italian study involving more than 1400 patients with systemic autoimmune diseases, including pSS, systemic lupus erythematosus (SLE) and systemic sclerosis, reinforced this hypothesis. Primary SS patients were characterized by having a significantly higher prevalence of CD in comparison to a wide general population (6.78% vs. 0.64%). Moreover, pSS patients with CD were younger at autoimmune disease diagnosis in comparison to a nonceliac group, thus suggesting that screening for CD may be considered in young pSS patients, especially at disease diagnosis [21].

It was revealed that patients with pancreatic involvement had a higher prevalence of central nervous system and renal involvement, Raynaud's phenomenon, lymphoma and hypocomplementemia in Sjogren's disease [24].

3.1.1. Gastroesophageal Reflux in Sjogren's Disease

As mentioned above, GERD was not mentioned when summarizing the results of the studies on gastrointestinal clinical manifestations in Sjogren's disease in the annual reviews of *Clinical and Experimental Rheumatology*. However, to summarize other published studies on the association between Sjogren's disease and GERD, they can be categorized as follows: GERD is a comorbidity of Sjogren's disease; GERD is an extraglandular manifestation of Sjogren's disease; and GERD is a risk factor for developing Sjogren's disease (Figure 2).

The exact mechanism of the link between SS and GERD is not fully understood. Several explanations are given for why GERD occurs in people with SS. We know that the pathophysiology of GERD is multifactorial. A variety of factors can cause GERD symptoms, such as gastric anatomy and motility, the antireflux barrier, reflux properties, clearance mechanisms and mucosal integrity. On the one hand, studies have shown that the pathophysiology of the gastroesophageal tract of patients with SjD is different, and on the other hand, studies do not always exclude confounding factors (e.g., medication), which can lead to a bias in the results. Moreover, the sequence of the development of SS and GERD is not definitively clear [11,25,26].

Gastroesophageal Reflux Disease as a Comorbidity of Sjogren's Disease

In this section, we will review publications listing GERD as a comorbidity in Sjögren's disease.

A Cox proportional hazards regression model was used to estimate the risk of gastroesophageal reflux disease in 4650 patients with Sjogren's disease from 2000 to 2011. This study demonstrated that the risk of GERD among SS patients is 2.41-fold greater than that for general population [25]. A review of the literature summarizes the possible association between GERD and rheumatoid arthritis, mixed connective tissue disorders, Sjogren's syndrome, systemic sclerosis and other diseases in which GERD is a comorbidity [26].

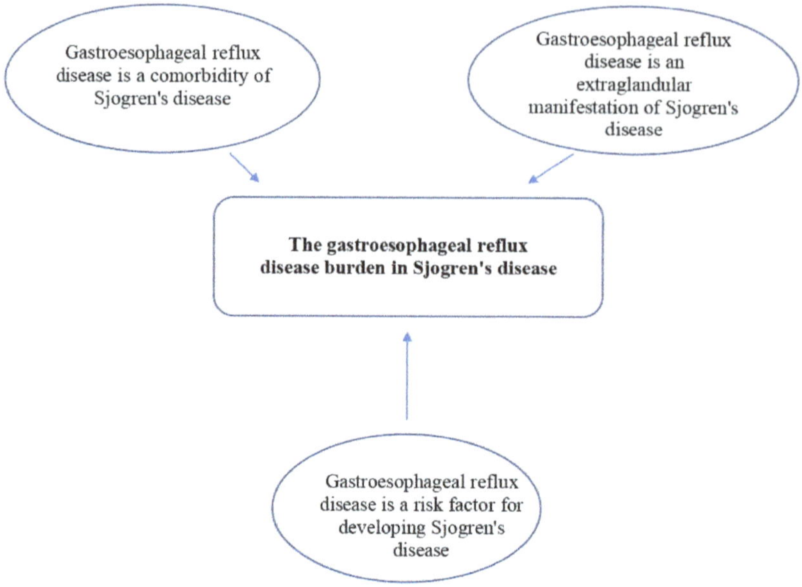

Figure 2. The association between Sjogren's disease and gastroesophageal reflux disease.

The results of the 2016 Sjögren's Foundation survey, with 25 questions designed in a collaborative effort between the Foundation, patients with SjD, SjD provider experts and a marketing research company, revealed that 48 percent of SjD patients have had GERD as a medical comorbidity [27].

A recent study to determine how pain, dryness and fatigue—the main symptoms of Sjögren's disease—contribute to cluster phenotypes identified GERD as a common comorbidity in Sjögren's disease patients. The 1454 participants from the Sjögren's International Collaborative Clinical Alliance (SICCA) Registry and 2920 participants of the Sjogren's Foundation survey were divided into the following groups: (1) low symptom burden across all categories (LSB); (2) dryness with low pain and low fatigue (DLP); (3) dryness with high pain and low-to-moderate fatigue (DHP); and (4) high symptom burden across all categories (HSB). The Sjogren's Foundation survey of 2920 people identified 1327 Sjogren's disease patients with comorbid gastroesophageal reflux disease. A significantly high prevalence of GERD as a comorbidity was found in group DHP and the lowest in group LSB, respectively, out of groups LSB (n = 665), DLP (n = 409), DHP (n = 611) and HSB (n = 1235), with n = 237 (39%), n = 155 (41%), n = 288(49%) and n = 647(54%) [28].

More recently, a large sample study, one of the aims of which was to determine the relationship between the diagnosis of SD and the comorbidities diagnosed in these patients, found that 60% of patients with Sjögren's disease reported oesophageal reflux as a comorbid condition [29].

The results of the study, which show that patients with Sjögren's disease have a higher risk of gastroesophageal reflux disease compared to the general population, suggest that reflux is a common extraglandular manifestation of Sjögren's disease [30]. The results of this study are flawed in that the prevalence may have been underestimated because only individuals who needed help were referred to the facility, the cross-sectional design used meant that a causal relationship based on the observed correlation between Sjögren's syndrome and gastroesophageal reflux disease may not have been established. Medication use was not assessed in this study. Finally, as this study was conducted in a Taiwanese population, the results of the study are generalizable to other ethnic populations. All of these studies described above did not assess the effect of drugs on the development of GERD, which can be considered a limitation of these studies.

Gastroesophageal Reflux Disease as an Extraglandular Manifestation of Sjogren's Disease

There is a dearth of scientific papers describing GERD as an extraglandular manifestation in Sjögren's disease. An early study found no association between swallowing disorders and esophageal motor function in patients with Sjogren's disease. The results of this study showed that pathological GERD, corresponding to the most common forms of dysmotility that are characteristic of GERD, was very common in SjD patients. These results underline the importance of an early and accurate diagnosis of GERD in SjD patients to prevent or correct esophageal pathology, as acid elimination from their esophagus is altered due to reduced saliva volume [30]. Also, another research study suggests that antibody-mediated disruption of M3-muscarinic receptor neurotransmission and the subsequent inhibition of smooth muscle contraction may lead to the gastrointestinal disturbances that are characteristic of Sjögren's disease [31,32].

In a study published more than a decade ago to assess the prevalence of gastroesophageal reflux disease (GERD) symptoms and tooth wear in patients with Sjögren's syndrome (SS) compared to controls, a statistically significantly higher proportion of SS patients reported suffering from heartburn and regurgitation compared to controls [33].

The review article highlights the problems that arise in the diagnosis of Sjogren's disease and the prognosis of the outcome of the disease, mentioning gastroesophageal reflux as an extra-glandular manifestation [34].

Gastroesophageal reflux (GER) has also been shown to be common in Sjogren's disease and can cause or contribute to a range of symptoms (such as heartburn, nausea, chronic cough, nausea, dysphagia). In this case–control study, the prevalence of GER was observed to be 60% in pSS patients compared to 23% in the control group [29]. A cross-sectional population-based study in Taiwan found that 4650 patients with SjD had a 2.4-fold higher risk of GERD compared to controls after adjusting for age, sex and comorbidities. Possible predictors of GERD in SjD may include reduced saliva volume, reduced esophageal motility, sphincter relaxation, slower gastric emptying time or side effects from medications [35].

Gastroesophageal reflux (GER) is present in 13 to 60% of pSS patients with gastrointestinal manifestations according to different researchers [7,36].

Chronic glandular inflammation impairs the protective function of the pharyngeal, laryngeal and esophageal mucosa against acid and gastric protease damage in Sjögren's disease. Tissue immunity depends on the protective mucin cell layer, which weakens the diffusion of hydrochloric acid and changes the pH. When the epithelium is under immune attack and inflammation develops, the pharynx, larynx and esophagus are unable to react adequately to the damaging effects of gastric reflux [35].

A survey of people claiming to have primary and secondary Sjogren's syndrome and sicca syndrome found that 86.97% of them experience intermittent/permanent dry mouth, and almost 80% of them experience GERD symptoms [37].

The study described in the previous section, in which the prevalence of GERD comorbidities was significantly highest in the dryness with high pain and low to moderate fatigue (DHP) group and lowest in the low symptom burden across all categories (dryness, pain, fatigue) (LSB) group [28], suggests that GERD is an extraglandular manifestation of Sjogren's disease.

Gastroesophageal Reflux Disease as a Risk Factor for Developing Sjogren's Disease: Insights from Mendelian Randomization Studies

There has been an observation that, in patients with Sjogren's disease, the SjD regimen did not improve GERD-related symptoms, and in some patients, reflux was exacerbated due to side effects of the drug. Surprisingly and inexplicably, when patients with SjD received medication for GERD, their condition improved at the same time. It was hypothesized that there might be a genetic link between GERD and SjDS, and that GERD might influence the onset and course of SjD [10]. To date, until this Mendelian study, there had been no evidence-based research on the role of GERD in determining the risk of developing SjD. The Mendelian randomized trial confirmed that there is a causal link between Sjögren's disease and gastroesophageal reflux disease, and that GERD is a risk factor for SjD, while Sjögren's disease itself has no effect on gastroesophageal reflux disease. This study is based on clinical observations and the authors hope that the results will also be used for clinical diagnosis and treatment. The authors emphasize that we should pay attention to the likelihood of SjD when diagnosing GERD, and that physicians can alleviate GERD symptoms in SS patients to control the progression of SS [11].

This study has limitations due to the sample size and the fact that only European populations were selected for the study. In the future, the authors of the mentioned study plan to expand the sample size and sample information to include more different ethnic groups in order to confirm a causal link between GERD and SjD.

The results of another recent Mendelian study suggest that some microorganisms may have a protective role against the development GERD, such as the *Family Clostridiales Vadin* BB60 group, *Genus Lachnospiraceae UCG004, Genus Methanobrevibacter* and *Phylum Actinobacteria*, whereas other microorganisms, such as the *Class Mollicutes*, *Genus Anaerostipes* and *Phylum Tenericutes*, may be risk factors for the development of GERD. With regard to reverse causality, where GERD is a consequence and the gut microbiota is a result, the studies show that GERD is caused by dysbiosis in 13 different classes of gut microbiota. This Mendelian study has shown a genetic link between changes in the abundance of gut microbiota and the risk of GERD. This not only supports the feasibility of gut microenvironmental treatment of GERD, but also lays the groundwork for advanced research into the role of the gut microbiota in the etiology of GERD [38].

Recently, it has been shown that the gut microbiota, metabolites and metabolic pathways in healthy children and children with GERD are different, and that differences in metabolites are associated with specific changes in bacterial abundance. In the future, this may provide new evidence on the pathogenesis of GERD, and possibly expand our knowledge of Sjogren's disease [38].

Helicobacter pylori is a Gram-positive bacterium and plays a role in the inflammation and carcinogenesis of the stomach lining. Helicobacter pylori infection is estimated to affect a large proportion of the world's population, with a prevalence ranging from 60.3 to 80% [39–48]. The results of two Mendelian randomization analyses reveal a causal link between H. pylori infection and an increased susceptibility to GERD, and may lead to a better understanding of the pathogenesis of GERD [44].

A bidirectional Mendelian randomized trial found that GERD may increase the likelihood of insomnia, snoring and obstructive sleep apnea, in addition to shortening sleep duration [45], and undoubtedly contributes to the increase in oral dryness and chronic fatigue in patients with SjD and GERD.

Characteristic Changes in Microbiota in Sjogren's Disease and Gastroesophageal Reflux Disease

GERD can increase the risk of SS due to changes in the gut and esophageal microbiota. A recent study shows that *Bacteroides* and *Prevotella* increase significantly in GERD patients, while *Actinobacteria, Lactobacilli, Micrococci, Rotella and Streptococci* decrease significantly in these patients [49]. Dysbiosis of the microbiota in the gastrointestinal tract due to gastroesophageal reflux disease may in turn increase the risk of Sjögren's syndrome [38,39]. The esophageal microbiome of GERD patients and healthy individuals has been studied and is characterized by two main types: a type I microbiome, which is associated with a healthy state and is dominated by Gram-positive bacteria, and a type II microbiome, which is associated with GERD and is characterized by the pronounced prevalence of Gram-negative and microaerophilic bacteria [50]. Recent evidence suggests that GERD may develop through an immunogenic pathway. The evidence shows that submucosal inflammation induced by cytokines with intact epithelial cells is observed in the distal esophagus of patients with GERD, likely due to an immunogenic pathway [40,51].

A recent study using 16S ribosomal RNA (16S rRNA) gene sequencing analysis investigated the association between salivary microbiota and GERD. GERD patients had a higher relative abundance of *Bacteroidetes phylum, Bacteroidia* class, *Bacteroidales* order, *Prevotellaceae* family and unidentified_*Prevotellaceae* genus. A comparison with individuals with undiagnosed GERD revealed a reduction in the *Actinobacteria phylum,* the unidentified *Actinobacteria* and *Bacilli* classes, the *Micrococcales* and *Lactobacillales* orders, the *Micrococcaceae* and *Streptococcaceae* families and the genuses *Rothia* and *Streptococcus* in the saliva of patients with GERD [39]. Although the authors of this study claim to have identified changes in salivary microbiota and biomarkers in GERD patients, the study is flawed due to the small sample size, the lack of healthy controls and the lack of an analysis of the effect of ph on oral microbiota.

Another recent study has identified distinct microbiota populations in the distal esophagus associated with different stages of gastroesophageal reflux disease [52]. A new study by the same authors shows that the oral microbiome differs significantly between acid reflux severity groups. This study suggests that excessive gastric acid reflux into the esophagus may lead to disturbances in the homeostasis of the oral microbiota, suggesting that the oral ecosystem of patients with GERD will be altered as a direct result of the gastric reflux and the alteration of saliva production. However, the design of this study is limited because oral saliva pH was not measured [53].

A recent Mendelian randomization (MR) analysis revealed a possible causal effect of specific microbial taxa on functional dyspepsia (FD) and irritable bowel syndrome (IBS), the symptoms of which are often overlapping with those of gastroesophageal reflux disease (GERD) [54]. The study has limitations in that potential causal relationships may not have been explored for all species, the European population studied may limit generalizability to other populations, and the small sample size studied.

Regarding the role of the microbiota, there is a lack of studies that simultaneously investigate the expression of the microbiota at different sites in the gastrointestinal tract of patients with GERD, Sjögren's disease. Further research into the links between GERD, Sjögren's disease and the microbiota on appropriate design will help to elucidate the pathogenesis of Sjögren's disease in the future, and will lead to the development of effective disease monitoring and treatment.

4. Conclusions

Overall, there is a lack of evidence-based studies assessing the association between GERD and Sjögren's disease and the changes in the microbiota associated with GERD in a multidisciplinary setting. Such studies are needed for the future, as this will improve the early diagnosis of Sjögren's disease and the personalized management of the disease.

Author Contributions: Conceptualization: D.M. and V.K.; Methodology, D.M.; Software, V.K.; Formal Analysis, D.M. and V.K.; Resources, D.M. and V.K.; Data Curation, D.M.; Writing—Original Draft Preparation, D.M. and V.K.; Writing—Review and Editing, D.M. and V.K.; Visualization, V.K.; Supervision, D.M. All authors have read and agreed to the published version of the manuscript.

Funding: This research received no external funding.

Institutional Review Board Statement: Not applicable.

Informed Consent Statement: Not applicable.

Data Availability Statement: Publicly available datasets were analyzed in this study and referred to in the list of references.

Conflicts of Interest: The authors declare no conflicts of interest.

References

1. Mieliauskaite, D.; Kontenis, V. Insights into Microbiota in Sjögren's Syndrome. *Medicina* **2023**, *59*, 1661. [CrossRef] [PubMed]
2. Thurtle, E.; Grosjean, A.; Steenackers, M.; Strege, K.; Barcelos, G.; Goswami, P. Epidemiology of Sjögren's: A Systematic Literature Review. *Rheumatol. Ther.* **2024**, *11*, 1–17. [CrossRef] [PubMed]
3. Wei, P.; Xing, Y.; Li, B.; Chen, F.; Hua, H. Proteomics-based analysis indicating α-enolase as a potential biomarker in primary Sjögren's syndrome. *Gland Surg.* **2020**, *9*, 2054–2063.
4. Li, X.X.; Maitiyaer, M.; Tan, Q.; Huang, W.H.; Liu, Y.; Liu, Z.P.; Wen, Y.Q.; Zheng, Y.; Chen, X.; Chen, R.L.; et al. Emerging biologic frontiers for Sjogren's syndrome: Unveiling novel approaches with emphasis on extra glandular pathology. *Front. Pharmacol.* **2024**, *15*, 1377055. [CrossRef]
5. Seror, R.; Bowman, S.J.; Brito-Zeron, P.; Theander, E.; Bootsma, H.; Tzioufas, A.; Gottenberg, J.E.; Ramos-Casals, M.; Dörner, T.; Ravaud, P.; et al. EULAR Sjögren's syndrome disease activity index (ESSDAI): A user guide. *RMD Open* **2015**, *1*, e000022. [CrossRef]
6. Ture, H.Y.; Kim, N.R.; Nam, E.J. EULAR Sjogren's Syndrome Patient Reported Index (ESSPRI) and Other Patient-Reported Outcomes in the Assessment of Glandular Dysfunction in Primary Sjögren's Syndrome. *Life* **2023**, *13*, 1991. [CrossRef]
7. Retamozo, S.; Acar-Denizli, N.; Rasmussen, A.; Horváth, I.F.; Baldini, C.; Priori, R.; Sandhya, P.; Hernandez-Molina, G.; Armagan, B.; Praprotnik, S.; et al. Systemic manifestations of primary Sjögren's syndrome out of the ESSDAI classification: Prevalence and clinical relevance in a large international, multi-ethnic cohort of patients. *Clin. Exp. Rheumatol.* **2019**, *37* (Suppl. 118), S97–S106.
8. Mihai, A.; Caruntu, C.; Jurcut, C.; Blajut, F.C.; Casian, M.; Opris-Belinski, D.; Ionescu, R.; Caruntu, A. The spectrum of extraglandular manifestations in primary Sjogren's syndrome. *J. Pers. Med.* **2023**, *13*, 961. [CrossRef] [PubMed]
9. Berry, J.; Tarn, J.; Lendrem, D.; Casement, J.; Ng, W.F. What can patients tell us in Sjögren's syndrome? *Rheumatol. Immunol. Res.* **2024**, *5*, 34–41. [CrossRef]
10. Zaterka, S.; Marion, S.B.; Roveda, F.; Perrotti, M.A.; Chinzonh, D. Historical perspective of gastroesophageal reflux disease clinical treatment. *Arq. Gastroenterol.* **2019**, *56*, 202–208. [CrossRef]
11. Liu, J.; Li, J.; Yuan, G.; Cao, T.; He, X. Relationship between Sjogren's syndrome and gastroesophageal reflux: A bidirectional Mendelian randomization study. *Sci. Rep.* **2024**, *14*, 15400.
12. Parisis, D.; Clara Chivasso, C.; Jason Perret, J.; Soyfoo, M.S.; Delporte, C. Current State of Knowledge on Primary Sjögren's Syndrome, an Autoimmune Exocrinopathy. *J. Clin. Med.* **2020**, *9*, 2299. [CrossRef] [PubMed]
13. Nguyen, Y.; Nocturne, G.; Henry, J.; Ng, W.F.; Belkhir, R.; Desmoulins, F.; Bergé, E.; Morel, J.; Perdriger, A.; Dernis, E.; et al. Identification of distinct subgroups of Sjögren's disease by cluster analysis based on clinical and biological manifestations: Data from the cross-sectional Paris-Saclay and the prospective ASSESS cohorts. *Lancet Rheumatol.* **2024**, *6*, e216–e225. [CrossRef] [PubMed]
14. Luciano, N.; Valentini, V.; Calabrò, A.; Elefante, E.; Vitale, A.A.; Baldini, C.C.; Bartoloni, E. One year in review 2015: Sjögren's syndrome. *Clin. Exp. Rheumatol.* **2015**, *33*, 259–271.
15. Ferro, F.; Vagelli, R.; Bruni, C.; Cafaro, G.; Marcucci, E.; Bartoloni, E.; Baldini, C. One year in review 2016: Sjögren's syndrome. *Clin. Exp. Rheumatol.* **2016**, *34*, 161–171.
16. Ferro, F.; Marcucci, E.E.; Orlandi, M.; Baldini, C.; Bartoloni-Bocci, E. One year in review 2017: Primary Sjögren's syndrome. *Clin. Exp. Rheumatol.* **2017**, *35*, 179–191.
17. Argyropoulou, O.D.; Valentini, E.E.; Ferro, F.F.; Leone, M.C.; Cafaro, G.G.; Bartoloni, E.; Baldini, C. One year in review 2018: Sjögren's syndrome. *Clin. Exp. Rheumatol.* **2018**, *36* (Suppl. 112), S14–S26.
18. Cafaro, G.; Croia, C.; Argyropoulou, O.D.; Leone, M.C.; Orlandi, M.; Finamore, F.; Cecchettini, A.A.; Ferro, F.; Baldini, C.; Bartoloni, E.E. One year in review 2019: Sjögren's syndrome. One year in review 2019: Sjögren's syndrome. *Clin. Exp. Rheumatol.* **2019**, *37* (Suppl. 118), S3–S15.
19. Manfre, V.; Cafaro, G.; Riccucci, I.; Zabotti, A.; Perricone, C.; Bootsma, H.; De Vita, S.; Bartoloni, E. One year in review 2020: Comorbidities, diagnosis and treatment of primary Sjogren's syndrome. *Clin. Exp. Rheumatol.* **2021**, *38*, S10–S22.
20. Cafaro, G.; Bursi, R.; Chatzis, L.G.; Fulvio, G.; Ferro, F.; Bartoloni, E.; Baldini, C. One year in review 2021: Sjögren's syndrome. *Clin. Exp. Rheumatol.* **2021**, *39* (Suppl. 133), S3–S13. [CrossRef]
21. Manfrè, V.; Chatzis, L.G.; Cafaro, G.; Fonzetti, S.; Calvacchi, S.; Fulvio, G.; Navarro Garcia, I.C.; La Rocca, G.; Ferro, F.; Perricone, C.; et al. Sjögren's syndrome: One year in review 2022. *Clin. Exp. Rheumatol.* **2022**, *40*, 2211–2224. [CrossRef] [PubMed]
22. Fass, R.; Boeckxstaens, G.E.; El-Serag, H.; Rosen, R.; Sifrim, D.; Vaezi, M.F. Gastro-oesophageal reflux disease. *Nat. Rev. Dis. Primers* **2021**, *7*, 55. [CrossRef] [PubMed]
23. Park, K.; Haberberger, R.V.; Gordon, T.P.; Jackson, M.W. Antibodies interfering with the type 3 muscarinic receptor pathway inhibit gastrointestinal motility and cholinergic neurotransmission in Sjogren's syndrome. *Arthritis. Rheum.* **2011**, *63*, 1426–1434. [CrossRef]
24. Longhino, S.; Chatzis, L.G.; Dal Pozzolo, R.; Peretti, S.; Fulvio, G.; La Rocca, G.; Navarro Garcia, I.C.; Orlandi, M.; Quartuccio, L.; Baldini, C.; et al. Sjögren's syndrome: One year in review 2023. *Exp. Rheumatol.* **2023**, *41*, 2343–2356. [CrossRef]
25. Chang, C.S.; Liao, C.H.; Muo, C.H.; Kao, C.H. Increased risk of concurrent gastroesophageal reflux disease among patients with Sjögren's syndrome: A nationwide population-based study. *Eur. J. Int. Med.* **2016**, *31*, 73–78. [CrossRef]
26. Akyuz, F.; Soyer, O.M. Which diseases are risk factors for developing gastroesophageal reflux disease? *Turk. J. Gastroenterol.* **2017**, *28*, S44–S47. [CrossRef] [PubMed]

27. McCoy, S.S.; Woodham, M.; Bunya, V.Y.; Saldanha, I.J.; Akpek, E.K.; Makara, M.A.; Baer, A.N. A comprehensive overview of living with Sjögren's: Results of a National Sjögren's Foundation survey. *Clin. Rheumatol.* **2022**, *41*, 2071–2078. [CrossRef]
28. McCoy, S.S.; Woodham, M.; Bartels, C.M.; Saldanha, I.J.; Bunya, V.Y.; Maerz, N.; Akpek, E.K.; Makara, M.A.; Baer, A.N. Symptom-Based Cluster Analysis Categorizes Sjögren's Disease Subtypes: An International Cohort Study Highlighting Disease Severity and Treatment Discordance. *Arthritis Rheumatol.* **2022**, *74*, 1569–1579. [CrossRef]
29. Felix Gomez, G.G.; Hugenberg, S.T.; Zunt, S.; Patel, J.S.; Wang, M.; Rajapuri, A.S.; Lembcke, L.R.; Rajendran, D.; Smith, J.C.; Cherlyan, B.; et al. Characterizing clinical findings of Sjogren's Disease patients in community practices using matched electronic dental-health record data. *PLoS ONE* **2023**, *18*, e0289335. [CrossRef]
30. Volter, F.O.; Fain, O.; Mathieu, E.; Thomas, M. Esophageal function and Sjogren's syndrome. *Dig. Dis. Sci.* **2004**, *49*, 248–253. [CrossRef]
31. Parka, K.; Parka, S.; Jacksonb, M.W. The inhibitory effects of antimuscarinic autoantibodies in the sera of primary Sjogren syndrome patients on the gastrointestinal motility. *Mol. Immunol.* **2013**, *56*, 583–587. [CrossRef] [PubMed]
32. Witas, R.; Peck, A.B.; Ambrus, J.L.; Nguyen, C.Q. Sjogren's Syndrome and TAM Receptors: A Possible Contribution to Disease Onset. *J. Immunol. Res.* **2019**, *2019*, 4813795. [CrossRef]
33. Nik, W.N.N.; Banerjee, A.; Moazzez, R. Gastro-oesophageal reflux disease symptoms and tooth wear in patients with Sjögren's syndrome. *Caries Res.* **2011**, *45*, 323–326. [CrossRef] [PubMed]
34. Maslinska, M.; Przygodzka, M.; Kwiatkowska, B.; Sikorska-Siudek, K. Sjögren's syndrome: Still not fully understood disease. *Rheumatol. Int.* **2015**, *35*, 233–241. [CrossRef]
35. Mandl, T.; Ekberg, O.; Wollmer, P.; Manthorpe, R.; Jacobsson, L.T. Dysphagia and dysmotility of the pharynx and oesophagus in patients with primary Sjogren's syndrome. *Scand. J. Rheumatol.* **2007**, *36*, 394–401.
36. Belafsky, P.C.; Postma, G.N. The laryngeal and esophageal manifestations of Sjögren's syndrome. *Curr. Rheumatol. Rep.* **2003**, *5*, 297–303. [CrossRef]
37. Rihab, B.; Lina, E.H.; Noémie, S.T.; Jean, S.; Marjolaine, G. The experience of dry mouth and screening for Sjogren's syndrome by the dentist: Patient-reported experiences. *BMC Oral Health* **2023**, *23*, 1010. [CrossRef]
38. Szymula, A.; Rosenthal, J.; Szczerba, B.M.; Bagavant, H.; Fu, S.M.; Deshmukh, U.S. T cell epitope mimicry between Sjögren's syndrome Antigen A (SSA)/Ro60 and oral, gut, skin and vaginal bacteria. *Clin. Immunol.* **2014**, *152*, 1–9. [CrossRef]
39. Qian, J.; Yang, M.; Xu, D.; Zhang, G.; Cai, Y.; Yang, B.; Wang, X.; Yu, Y. Alterations of The Salivary microbiota in gastroesophageal reflux disease. *J. Oral. Biosci.* **2023**, *65*, 280–286. [CrossRef]
40. Mazgaeen, L.; Gurung, P. Recent advances in lipopolysaccharide recognition systems. *Int. J. Mol. Sci.* **2020**, *21*, 379. [CrossRef]
41. Ye, X.; Yu, F.; Zhou, J.; Zhao, C.; Wu, J.; Ni, X. Analysis of the gut microbiota in children with gastroesophageal reflux disease using metagenomics and metabolomics. *Front. Cell. Infect. Microbiol.* **2023**, *13*, 1267192. [CrossRef] [PubMed]
42. van der Meulen, T.A.; Harmsen, H.J.M.; Vila, A.V.; Kurilshikov, A.; Liefers, S.C.; Zhernakova, A.; Fu, J.; Wijmenga, C.; Weersma, R.K.; de Leeuw, K.; et al. Shared gut, but distinct oral microbiota composition in primary Sjögren's syndrome and systemic lupus erythematosus. *J. Autoimmun.* **2019**, *97*, 77–87. [CrossRef] [PubMed]
43. van der Meulen, T.A.; Harmsen, H.; Bootsma, H.; Spijkervet, F.; Kroese, F.; Vissink, A. The microbiome-systemic diseases connection. *Oral. Dis.* **2016**, *22*, 719–734. [CrossRef]
44. Wang, K.; Wang, S.; Chen, Y.; Lu, X.; Wang, D.; Zhang, Y.; Pan, W.; Zhou, C.; Zou, D. Causal relationship between gut microbiota and risk of gastroesophageal reflux disease: A genetic correlation and bidirectional Mendelian randomization study. *Front. Immunol.* **2024**, *15*, 1327503. [CrossRef]
45. Qin, S.; Wang, C.; Wang, X.; Wu, W.; Liu, C. Causal association of gastroesophageal reflux disease with obstructive sleep apnea and sleep-related phenotypes: A bidirectional two-sample Mendelian randomization study. *Front. Neurol.* **2023**, *14*, 1283286. [CrossRef] [PubMed]
46. Malfertheiner, P.; Megraud, F.; O'Morain, C.A.; Gisbert, J.P.; Kuipers, E.J.; Axon, A.T.; Bazzoli, F.; Gasparini, A.; Atherton, J.; Graham, D.Y.; et al. Management of Helicobacter pylori infection-the Mastricht V/Florence Consensus Report. *Gut* **2017**, *66*, 6–30. [CrossRef]
47. Wang, L.; Cao, Z.M.; Zhang, L.L.; Dai, X.C.; Liu, Z.J.; Zeng, Y.X.; Li, X.Y.; Wu, Q.J.; Lv, W. Helicobacter pylori and autoimmune diseases: Involving multiple systems. *Front. Immunol.* **2022**, *13*, 833424. [CrossRef] [PubMed]
48. Chen, J.; Zhang, J.; Ma, X.; Ren, Y.; Tang, Y.; Zhang, Z.; Ye, W.; Zhang, Z.; Lin, Z.; Wang, L.; et al. Causal relationship between Helicobacter pylori antibodies and gastroesophageal reflux disease (GERD): A Mendelian study. *PLoS ONE* **2023**, *18*, e0294771. [CrossRef]
49. Vivino, F.B.; Bunya, V.Y.; Massaro-Giordano, G.; Johr, C.R.; Giattino, S.L.; Schorpion, A.; Shafer, B.; Peck, A.; Sivils, K.; Rasmussen, A.; et al. Sjogren's syndrome: An update on disease pathogenesis, clinical manifestations and treatment. *Clin. Immunol.* **2019**, *203*, 81–121. [CrossRef]
50. Lopetuso, L.R.; Severgnini, M.; Pecere, S.; Ponziani, F.R.; Boskoski, I.; Larghi, A.; Quaranta, G.; Masucci, L.; Ianniro, G.; Camboni, T.; et al. Esophageal microbiome signature in patients with Barrett's esophagus and esophageal adenocarcinoma. *PLoS ONE* **2020**, *15*, e0231789. [CrossRef]
51. D'Souza, S.M.; Houston, K.; Keenan, L.; Yoo, B.S.; Parekh, P.J.; Johnson, D.A. Role of microbial dysbiosis in the pathogenesis of esophageal mucosal disease: A paradigm shift from acid to bacteria? *World. J. Gastroenterol.* **2021**, *27*, 2054–2072. [CrossRef] [PubMed]

52. Zhou, J.; Shrestha, P.; Qiu, Z.; Harman, D.G.; Teoh, W.-C.; Al-Sohaily, S.; Liem, H.; Turner, I.; Ho, V. Distinct microbiota dysbiosis in patients with non-erosive reflux disease and esophageal adenocarcinoma. *J. Clin. Med.* **2020**, *9*, 2162. [CrossRef] [PubMed]
53. Power, D.J.; Ho, V.; Zhou, J. Association between Oral Microbiome and Gastroesophageal Reflux Severity. *J. Clin. Med.* **2024**, *13*, 4479. [CrossRef]
54. Huang, Y.; Kang, Z.; He, Y.; Qiu, Y.; Song, Y.; Liu, W. Association between gut microbiota and common overlapping gastrointestinal disorders: A bidirectional two-sample Mendelian randomization study. *Front. Microbiol.* **2024**, *15*, 1343564. [CrossRef] [PubMed]

medicina

MDPI

Article

Integrating Rehabilitation Services into Routine Care of Rheumatoid Arthritis May Reduce the Inflammatory Response: A Hospital-Based Follow-Up Study in Taiwan

Hui-Ju Huang [1,†], Wei-Jen Chen [2,3,4,†], Hanoch Livneh [5,†], Hua-Lung Huang [6], Ming-Chi Lu [7,8,9,*] and Tzung-Yi Tsai [9,10,*]

1 Department of Nursing, Dalin Tzu Chi Hospital, Buddhist Tzu Chi Medical Foundation, Chiayi 62247, Taiwan; df778383@tzuchi.com.tw
2 Center of Sports Medicine, Dalin Tzu Chi Hospital, Buddhist Tzu Chi Medical Foundation, Chiayi 62247, Taiwan; tough2915@hotmail.com
3 Graduate Institute of Sports Science, National Taiwan Sport University, Taoyuan 333325, Taiwan
4 School of Post-Baccalaureate Chinese Medicine, Tzu Chi University, Hualien 970374, Taiwan
5 Rehabilitation Counseling Program, Portland State University, Portland, OR 97207-0751, USA; livnehh@pdx.edu
6 Department of Rehabilitation, Dalin Tzu Chi Hospital, Buddhist Tzu Chi Medical Foundation, Chiayi 62247, Taiwan
7 School of Medicine, Tzu Chi University, Hualien 97004, Taiwan
8 Division of Allergy, Immunology and Rheumatology, Dalin Tzu Chi Hospital, Buddhist Tzu Chi Medical Foundation, Dalin Township, Chiayi 62247, Taiwan
9 Department of Medical Research, Dalin Tzu Chi Hospital, Buddhist Tzu Chi Medical Foundation, Chiayi 62247, Taiwan
10 Department of Environmental and Occupational Health, College of Medicine, National Cheng Kung University, Tainan 333325, Taiwan
* Correspondence: dm252940@tzuchi.com.tw (M.-C.L.); dm732024@tzuchi.com.tw (T.-Y.T.); Tel.: +886-5-2648000 (ext. 8713) (M.-C.L.); +886-5-2648000 (ext. 3209) (T.-Y.T.); Fax: +886-5-2648006 (M.-C.L. & T.-Y.T.)
† These authors contributed equally to this work.

Abstract: *Background and Objectives:* For persons with rheumatoid arthritis (RA), the accompanying systemic inflammatory conditions often insidiously damage extra-glandular organs, causing poor outcomes. Despite evidence manifesting the application of rehabilitation services (RSs), the association between RSs use and changes in the inflammatory response among persons with RA has not yet been established. With that in mind, this study aimed to evaluate changes in C-reactive protein (CRP) and erythrocyte sedimentation rate (ESR) before and after long-term RSs use. *Materials and Methods:* For this two-group pre and posttest study, medical data of 4505 persons with RA aged 20–70 years between 2012 and 2017 were retrieved from an electronic medical record database held by a hospital in Taiwan. Of them, 1387 subjects were categorized as RSs users, who received RSs at least six times within the first year of RA onset. Generalized estimating equations analysis was then employed to compare the changes in ESR and CRP at baseline, and at 12, 18, 24, 30, and 36 months after RA onset. *Results:* After adjusting for inherent differences and mature impact, those receiving standard care plus RSs were found to have a lower CRP level than those without receiving RSs. This benefit was maintained within a 3-year follow-up period. Additionally, a slight but nonsignificant reduction in ESR existed over the same timeframe. *Conclusions:* Integrating RSs into conventional care may be helpful to modulate the inflammation for RA patients, but further research via randomized controlled trials is needed to validate the application of RSs.

Keywords: rheumatoid arthritis; rehabilitation services; inflammatory response; generalized estimating equations; follow-up study

1. Introduction

Rheumatoid arthritis (RA) is an autoimmune disorder featuring progressive joint destruction resulting from chronic synovial inflammation. RA mainly affects working age people, thus imposing significant consequences on physical functioning and working capacity [1]. One estimate indicated that within the first 3 years after RA onset, approximately 30% of affected people become disabled, thus leading to a socioeconomic burden [2]. According to a recent report, the all-cause societal costs for RA annually is approximately USD 40 billion; likewise, the per-capita healthcare costs for RA patients is USD 20,919, triple that of those without RA [3].

Today, a growing body of evidence supports the notion that the inner inflammation accompanying RA may threaten other organs and systems beyond the joints, and increase risks of cardiovascular disease, pulmonary disease, and cancer [4,5]. In response to inflammation from RA, the body produces C-reactive protein (CRP), and the erythrocyte sedimentation rate (ESR) would increase throughout the body. In clinical practice, therefore, measuring these parameters in the serum can assist to diagnose and monitor related symptoms for persons with RA [6,7]. On top of that, both indicators have been incorporated into disease activity composite scores, including the 28-joint disease activity score (DAS 28). In a study that followed patients with inflammatory arthritis for ten years, it showed that an elevated CRP level ($\geqq$5 mg/L) was correlated with a three-fold increase in death due to cardiovascular disease, independent of conventional risk factors [8]. Given that the persistent inflammatory condition significantly worsens outcomes for those afflicted with RA, efforts focusing on breaking the loop of inflammation driven by RA are of paramount importance.

Currently, rehabilitation services (RSs) have been proposed as a potential for restoring RA patients' functional independence and improving their psychophysical function [7]. The application of RSs in the field of rheumatology mainly covers non-pharmacological therapy and also includes therapeutic patient education, exercises, physical modalities, orthoses, assistive devices, hydrotherapy, and dietary interventions [7]. Former evidence has indicated that hydrotherapy may reduce disease activity, improve mood, and mitigate joint tenderness as compared to no intervention via regulating the inflammatory milieu and oxidative stress [7,9]. Additionally, a recent study of 40 people with RA found that a combined treatment approach of medication and hydrotherapy remarkably abated damage from reactive oxygen species [10]. Some studies using both animal models and human experiments further documented that the use of RSs could be one way to enhance physical function via suppressing the release of bodily inflammatory cytokines, particularly interleukin (IL)-6, IL-1, and tumor necrosis factor-á [11,12], all of which are correlated with the production of acute-phase reactants and rheumatoid cachexia, which impair physical performance [6,7,13].

While there is growing evidence for the benefits of RSs, no concrete, large-scale follow-up data are available to investigate the specific effects of adding RSs into routine care on changes in CRP and ESR in RA patients. A long-term assessment towards this neglected area not only adds to the body of evidence regarding specific therapeutic effects, but also provides novel information for decision makers involved in healthcare services for RA patients. Therefore, to address this gap, we carried out a pretest–posttest follow-up experimental design study to clarify the association between RSs use and changes in CRP and ESR in RA patients.

2. Materials and Methods

2.1. Research Design and Participants

The retrospective observational study focused on RA patients seen at the rheumatology clinic in a 900-bed regional hospital in Taiwan. Since 2012, the target hospital set up an electronic medical record database (EMRD) to store healthcare claim data, including records of patients' demographics, diagnoses, prescriptions, and hospitalizations that occurred in the target hospital. The identification numbers of patients in the datasets were encrypted to protect privacy. As the encryption is consistent across all datasets, the encrypted identification numbers remain unique, which makes it feasible to conduct longitudinal follow-up investigations. Prior to commencement, this study was approved by the institutional review board and ethics committee of Buddhist Dalin Tzu Chi Hospital and conducted in accordance with the declaration of Helsinki (No. B11002011).

Herein, we recruited patients aged 20–70 years old who were seen both in outpatient and inpatient settings, diagnosed by the International Classification of Diseases, Ninth Revision, Clinical Modification (ICD-9-CM) with a category of 714.0, from January 2012 to December 2017. The date when each RA patient received the relevant treatments in the target hospital was deemed the index date. In order to improve the accuracy of the RA diagnosis, we only selected RA patients who received treatments from rheumatologists. A total of 6518 RA patients were initially identified for the study. The patients' relevant disease activity must be evaluated at baseline by their treating rheumatologist and rheumatology nurse and monitored at least every three months thereafter. We excluded persons who did not complete scheduled laboratory tests, or who were followed for less than one year and had incomplete data (n = 2013). A total of 4505 RA subjects were included in the final analysis.

2.2. Exposure of Rehabilitation Services Usage

Following the abovementioned filtering process, study participants were further linked to the ambulatory care visit claims to identify their pattern of RSs use after the RA episode. We searched for relevant RSs codes, which comprised 42007A, 42010A9, 42010A7, 42004A2, 42010AD, 42010A5, 42004A8, 42004A, 42010A6, 42004A1, 42016C, 42004A9, 42013A, 42001A, 42013A2, 42013A6, 43026C, 42004A5, 43007A8, 43007A4, 43029A, 43011C, 43010C, 43016C, 43017C, 43007A1, 42107A, 43007AA, 42010A, 44010C, 43015C, 43014C, 42013A1, 44007A2, 44007A9, 44007A, 43007A7, 44007AA, 42004A4, 43007A2, 43012C, 43013C, 42010AB, 44007A8, 43007AF, 43004A, 43007AB, 44004A, 42004A3, and 43007A. In Taiwan, all RSs covered by the National Health Insurance (NHI) are provided only by board-certified physical therapists who received rigorous training in medical schools and through relevant accredited hospital programs. Additionally, the guideline by the NHI indicated that six adjunctive treatments, like acupuncture, had to be delivered every week for six weeks in total to each patient, and are, accordingly, defined as one complete RSs treatment [14]. Accordingly, the participants were identified as RSs users if their records included any of the above codes and had at least six sessions within the timeframe after the onset of RA, and the remaining cases were classified as non-RSs users.

2.3. Measurement of Primary Outcomes

Primary outcomes in this work focus on the changes in CRP and ESR. For CRP, the hospital used an automated latex particle-enhanced immunoturbidimetric assay to calculate the CRP level in serum or plasma (Beckman Coulter DxC 700 AU analyzers, Brea, CA, USA). As for ESR, it was measured with quantitative capillary photometry (Sysmex, ESR Analyzer Alifax Test 1, Kobe, Japan). Because the two inflammatory indicators must be regularly monitored for RA patients, we were able to retrieve these records from the EMRD at the following times: baseline (T0), 12 (T1), 18 (T2), 24 (T3), 30 (T4), and 36 (T5) months after the index date (Figure 1).

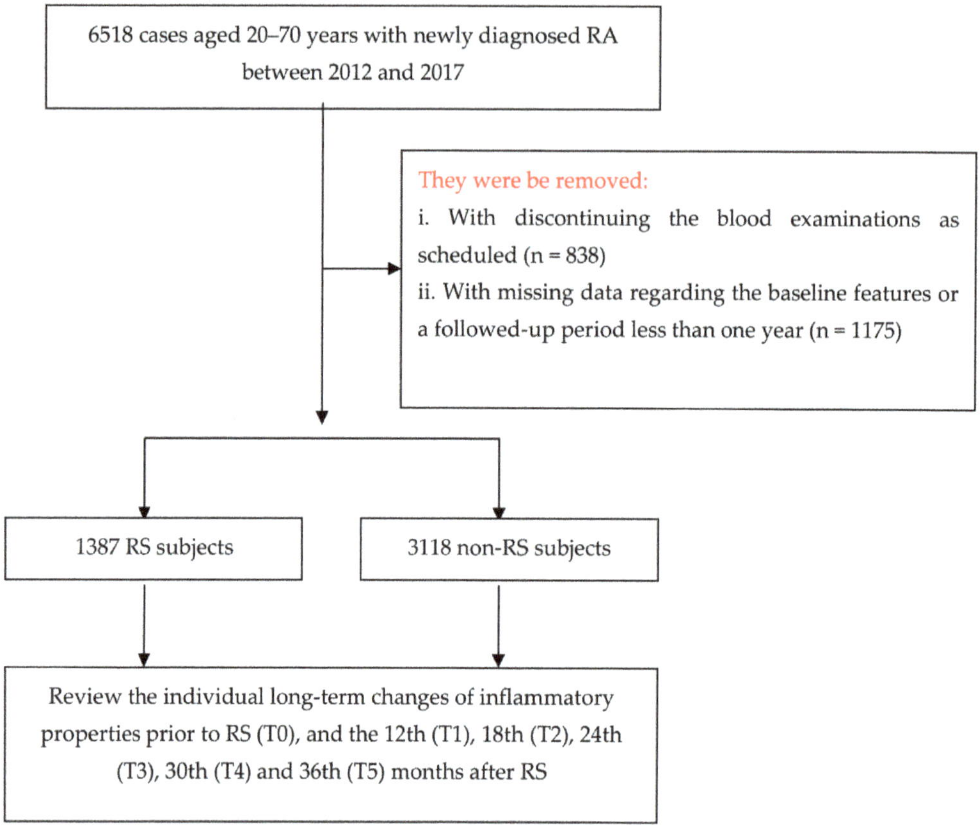

Figure 1. Flowchart showing the method of selecting and following study subjects. RSs, rehabilitation services; RA, rheumatoid arthritis.

2.4. Covariates

Covariates considered for the study included gender, age, height, body weight, and smoking status [15]. Subjects who reported "currently" or "yes/past" to smoking were classified as users. Comorbid medical conditions for each individual was assessed using the established Charlson–Deyo comorbidity index (CCI) [16]. The CCI contains 17 chronic diseases, with a score between 1 and 6 points, and the sum of these scores is regarded as a measure of comorbidity burden. The comorbidities identified for the CCI included myocardial infarction, congestive heart failure, peripheral vascular disease, cerebrovascular disease, dementia, chronic pulmonary disease, rheumatological disease, peptic ulcer disease, mild liver disease, moderate or severe liver disease, diabetes mellitus (DM), DM with chronic complications, renal diseases, any malignancy, metastatic solid tumor, and HIV infection. To avoid double counting and possible over-adjustment in a regression equation, the diagnosis of RA was excluded from the CCI score in this work. Additionally, medication use was separated into two groups based on whether the patient ever took corticosteroids or disease-modifying anti-rheumatic drugs for more than 6 months after the index date.

2.5. Statistical Modeling

We used SAS 9.3 (SAS Institute, Cary, NC, USA) to link the data, and SPSS 22.0 (Chicago, IL, USA) to perform all statistical tests. At the beginning of the analysis, we employed descriptive statistics, including the mean, standard deviation (SD), and percentage, to describe the distributions for participants. Then, the distributions of baseline characteristics for both RSs users and non-RSs users were compared using the Student's t-test and $\div^2$ test, as applicable. Additionally, intergroup differences before and after RSs involvement, for each of the outcomes, were studied using the generalized estimating equation (GEE) model, which is a statistical procedure that extends the capabilities of generalized linear models for analyzing longitudinal data or other clustered response data [17]. Each GEE model produces estimates in terms of the main effect of time (baseline as the reference category), intervention effect (control group as the reference category), and the effect of one interaction term between the intervention and time after covariate adjustment [18]. The changes in intervention effects over time can then be confirmed from the interaction term providing it was pronounced. Covariates in which the difference reached statistical significance at baseline were regarded as the control variables while using the multivariate GEE model [19]. Robust standard errors were selected to calculate the significance of parameter estimates, and the autoregressive first-order working correlation matrix was utilized to adjust for the time effect [18].

Meanwhile, we also conducted one sensitivity analysis to verify the exposure–response impact of RSs. In this sensitivity analysis, we included the values of ESR and CRP at T0 and T1, and further examined the amplitude of change after separating the use patterns of RSs that occurred within the first year after RA onset, according to their placement in either above or below the 50th percentile of the frequency of RSs use. All statistical significance levels were determined at a two-tailed significance level of less than 0.05.

3. Results

3.1. Baseline Characteristics for All Participants

Demographic and clinical characteristics of the study sample are given in Table 1. During the study period, a total of 4505 RA patients were recruited, consisting of 1387 in the RSs group and 3118 in the non-RSs group. The mean age of enrollees was 54.2 years. Over half of the enrollees were female and nonsmokers. Significant differences were detected in age, cigarette smoking, weight, and baseline CCI scores between the two groups (all $p \leq 0.05$).

Table 1. Demographic and clinical characteristics of study participants by group.

Variables	All Enrollees (*n* = 4505)		RSs Group (*n* = 1387)		Non-RSs Group (*n* = 3118)		*p*
	N	%	N	%	N	%	
Demographic data							
Sex							<0.01
Female	3443	76.4	1109	80.0	2334	74.9	
Male	1062	23.6	278	20.0	784	25.1	
Cigarette smoking							0.001
Yes	63	1.4	31	2.2	32	1.0	
NO	4442	98.6	1356	97.8	3086	99.0	
Age (mean ± SD)	54.2 ± 13.1		56.2 ± 12.7		53.25 ± 13.1		<0.01
Height	156.6 ± 7.4		156.9 ± 7.6		156.3 ± 7.3		0.65
Weight	59.9 ± 10.9		62.7 ± 11.3		57.6 ± 10.0		0.01
Clinical characteristics							
Medication use							0.06
Yes	3090	68.6	923	66.5	2167	69.5	
No	1415	31.4	464	33.5	951	30.5	
CCI (mean ± SD)	2.56 ± 1.32		3.17 ± 1.34		2.29 ± 1.30		<0.01
Baseline CRP (mean ± SD)	1.14 ± 2.91		1.63 ± 3.38		0.92 ± 2.13		<0.01
Baseline ESP (mean ± SD)	20.37 ± 11.42		21.46 ± 14.10		19.86 ± 10.02		0.03

SD, standard deviation; CCI, Charlson–Deyo comorbidity index; CRP, C-reactive protein; ESR, erythrocyte sedimentation rate; RSs, rehabilitation services.

3.2. Comparisons of Levels of CRP and ESR in the RSs Groups Versus Non-RSs Groups

After adjusting for the variables found to be significant in the univariate analysis, including age, cigarette smoking, weight, and baseline CCI scores, the multivariate analysis with the GEE procedure revealed a baseline difference in the CRP score between the RSs and the non-RSs groups ($p < 0.01$) (Table 2). Meanwhile, CRP levels at T1, T2, T3, T4, and T5 were similar to those measured at T0, implying a nonsignificant maturation effect across follow-up times. After considering the baseline differences of CRP between two groups using the multivariate GEE model, we noted that the reduction slope in the CRP level was still larger in the RSs group compared to the non-RSs group, regardless of the time assessed, with T1, T2, T3, and T4, yielding $\hat{a} = -0.77$ (T1), $\hat{a} = -1.25$ (T2), $\hat{a} = -2.13$ (T3), $\hat{a} = -3.44$ (T4), and $\hat{a} = -3.93$ (T5), respectively (Table 2 and Figure 2).

Table 2. Effects of RSs on inflammation level in the participants by GEE model.

Variables	CRP		ESR	
	Regression Coefficient +	p	Regression Coefficient +	p
Intercept	0.79	<0.01	9.80	<0.01
RSs vs. non-RSs	0.73	<0.01	1.56	0.04
T1 vs. T0	−0.15	0.07	−4.0	<0.01
T2 vs. T0	−0.09	0.10	−3.83	0.02
T3 vs. T0	0.24	0.22	−1.39	0.14
T4 vs. T0	0.85	0.09	−0.89	0.49
T5 vs. T0	1.08	0.06	−0.41	0.16
Interaction of T1×Group	−0.22	0.04	1.81	0.22
Interaction of T2×Group	−1.06	0.01	1.09	0.18
Interaction of T3×Group	−2.13	<0.01	0.27	0.14
Interaction of T4×Group	−3.02	<0.01	−0.11	0.08
Interaction of T5×Group	−2.72	<0.01	−0.20	0.07

RSs, rehabilitation services; T0, date of first diagnosis of RA; T1, 12 months after RA onset; T2, 18 months after RA onset. T3, 24 months after RA onset. T4, 30 months after RA onset. T5, 36 months after RA onset. RSs vs. non-RSs represents the baseline difference between two groups. T1 vs. T0, change between T0 and T1; T2 vs. T0, change between T0 and T2; T3 vs. T0, change between T0 and T3; T4 vs. T0, change between T0 and T4; T5 vs. T0, change between T0 and T5. Interaction of T1×Group, difference between RSs and non-RSs groups within the period of T0–T1; Interaction of T2×Group, difference between RSs and non-RSs groups within the period of T0–T2; Interaction of T3×Group, difference between RSs and non-RSs groups within the period of T0–T3; Interaction of T4×Group, difference between RSs and non-RSs groups within the period of T0–T4; and Interaction of T5×Group, difference between RSs and non-RSs groups within the period of T0–T5. + adjustment for age, cigarette smoking, weight, and baseline CCI scores.

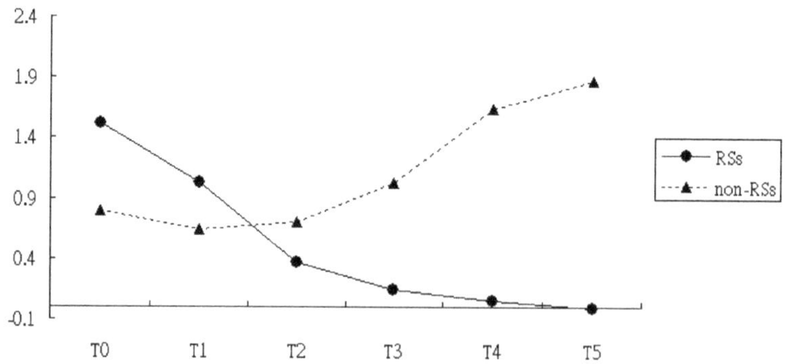

Figure 2. CRP measure over time among patients with and without RSs use. T0, date of first diagnosis of RA; T1, 12 months after RA onset; T2, 18 months after RA onset. T3, 24 months after RA onset; T4, 30 months after RA onset; and T5, 36 months after RA onset.

For ESR, the GEE model reported that a baseline difference existed between the group treated with RSs and the nontreated group, supporting estimates calculated from the Student's t-test. On top of that, the ESR levels at T1 and T2 were remarkably different from those at T0, implying a maturation effect might have emerged. In other words, the mean ESR level at T1 and T2 was significantly lower than the mean ESR at T0, even without the RSs intervention. After corrections for baseline differences along with the maturation effect, we found that the reduction in ESR was larger in the RSs group than the non-RSs group during the study timeframe, although the difference did not reach statistical significance (Table 2 and Figure 3).

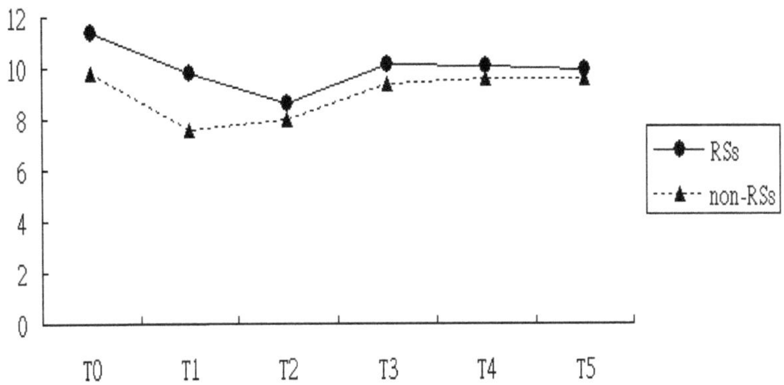

Figure 3. ESR measure over time among patients with and without RSs use. T0, date of first diagnosis of RA; T1, 12 months after RA onset; T2, 18 months after RA onset; T3, 24 months after RA onset; T4, 30 months after RA onset; and T5, 36 months after RA onset.

After carrying out a sensitivity analysis, where only the values of ESR and CRP at T0 and T1 among subjects were used, it was revealed that RSs use intensity was inversely correlated with CRP level, but not for ESR (Table 3). In a nutshell, for RA subjects, the more frequent usage of RSs was associated with a lower the CRP level after RA onset.

Table 3. Sensitivity analysis regarding the effect of RSs on inflammation properties by different usage pattern.

RSs Usage Pattern	CRP		ESR	
	Regression Coefficient	p	Regression Coefficient	p
Non-RSs group	1		1	
RSs group	−0.54	<0.01	1.33	0.52
Low intensity	−0.37	0.003	1.74	0.29
High intensity	−0.69	<0.01	1.26	0.08

CRP, C-reactive protein; ESR, erythrocyte sedimentation rate; RSs, rehabilitation services.

4. Discussion

RSs use has long been a frequently employed complementary approach for the management of RA. Despite this, our current understanding of the relationships between RSs application and changes in inflammatory indicators is still lacking, and previous studies have either used small samples or have been cross-sectional in nature [9,10]. To our knowledge, this is the first study to directly examine the relationships between RSs use and the subsequent changes in inflammatory properties among RA persons. Over the 3-year follow-up period, we noted that the integration of RSs to standard care did ameliorate inflammation in RA patients, especially as measured by CRP levels. The merit of this study is that we capitalized on empirical research using follow-up measures, which allowed us to deliberately clarify the potential causal relationship [20]. This provides for robust and empirically informed guidance for healthcare providers while managing RA patients.

After fitting the GEE multivariate model on the basis of the first-order autoregressive procedure, we found that integrating RSs into routine care substantially reduced CRP levels, supporting previous research, which found that receiving 3-month hydrotherapy sessions in addition to conventional treatment substantially reduced levels of reactive oxygen species among RA patients [10]. We speculated that direct participation in the relevant RSs programs may simultaneously provide intangible benefits as well, such as allowing patients to socialize and share joyous moments during RSs sessions, which in turn may reduce stress, and consequently decrease the expression of serum inflammatory mediators like IL-6, IL-1, and tumor necrosis factor-á [11,21]. In a prior murine model with collagen-induced arthritis, the authors observed that the rats, which were placed on a treadmill to exercise for 15 min per day for three weeks, had markedly reduced levels of inflammatory factors, thus improving the inflammation-related joint damage via the suppression of NFATc1and NF-êB luciferase activities [12]. It is well known that inflammatory markers are deeply involved in the production of CRP in hepatocytes [6,7]. Since downregulated NF-êB expression has been implicated in various inflammatory diseases [7,22], instituting several novel RSs approaches targeting this intracellular pathway may be considered, especially in the management of patients with rheumatic diseases.

Unlike the positive impact of RSs on CRP, our findings indicated a recognizable, yet not statistically significant, decrease in the ESR in the RSs group. In clinical practice, these two acute phase reactants are frequently used as markers for clinical signs and symptoms of inflammation. We speculate that the ESR measure is more likely to be influenced by the concentrations of fibrinogen and alpha globulins [23]. Fibrinogen is a fibrous protein known to be a slow-reacting positive acute phase reactant [24]. Therefore, ESR is relatively insensitive to the inflammatory process, especially for patients with systemic rheumatic diseases and those with concomitant renal insufficiency, low albumin, and anemia [25,26]. Thus, of studies conducted thus far, CRP has been acknowledged to be a better indicator of the acute inflammation phase, and has yielded a sensitivity of 0.86, specificity of 0.67, and summary receiver operating characteristic curve (SROC) of 0.86, as compared with a sensitivity of 0.77, specificity of 0.59, and SROC of 0.75 for ESR [27]. This, in a nutshell, is the reason that a nonsignificant ESR reduction was observed for the RSs group.

Limitations

The GEE approach, an enlargement of the generalized linear model approach, can model the correlated data via the introduction of second-order variance components. To our knowledge, this was the first evidence-based longitudinal study to explore the association between RSs use and changes in CRP and ESR among RA patients after fitting the GEE procedure, thereby allowing us to clarify the magnitude of RSs effect. While considerable efforts were made in the design of this study, there were several drawbacks related to the sample selection process, ability to generalize findings, and research design. First and foremost, patients from a single center were enrolled; therefore, our results may not generalize to groups with different demographic and geographic features. Additional research focusing on more targets should be considered in heterogeneous populations to confirm the replicability of present findings. Second, since all analytical data were extracted from a claims-based database, several key factors, such as lifestyle behaviors, family history, and biochemical data, were not available. To minimize the effect of confounding during the statistical analysis, we set objective criteria to balance differences between groups treated or not treated with RSs via assessments of demographic and disease variables, as shown in Table 1. In addition to utilizing multivariate analysis to control for inherent baseline differences between patients, we further considered the potential maturation effect via the GEE procedure, thus minimizing the probability of an inflated type I error [18]. Third, the related RSs received during treatment were integrated in one consolidated column of the database. In such a case, we merely abstracted the corresponding fees from this to ascertain the RSs exposure and were unable to clarify the specific RSs type. Future works, through the applications of various recruitment methods in ethnically diverse populations, are recommended. Fourth, although our study revealed a substantial beneficial association between RSs use and a decreased CRP level among RA patients, it must be recognized that participants were not initially randomly categorized into users and nonusers and were recruited from a single country only. Even so, preceding the RSs intervention, we observed that RSs subjects possessed higher levels of CCI, CRP, and ESR than did non-RSs users at the index date (Table 1), which implies that the conclusions reported would underestimate, rather than overestimate, the effects of RSs. That being said, a study adopting a larger cohort of RA patients using a randomized clinical trial design is still needed to minimize confounding by covariates not explicitly accounted for in the present design.

5. Conclusions

Faced with the dire harmful manifestations caused by inflammation, it is of importance to extend the horizons of traditional therapy procedures and explore the role of RSs in alleviating inflammation among RA patients. The findings of the present study suggest that integrating RSs into standard care may partially lower the subsequent systemic inflammation response, especially in CRP levels. This benefit is sustained over a 3-year follow-up period. Our findings support the integration of RSs into routine disease management for those with rheumatological disorders. This study not only bridges the chasm regarding the long-term assessment of RSs usage to changes in inflammatory parameters, but also provides an impetus for further in vivo research that focuses on the exploration of the beneficial mechanisms of RSs in the treatment of chronic diseases. Therefore, we recommend that healthcare providers proactively assess patients' inflammatory status and implement this novel and safe regimen in managing RA.

Author Contributions: Conceptualization, H.-J.H. and T.-Y.T.; methodology, W.-J.C., H.L. and H.-L.H.; software, T.-Y.T.; validation, W.-J.C. and H.L.; formal analysis, M.-C.L. and T.-Y.T.; investigation, H.-J.H., W.-J.C., H.-L.H. and T.-Y.T.; resources, M.-C.L.; writing—original draft, H.-J.H., W.-J.C., H.L., M.-C.L. and T.-Y.T. All authors have read and agreed to the published version of the manuscript.

Funding: This research received no funding.

Institutional Review Board Statement: The study was approved by the Institutional Review Board and ethics committee of Buddhist Dalin Tzu Chi Hospital (Approval code: No. B11002011 Approval date: 21 June 2021).

Informed Consent Statement: The study was approved by the facility's institutional review board to be exempt from the requirement for written informed consent and conducted in accordance with the Declaration of Helsinki.

Data Availability Statement: The data presented in this study are available on request from the corresponding author.

Acknowledgments: This study was supported by Grant DTCRD112(2)-I-27 from the Buddhist Dalin Tzu Chi Hospital.

Conflicts of Interest: The authors declare no conflicts of interest.

References

1. Kirkeskov, L.; Bray, K. Employment of patients with rheumatoid arthritis—A systematic review and meta-analysis. *BMC Rheumatol.* **2023**, *7*, 41. [CrossRef] [PubMed]
2. Sokka, T. Work disability in early rheumatoid arthritis *Clin. Exp. Rheumatol.* **2003**, *21*, S71–S74.
3. Chen, C.I.; Wang, L.; Wei, W.; Yuce, H.; Phillips, K. Burden of rheumatoid arthritis among US medicare population: Co-morbidities, health-care resource utilization and costs. *Rheumatol. Adv. Pract.* **2018**, *2*, I1–I9. [CrossRef] [PubMed]
4. Burska, A.; Boissinot, M.; Ponchel, F. Cytokines as biomarkers in rheumatoid arthritis. *Mediat. Inflamm.* **2014**, *2014*, 545493. [CrossRef]

[20] Rheumatology Unit, ASL VC Sant'Andrea Hospital, 13100 Vercelli, Italy; rosetta.vitetta@aslvc.piemonte.it (R.V.); alessia.fiorenza@aslvc.piemonte.it (A.F.); guido.rovera.gr@gmail.com (G.R.)
[21] Rheumatology Unit, IRCCS Sacro Cuore Don Calabria Hospital, 37024 Negrar di Valpolicella, Italy; avolpe127@gmail.com (A.V.); antonio.marchetta@sacrocuore.it (A.M.)
[22] Internal Medicine and Rheumatology Unit, ASL Romagna—Rimini, 47924 Rimini, Italy; mariacristina.focherini@auslromagna.it (M.C.F.); fabio.mascella@auslromagna.it (F.M.)
[23] Rheumatology Unit, G.B. Morgagni—L. Pierantoni Hospital, 47121 Forli, Italy; francesco.girelli@auslromagna.it (F.G.); siiberna@yahoo.it (S.B.)
[24] Rheumatology Unit, Division of Internal Medicine, A.O. Papardo, 98158 Messina, Italy; aldomolica@alice.it
[25] Rheumatology Department, Azienda Ospedaliero-Universitaria Città della Salute e della Scienza di Torino, 10126 Torino, Italy; fusaro.reumatorino@gmail.com (E.F.); mariachiaraditto@gmail.com (M.C.D.); simone.parisi@hotmail.it (S.P.)
[26] Rheumatology Unit, University of Modena and Reggio Emilia, 41125 Modena, Italy; gilda.sandri@unimore.it (G.S.); dilia.giuggioli@unimore.it (D.G.); carlo.salvarani@unimore.it (C.S.)
[27] Medical Oncology Unit, A.O. Papardo, 98158 Messina, Italy; verifra82@yahoo.it
[28] Internal Medicine Unit, Milano-Bicocca University, 20126 Milano, Italy; francesco.molica3@gmail.com
[29] Unit of Diagnostic and Interventional Radiology, Santa Corona Hospital, 17027 Pietra Ligure, Italy; giulio.ferrero@gmail.com
* Correspondence: cellettieleonora@gmail.com

Abstract: *Background and Objectives:* The treatment landscape for Rheumatoid Arthritis (RA) has evolved significantly with the introduction of Janus kinase inhibitors (JAKi), such as Tofacitinib (TOFA), which offer a new therapeutic option for patients who have failed or are intolerant to conventional synthetic disease-modifying antirheumatic drugs (csDMARDs). Safety concerns, particularly related to cardiovascular and cancer risks, prompted a need for additional investigation in real-world clinical settings. This study aimed to evaluate the long-term effectiveness and predictors of response to TOFA in two subpopulations of RA patients, categorized by differing cardiovascular risk profiles. *Materials and Methods:* This was a retrospective, multicenter observational study conducted as part of the BIRRA project, involving 23 Italian rheumatological referral centers. A total of 213 patients diagnosed with RA and treated with TOFA were included, with data collected on baseline demographics, clinical history, disease activity, and comorbidities. Patients were divided into high-risk and low-risk cardiovascular groups based on age ($\geq$65 years) and the presence of at least one cardiovascular risk factor. Disease activity was assessed at baseline, 6 months, and 12 months using DAS28-ESR and DAS28-CRP. Treatment response was evaluated using intention-to-treat (ITT) and per-protocol (PP) approaches. Predictors of low disease activity (LDA) and remission were assessed through logistic regression, and clustering analyses were used to identify subgroups of patients with different therapeutic responses. *Results:* The study included 213 patients, with 129 classified as high-risk. For the overall cohort, patients achieving LDA and remission at 6 months were 20% and 12%, respectively, for the ITT analysis, and 29% and 14% for the PP analysis. At 12 months, 26% of patients reached LDA, and 17% achieved remission according to ITT, while for the PP analysis, these rates were 30% and 19%, respectively. No significant differences in remission or LDA rates were observed between the high-risk and low-risk groups. In the high-risk subgroup, 17% of patients reached LDA and 9% achieved remission at 6 months (ITT analysis), while these rates increased to 22% and 13%, respectively, in the PP analysis. At 12 months, 22% achieved LDA and 13% achieved remission in the ITT analysis, while 28% and 17% did so in the PP analysis. The reduction in DAS28-ESR and DAS28-CRP scores was significant ($p < 0.001$) across all time points for both high-risk and low-risk patients. Logistic regression analyses revealed that none of the baseline characteristics—including age, sex, comorbidities, rheumatoid factor, anti-citrullinated protein antibody (ACPA) positivity, initial disease severity, or treatment history—were significant predictors of remission or LDA at 6 or 12 months. The clustering analysis suggested that older patients, particularly those with worse baseline DAS28 scores, tended to show a less favorable response to treatment, potentially indicating impacts of age-related factors such as immunosenescence on therapeutic outcomes. *Conclusions:* Tofacitinib demonstrated similar effectiveness in both high- and low-risk cardiovascular subgroups of RA patients, with significant reductions in disease activity observed at both 6 and 12 months. Despite safety concerns related to cardiovascular risk, TOFA remained an effective treatment option across patient subgroups, with no significant differences in remission or LDA rates based on cardiovascular risk profiles. Age appeared to negatively impact treatment response, highlighting the role of immunosenescence in RA management. These findings support the use of TOFA as a personalized therapeutic option for RA, emphasizing the need for careful evaluation of cardiovascular and age-related risks in clinical decision-making.

Keywords: rheumatoid arthritis; tofacitinib; cardiovascular risk

1. Introduction

Rheumatoid arthritis (RA) is a chronic disease that belongs to the group of adult chronic inflammatory rheumatisms that lead to a progressive disability. If left untreated, rheumatoid arthritis can cause joint erosions and deformities that can lead to severe disability. In addition, extra-articular manifestations of RA, such as interstitial lung disease, vasculitis, and lymphoma, can be very serious and even life-threatening. In 2019, 18 million people worldwide were living with rheumatoid arthritis. About 70% of people living with rheumatoid arthritis are women, and 55% are older than 55 years [1]. Treatment options available today for RA have been greatly increased compared to the first class of conventional synthetic disease-modifying antirheumatic drugs (csDMARDs). Therefore, aiming for remission with the 'treat-to-target' attitude has become realistically more achievable at the present time. The most recent therapeutic option landed in clinical practice to patients with RA are oral small-molecule Janus kinase inhibitors (JAKi). Tofacitinib (TOFA) was the first JAKi to be approved in 2012 by the US Food and Drug Administration (FDA) and in 2017 by the European Medicines Agency (EMA) for the treatment, with or without methotrexate (MTX), of moderate to severe active RA in adult patients who have inadequately responded to or cannot tolerate one or more csDMARDs [1].

TOFA, inhibiting several JAK subtypes, especially JAK3 and JAK1, acts on synovial JAK/STAT targets through JAK-mediated IFN and IL-6 signaling pathways, thus blocking the role of JAK in synovial responses from playing a therapeutic role in RA [2,3].

Both the European Alliance of Associations for Rheumatology (EULAR) and the American College of Rheumatology (ACR) recommend JAKi as a second- and third-line treatment for RA [4,5]. Randomized controlled trials (RCTs) involving JAKi for the treatment of RA patients have demonstrated favorable outcomes [6]. In a series of phase II and phase III RCTs, the efficacy of TOFA has been extensively evaluated, demonstrating the efficacy profile of these small-molecule oral agents, prescribed either as monotherapy or in combination with MTX or other csDMARDs [7,8].

After the FDA approval of TOFA, concerns over a potential increased risk of serious infections, cardiovascular events, and cancers were raised. This finding prompted the FDA to require a post-marketing head-to-head safety trial [9] comparing the risk of major adverse cardiovascular events and cancers in patients with RA between TOFA 5 and 10 mg twice a day, and a tumor necrosis factor inhibitor (TNFi) among adalimumab or etanercept. Patient inclusion criteria were age $\geq$ 50 years and a medical history with at least one cardiovascular risk factor [9,10] from the ORAL Surveillance study, which in 2021 caused the FDA to require boxed warnings for TOFA to include risk information on serious heart-related events, cancer, blood clots, and death [3]. This study identified a high-risk and low-risk tofacitinib population with different relative risk vs TNFi. In 2023, the study results caused restrictions by EMA on the use of most oral JAKis by specific patient populations [11]. Thus, a posthoc analysis of ORAL Surveillance [10] allowed two subgroups of patients to be identified: a high-risk population, including patients aged $\geq$ 65 years and with at least one cardiovascular risk; and a low-risk population, including patients younger than 65 without any risk of major adverse cardiovascular events.

Today, due to all these evolutions in the history of this drug, extensive observational research on JAKi in RA is expanding, with particular attention to real-world clinical settings [12–15]. The aim of the present study is to evaluate the effectiveness and the predictors of clinical response in a large multicenter observational retrospective cohort of patients with RA, treated with Tofacitinib, considering the two different subpopulations, with different relative cardiovascular risks. Thus, data concerning the efficacy of this drug, extrapolated considering the two easily identifiable and clinically practical populations, can further improve the individualized benefit/risk assessment and clinical decision making regarding the treatment with TOFA.

2. Materials and Methods

2.1. Patients

As a part of the BIRRA (BIologics Retention Rate Assessment) project, this retrospective study was designed to evaluate the effectiveness of TOFA in RA patients. The study was performed according to the Declaration of Helsinki principles, and it was approved by the local ethics committees. Patients with confirmed diagnosis of RA who received TOFA were enrolled from 23 Italian rheumatological referral centers. The enrollment period extended from April 2019 to April 2023 with a maximum observation period of one year. Clinical history, treatment history and RA disease activity at baseline were recorded. For each patient, the following baseline data were recorded: general characteristics (age, sex, body mass index—BMI), smoking habit, disease duration, positivity for rheumatoid factor—RF, anti-citrullinated protein antibody -ACPA positivity, swollen and tender joint count—SJC and TJC, ESR, CRP, patient Visual Analogue Scale, disease activity, line of treatment, concomitant csDMARD use, concomitant steroids use, steroids dose (PDN-Eq), prior bDMARD use, prior tsDMARD use, and concomitant relevant disease. Disease activity was assessed in all patients by calculating both the DAS28-ESR and DAS28-CRP. Relevant comorbidities considered included diabetes, dyslipidemia, history of major adverse cardiovascular events (MACE), cancer, and arterial hypertension.

2.2. Statistical Analysis

Descriptive statistics of clinical and laboratory demographic characteristics were provided as medians with interquartile range (IQR) or percentage. Response to TOFA was assessed with an "intention to treat" (ITT) and "per protocol" (PP) analysis. The use of ITT and PP analyses in this study on the treatment of RA patients with TOFA is valuable for providing a comprehensive and accurate assessment of treatment efficacy. The ITT analysis includes all patients originally enrolled in the study, regardless of whether they completed the treatment or strictly adhered to the study protocol. This approach reflects the effectiveness of the treatment in real-world clinical practice, where some patients may discontinue or modify their treatment. In contrast, the PP analysis considers only those patients who completed the treatment as per the planned protocol, offering an estimate of the maximum efficacy of the treatment under ideal conditions. Using both analyses allows for an evaluation of both the real-world impact of the drug on the general population and its potential efficacy in patients with optimal adherence to the treatment.

DAS28-ESR/DAS28-CRP values at baseline, after 6 and 12 months of treatment were compared by Wilcoxon's test and for paired nonparametric variables.

Logistic regressions tested which of the following factors were associated with achieving remission and/or LDA at 6 months and 12 months: age, sex, body mass index, smoking habit, duration of disease, presence of RF and/or ACPA, line of treatment, concomitant treatment with both steroids and csDMARDs, and DAS28-ESR/DAS28-CRP at baseline.

We also analyzed a subgroup of patients (high-risk group) who had at least one relevant comorbidity/risk factor among those considered by EMA (Table 1), including diabetes, dyslipidemia, hypertension, history or family history of coronary heart disease, history of venous thromboembolism, or history of cancer. The study was designed to focus on the extrapolation of data related to the high-cardiovascular-risk population, defined by the presence of at least one cardiovascular risk factor or age $\geq$ 65 years. While data from the overall group were used as a broader reference context, the primary aim was to specifically evaluate the characteristics and therapeutic response of this subgroup, without direct comparison to the low-risk population.

Table 1. Risks of major adverse cardiovascular events considered by EMA's Pharmacovigilance Risk Assessment Committee (PRAC) [11].

- Aged 65 years or older
- Long-term smokers or former smokers
- History of hypertension
- History of coronary heart disease
- Family history of coronary heart disease
- Dyslipidemia
- History of diabetes mellitus
- History of venous thromboembolism
- History of cancer

We used logistic regression to identify predictor variables of low disease activity and/or remission and clustering analysis to identify potential subgroups of patients with characteristics that influence therapeutic response.

All tests performed were two-tailed, and the significance level was set at 0.05 (with a 95% confidence interval).

3. Results

A total of 213 patients were included in the study. Their baseline characteristics are shown in Table 2.

Table 2. Baseline characteristics split between the overall patient population and high-risk patients.

Characteristics		Overall Group	High-Risk Group
N		213	129
M:F n (%)		39 (18.3):174 (81.7)	12 (9.3):117 (90.7)
Age, median [IQR] yrs		60 [51–82] *	72 [61–86] *
Smokers, n (%)	Yes	42 (19.7)	23 (17.8)
	Former	44 (20.6)	22 (17.1)
	No	127 (66.3)	84 (65.1)
Body mass index, median [IQR] kg/m^2		24.8 [22.0–42.7]	24.3 [21.0–39.7]
Disease duration, median [IQR], months		123 [78–532]	158 [82–402]
RF positivity, n (%)		140 (65.7)	81 (62.7)
ACPA positivity, n (%)		131 (61.5)	80 (62)
SJC, median [IQR]		6 [4–26]	5 [4–27]
TJC, median [IQR]		4 [2–22]	4 [2–24]
ESR, median [IQR], mm/h		32 [19.5–98]	36 [21–75]
CRP, median [IQR], mg/dL		1.4 [0.5–19]	1.9 [0.6–20]
VAS patient (0–100), median [IQR]		70 [50–100]	65 [45–100]
DAS28 (ESR), median [IQR]		5.3 [4.2–7.0]	5.6 [2.8–7.2]
DAS28 (CRP), median [IQR]		5.3 [3.6–6.6] *	5.0 [2.3–6.9] *
Line of treatment, [IQR]		2 [1–9]	2 [1–8]

Table 2. *Cont.*

Characteristics		Overall Group	High-Risk Group
Concomitant csDMARD use, n (%)	MTX	54 (25.3)	12 (19.4)
	LFN	4 (1.9)	3 (4.8)
	SSZ	2 (0.9)	0 (0.9)
	HCQ	10 (4.7)	3 (4.8)
Concomitant steroids use, n (%)		104 (48.8)	56 (43.4)
Steroids dose (PDN-Eq), median, mg/die		4 [5–25]	4 [5–25]
Prior bDMARD use, n (%)	TNFi	110 (50.2)	63 (48.9)
	IL6i	50 (23.5)	31 (24.0)
	IL1i	3 (1.4)	1 (0.8)
	CD20i	16 (7.5)	11 (8.5)
	CD80i	34 (16.0)	23 (17.8)
Prior tsDMARD use, n (%)		60 (28.2)	46 (35.6)
JAKi-naive, n (%)		58 (27.2)	16 (12.4)
Concomitant relevant disease, n (%)	Diabetes	12 (5.6)	6 (9.7)
	Hypercholesterolemia	39 (18.3)	16 (25.8)
	MACE	9 (4.2)	6 (9.7)
	Arterial hypertension	61 (28.6)	19 (30.6)
	Cancer	11 (5.1)	3 (4.8)

RF, rheumatoid factor; ACPA, anti-citrullinated protein antibodies; SJC, swollen joints count; TJC, tender joints count; ESR, erythrocyte sedimentation rate; CRP, C-reactive protein, VAS, visual analogic scale; DAS28, disease activity score 28; csDMARD, conventional synthetic modified antirheumatic drugs; PDN-Eq, prednisone equivalent; bDMARD, biological modified antirheumatic drugs; tsDMARD, targeted synthetic modified antirheumatic drugs; TNFi, TNF inhibitors; IL-6i, IL-6 inhibitors; IL-1i, IL-1 inhibitors; CD20i, CD20 inhibitors; CD80i, CD80inhibitors; MACE, major adverse cardiovascular events. * significant difference.

Patients in LDA and in remission at 6 months were 20% and 12%, respectively, for the ITT analysis and 29% and 14%, respectively, for the PP analysis (Figure 1). Patients with LDA and in remission at 12 months were 26% and 17%, respectively, for the ITT analysis and 30% and 19%, respectively, for the PP analysis (Figure 1). There was no significant difference between the two analysis groups.

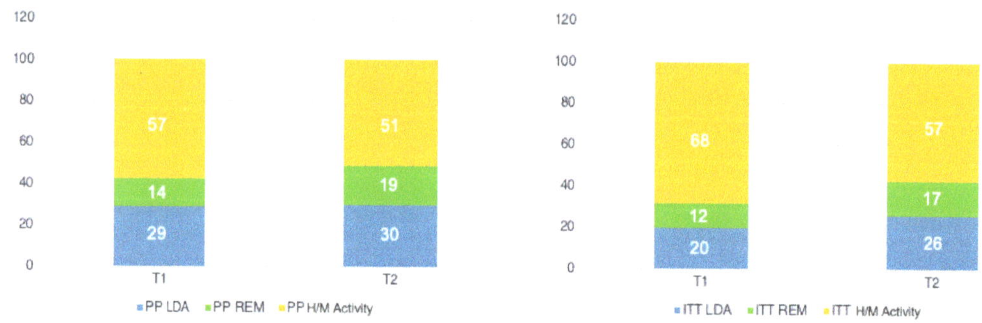

Figure 1. Patients achieving remission (REM), low disease activity (LDA), high/moderate (H/M) disease activity (Percentage) at T1 (6 months) and T2 (12 months). Intention to treat (ITT) and per protocol (PP) analysis.

The analysis of the population considered at risk (129 patients; Table 2) according to the factors highlighted by EMA (Table 1) did not highlight substantial differences compared to overall patients, except for age (p: 0.000) and DAS28CRP (p: 0.000). No significant differences emerged either in terms of remission rate or in LDA.

Patients considered at high risk in LDA and in remission at 6 months were 17% and 9%, respectively, for the ITT analysis and 22% and 13%, respectively, for the PP analysis

(Figure 2). Patients considered at high risk in LDA and in remission at 12 months were 22% and 13%, respectively, for the ITT analysis and 28% and 17%, respectively, for the PP analysis (Figure 3). There was no significant difference between the two analysis groups.

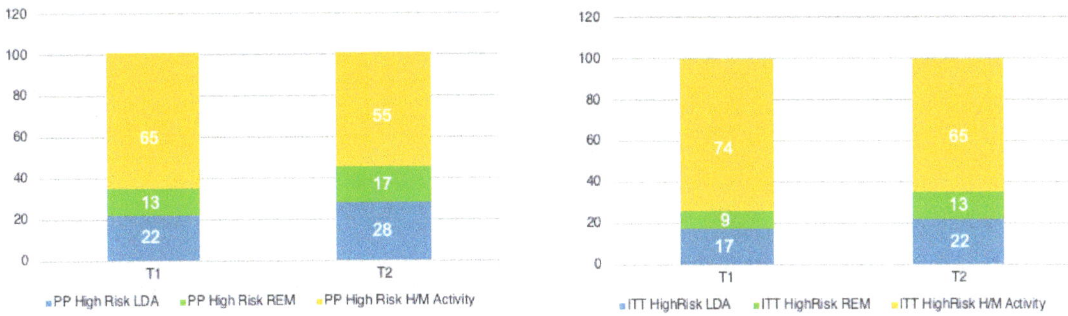

Figure 2. High-risk patients achieving remission (REM), low disease activity (LDA), high/moderate (H/M) disease activity (Percentage) at T1 (6 months) and T2 (12 months). Intention to treat (ITT) and per protocol (PP) analysis.

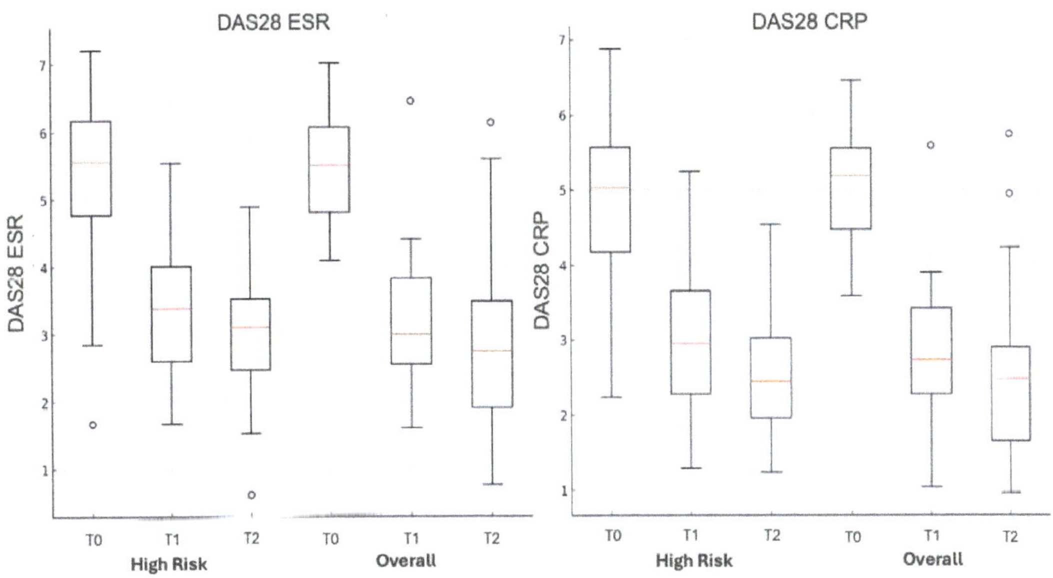

Figure 3. Comparison of the DAS28 ESR and DAS28 CRP trend between a group of high-risk patients (according to EMA) and overall at T0 (baseline), T1 (6 months) and T2 (12 months).

In the overall group, a significant reduction ($p < 0.001$) was observed in DAS28-ESR and DAS28-CRP (DAS28-ESR ΔT0–T1: 2.3; ΔT0–T2: 2.6 and DAS28-CRP ΔT0–T1: 2.5; ΔT0–T2: 2.7) at both time points (T1 and T2) (Figure 3).

Similarly, in the high-risk group, a significant reduction ($p < 0.001$) was observed in DAS28-ESR and DAS28-CRP (DAS28-ESR ΔT0–T1: 1.9; ΔT0–T2: 2.2 and DAS28-CRP ΔT0–T1: 2.1; ΔT0–T2: 2.6) at both time points (T1 and T2) (Figure 3).

Logistic regressions showed no predictors of remission or LDA at 6 months or 12 months. In particular, sex, age, seropositivity, presence of comorbidities, initial ESR and CRP values, line of therapy, association with csDMARDs and/or steroids did not show any significant correlation.

The clustering analysis highlighted the presence of a small group of patients, markedly older, who tend to have a worse DAS28 trend than the remainder of younger patients. In this group of patients, age is the variable that has the greatest impact on the improvement of the DAS28 among the patients in the cluster ($p = 0.023$). The other variables do not show a significant impact. Age is therefore moderately negatively correlated with improvement in DAS28. The results also highlighted that older patients tend to have a longer disease duration, but the data do not correlate with the number of treatment failures ($p > 0.05$). Thus, the duration of the disease does not seem to reflect (or in any case itself alone) a prolonged lack of therapeutic response over time.

However, the presence of multicollinearity and the limited number of observations suggest the need for additional data to obtain more robust results.

4. Discussion

In this study, a significant reduction in disease activity, assessed with DAS28-ESR and DAS28-CRP, was reported both at 6 and 12 months in RA patients after the start of therapy with TOFA.

The analysis of the subpopulation considered at higher risk according to the factors highlighted by EMA did not highlight substantial differences compared to the low-risk population, neither in terms of difference in reaching LDA nor in remission rate according to other data in the literature referring to other JAK inhibitors such as baricitinib [16].

None among the predictor factors assessed in this study (sex, age, seropositivity, presence of comorbidities, initial ESR and CRP values, line of therapy, association with csDMARDs and/or steroids), has shown a correlation with remission or LDA rates at 6 months or 12 months, in any of the two relative-risk subpopulations.

If a careful evaluation of cardiovascular risk is essential with regards to safety of TOFA, this humble study seems to bear witness to how this evaluation may not be equally valid for the evaluation of the effectiveness of the drug, since it resulted in a valid therapeutic option in both risk subgroups of the population examined.

To date, following the increasing attention to cardiovascular risk profiling with JAKi therapy, there are growing studies concerning many different safety aspects of the drugs [17–19].

Not so frequent are studies which, considering the profiling of cardiovascular risk and the clinical division into high- or low-risk subgroups, verify the possible differential rates of effectiveness.

We considered worthy of reflection a result highlighted by the clustering analysis, whereby a small group of patients with a worse DAS28 trend correlates with older age. Contextually, all the other variables do not show a significant impact. The presence of multicollinearity and the limited number of observations do not justify considering this data as having a strong scientific meaning; in any case, these results lead us to some reflections and insights.

Over the last decade, evidence has accumulated that, with progressive age, the immune system and the propensity for abnormal immunity change fundamentally, thus increasing the risk of infection, cancer and immune-mediated tissue damage. Senescence-related changes in innate and adaptive immune responses observed in healthy adults > 50 years of age are found to be anticipated and accelerated in chronic inflammatory conditions [20,21]. RA has been considered a model of premature senescence because, as the disease progresses, there is a higher prevalence of age-related diseases.

Senescent immune cells acquire the "senescence-associated secretory phenotype" which promotes and sustains tissue inflammation and is defective in balancing cytoplasmic kinase and phosphatase activities, changing their activation thresholds, weakening DNA repair and compromising the telomeric maintenance [22,23]. More than just epiphonema, in RA populations, these changes have been implicated in poor disease outcomes: they may contribute to the aggravation of both articular and extra-articular manifestations and may implicate a reduced response to standard treatments [24–26].

This study has some limitations that should be considered when interpreting the results. The retrospective observational design may introduce selection bias and limit the ability to establish direct causal relationships between treatment and outcomes. Data collection from multiple centers could lead to some heterogeneity in patient management. Finally, the relatively limited number of patients may reduce the statistical power of certain analyses, necessitating further prospective studies to confirm and expand upon the observed results.

5. Conclusions

In conclusion, the rheumatological population, as well as the global one, has been experiencing an aging trend. Results like those of the present study, by which the effectiveness of a drug seems to negatively correlate with age, lead us to imagine a deep interconnection between systemic inflammation, immunosenescence and age-related disease, worthy of consideration in those RA patients difficult to treat.

Author Contributions: Writing—original draft, M.P. (Marta Priora) and A.B. (Andrea Becciolini); Writing—review and editing, E.C., A.L.G., M.P. (Marino Paroli), E.B., R.A., V.N., F.O., F.L., A.F. (Antonella Farina), P.D.M., M.C., V.R., P.S., M.L., E.V., O.A., R.V., A.V., A.B. (Alessandra Bezzi), F.G., A.B.M.C., R.C., E.D.D., G.A. (Giuditta Adorni), D.S., G.L., E.A., I.P., N.M., A.I., E.F., M.C.D., V.B., D.C., G.B., F.S., Y.D.B., R.F. (Rosario Foti), G.A. (Giorgio Amato), F.D.L., R.F. (Roberta Foti), M.R., A.F. (Alessia Fiorenza), G.R., A.M., M.C.F., F.M., S.B., G.S., D.G., C.S., V.F., F.M.C., G.F., A.A. and S.P.; Visualization, M.D.P. and E.S. All authors have read and agreed to the published version of the manuscript.

Funding: This research received no external funding.

Institutional Review Board Statement: The study was carried out following the Declaration of Helsinki principles and approved by the local Ethics Committees (the main is the Comitato Etico dell'Area Vasta Emilia Nord, protocol code 34,713, approved on 28 August 2019).

Informed Consent Statement: Informed consent was obtained from all subjects involved in the study.

Data Availability Statement: The data presented in this study are available on request from the corresponding author. The data are not publicly available due to privacy.

Conflicts of Interest: The authors declare no conflicts of interest.

References

1. Mortezavi, M.; Mysler, E.F. Clinical scenarios-based guide for tofacitinib in rheumatoid arthritis. *Ther. Adv. Chronic Dis.* **2023**, *14*, 20406223231178270. [CrossRef] [PubMed]
2. Gao, Y.; Gao, Y.N.; Wang, M.J.; Zhang, Y.; Zhang, F.Q.; He, Z.X.; Chen, W.; Li, H.C.; Xie, Z.J.; Wen, C.P. Efficacy and safety of tofacitinib combined with methotrexate in the treatment of rheumatoid arthritis: A systematic review and meta-analysis. *Heliyon* **2023**, *9*, e15839. [CrossRef] [PubMed]
3. Fleischmann, R.; Mysler, E.; Hall, S.; Kivitz, A.J.; Moots, R.J.; Luo, Z.; DeMasi, R.; Soma, K.; Zhang, R.; Takiya, L.; et al. Efficacy and safety of tofacitinib monotherapy, tofacitinib with methotrexate, and adalimumab with methotrexate in patients with rheumatoid arthritis (ORAL Strategy): A phase 3b/4, double-blind, head-to-head, randomised controlled trial. *Lancet* **2017**, *390*, 457–468. [CrossRef]
4. Smolen, J.S.; Landewé, R.B.M.; Bergstra, S.A.; Kerschbaumer, A.; Sepriano, A.; Aletaha, D.; Caporali, R.; Edwards, C.J.; Hyrich, K.L.; Pope, J.E.; et al. EULAR recommendations for the management of rheumatoid arthritis with synthetic and biological disease-modifying antirheumatic drugs: 2022 update. *Ann. Rheum. Dis.* **2023**, *82*, 3–18. [CrossRef]
5. Fraenkel, L.; Bathon, J.M.; England, B.R.; St Clair, E.W.; Arayssi, T.; Carandang, K.; Deane, K.D.; Genovese, M.; Huston, K.K.; Kerr, G.; et al. 2021 American College of Rheumatology Guideline for the Treatment of Rheumatoid Arthritis. *Arthritis Care Res.* **2021**, *73*, 924–939. [CrossRef]
6. Singh, J.A.; Hossain, A.; Tanjong Ghogomu, E.; Mudano, A.S.; Tugwell, P.; Wells, G.A. Biologic or tofacitinib monotherapy for rheumatoid arthritis in people with traditional disease-modifying anti-rheumatic drug (DMARD) failure: A Cochrane Systematic Review and network meta-analysis (NMA). *Cochrane Database Syst. Rev.* **2016**, *11*, CD012437. [CrossRef] [PubMed]
7. Tasso, M.; Bertolini, N.; Mostacciuolo, E.; Passavanti, S.; Luppino, J.M.E.; Del Puente, A.; Peluso, R.; Santelli, F.; Scarpa, R.; Costa, L.; et al. Effectiveness and safety profile of tofacitinib and baricitinib in rheumatoid arthritis patients: Results from a 24-month real-life prospective study in Southern-Italy. *Reumatismo* **2022**, *74*, 131–136. [CrossRef]

8. Burmester, G.R.; Blanco, R.; Charles-Schoeman, C.; Wollenhaupt, J.; Zerbini, C.; Benda, B.; Gruben, D.; Wallenstein, G.; Krishnaswami, S.; Zwillich, S.H.; et al. Tofacitinib (CP-690,550) in combination with methotrexate in patients with active rheumatoid arthritis with an inadequate response to tumour necrosis factor inhibitors: A randomised phase 3 trial. *Lancet* **2013**, *381*, 451–460. [CrossRef]
9. Ytterberg, S.R.; Bhatt, D.L.; Mikuls, T.R.; Koch, G.G.; Fleischmann, R.; Rivas, J.L.; Germino, R.; Menon, S.; Sun, Y.; Wang, C.; et al. Cardiovascular and Cancer Risk with Tofacitinib in Rheumatoid Arthritis. *N. Engl. J. Med.* **2022**, *386*, 316–326. [CrossRef]
10. Kristensen, L.E.; Danese, S.; Yndestad, A.; Wang, C.; Nagy, E.; Modesto, I.; Rivas, J.; Benda, B. Identification of two tofacitinib subpopulations with different relative risk versus TNF inhibitors: An analysis of the open label, randomised controlled study ORAL Surveillance. *Ann. Rheum. Dis.* **2023**, *82*, 901–910. [CrossRef]
11. European Medicines Agency. Pharmacovigilance Risk Assessment Committee (PRAC) 24–27 October 2022. Available online: https://www.ema.europa.eu/en/news/meeting-highlights-pharmacovigilance-risk-assessment-committee-prac-24-27-october-2022 (accessed on 10 September 2024).
12. Charles-Schoeman, C.; Buch, M.H.; Dougados, M.; Bhatt, D.L.; Giles, J.T.; Ytterberg, S.R.; Koch, G.G.; Vranic, I.; Wu, J.; Wang, C.; et al. Risk of major adverse cardiovascular events with tofacitinib versus tumour necrosis factor inhibitors in patients with rheumatoid arthritis with or without a history of atherosclerotic cardiovascular disease: A post hoc analysis from ORAL Surveillance. *Ann. Rheum. Dis.* **2023**, *82*, 119–129. [CrossRef] [PubMed]
13. Buch, M.H.; Bhatt, D.L.; Charles-Schoeman, C.; Giles, J.T.; Mikuls, T.; Koch, G.G.; Ytterberg, S.; Nagy, E.; Jo, H.; Kwok, K.; et al. Risk of extended major adverse cardiovascular event endpoints with tofacitinib versus TNF inhibitors in patients with rheumatoid arthritis: A post hoc analysis of a phase 3b/4 randomised safety study. *RMD Open* **2024**, *10*, e003912. [CrossRef] [PubMed]
14. Szekanecz, Z.; Buch, M.H.; Charles-Schoeman, C.; Galloway, J.; Karpouzas, G.A.; Kristensen, L.E.; Ytterberg, S.R.; Hamar, A.; Fleischmann, R. Efficacy and safety of JAK inhibitors in rheumatoid arthritis: Update for the practising clinician. *Nat. Rev. Rheumatol.* **2024**, *20*, 101–115. [CrossRef] [PubMed]
15. Paroli, M.; Becciolini, A.; Bravi, E.; Andracco, R.; Nucera, V.; Parisi, S.; Ometto, F.; Lumetti, F.; Farina, A.; Del Medico, P.; et al. Long-Term Retention Rate of Tofacitinib in Rheumatoid Arthritis: An Italian Multicenter Retrospective Cohort Study. *Medicina* **2023**, *59*, 1480. [CrossRef] [PubMed]
16. Parisi, S.; Andrea, B.; Chiara, D.M.; Alberto, L.G.; Maddalena, L.; Palma, S.; Olga, A.; Massimo, R.; Marino, P.; Rosalba, C.; et al. Analysis of survival rate and persistence predictors of baricitinib in real-world data from a large cohort of rheumatoid arthritis patients. *Curr. Res. Pharmacol. Drug Discov.* **2024**, *6*, 100178. [CrossRef] [PubMed] [PubMed Central]
17. Haraoui, B.; Khraishi, M.; Choquette, D.; Fortin, I.; Kinch, C.D.; Galos, C.; Roy, P.; Gruben, D.; Vaillancourt, J.; Sampalis, J.S.; et al. Tofacitinib Safety and Effectiveness in Canadian Patients with Rheumatoid Arthritis by Cardiovascular Risk Enrichment: Subanalysis of the CANTORAL Study. *Rheumatol. Ther.* **2024**, *11*, 1629–1648. [CrossRef]
18. Taylor, P.C.; Balsa, A.; Mongey, A.B.; Filková, M.; Chebbah, M.; Le Clanche, S.; Verhagen LA, W.; Witte, T.; Opris-Belinski, D.; Marotte, H.; et al. Does Concomitant Use of Methotrexate with JAK Inhibition Confer Benefit for Cardiovascular Outcomes? A Commentary. *Rheumatol. Ther.* **2024**, *11*, 1425–1435. [CrossRef]
19. Pugliesi, A.; Oliveira, D.G.C.; Filho, V.A.S.; Machado, J.O.; Pereira, A.G.; Bichuette, J.C.S.; Sachetto, Z.; de Carvalho, L.S.F.; Bertolo, M.B. Cardiovascular safety of the class of JAK inhibitors or tocilizumab compared with TNF inhibitors in patients with rheumatoid arthritis: Systematic review and a traditional and Bayesian network meta-analysis of randomized clinical trials. *Semin. Arthritis Rheum.* **2024**, *69*, 152563. [CrossRef]
20. Weyand, C.M.; Yang, Z.; Goronzy, J.J. T-cell aging in rheumatoid arthritis. *Curr. Opin. Rheumatol.* **2014**, *26*, 93–100. [CrossRef]
21. Li, X.; Li, C.; Zhang, W.; Wang, Y.; Qian, P.; Huang, H. Inflammation and aging: Signaling pathways and intervention therapies. *Signal Transduct. Target. Ther.* **2023**, *8*, 239. [CrossRef]
22. Barbé-Tuana, F.; Funchal, G.; Schmitz, C.R.R.; Maurmann, R.M.; Bauer, M.E. The interplay between immunosenescence and age-related diseases. *Semin. Immunopathol.* **2020**, *42*, 545–557. [CrossRef] [PubMed]
23. Furman, D.; Campisi, J.; Verdin, E.; Carrera-Bastos, P.; Targ, S.; Franceschi, C.; Ferrucci, L.; Gilroy, D.W.; Fasano, A.; Miller, G.W.; et al. Chronic inflammation in the etiology of disease across the life span. *Nat. Med.* **2019**, *25*, 1822–1832. [CrossRef] [PubMed]
24. Franceschi, C.; Garagnani, P.; Vitale, G.; Capri, M.; Salvioli, S. Inflammaging and 'Garb-aging'. *Trends Endocrinol. Metab.* **2017**, *28*, 199–212. [CrossRef]
25. Bauer, M.E. Accelerated immunosenescence in rheumatoid arthritis: Impact on clinical progression. *Immun. Ageing* **2020**, *17*, 6. [CrossRef] [PubMed]
26. Franceschi, C.; Bonafè, M.; Valensin, S.; Olivieri, F.; de Luca, M.; Ottaviani, E.; de Benedictis, G. Inflamm-aging: An evolutionary perspective on Immunosenescence. *Ann. N. Y. Acad. Sci.* **2000**, *908*, 244–254. [CrossRef]

medicina MDPI

Article

Circulating B Lymphocyte Subsets in Patients with Systemic Lupus Erythematosus

Joanna Kosałka-Węgiel [1,2,*], Bogdan Jakieła [3], Radosław Dziedzic [4], Mamert , Lech Zaręba [5], Stanisława Bazan-Socha [2,3], Marek Sanak [3], Jacek Musiał [3] and Mariusz Korkosz [1,2]

1 Jagiellonian University Medical College, Department of Rheumatology and Immunology, Jakubowskiego 2, 30-688 Kraków, Poland; mariusz.korkosz@uj.edu.pl
2 University Hospital, Department of Rheumatology, Immunology and Internal Medicine, Jakubowskiego 2, 30-688 Kraków, Poland; mamert.mmm@gmail.com (M.M.); lek.andzelika.siwiec@gmail.com (A.S.-K.); stanislawa.bazan-socha@uj.edu.pl (S.B.-S.)
3 Jagiellonian University Medical College, Department of Internal Medicine, Faculty of Medicine, Jakubowskiego 2, 30-688 Kraków, Poland; b.jakiela@uj.edu.pl (B.J.); marek.sanak@uj.edu.pl (M.S.); jacek.musial@uj.edu.pl (J.M.)
4 Jagiellonian University Medical College, Doctoral School of Medical and Health Sciences, Św. Łazarza 16, 31-530 Kraków, Poland; radoslaw.dziedzic@doctoral.uj.edu.pl
5 University of Rzeszów, College of Natural Sciences, Institute of Computer Science, Pigonia 1, 35-310 Rzeszów, Poland; lzareba@ur.edu.pl
* Correspondence: joanna.kosalka@uj.edu.pl; Tel.: +48-12-400-31-10

Abstract: *Background/Objectives*: Systemic lupus erythematosus (SLE) is an autoimmune disease characterized by the abnormal activation of autoreactive T and B cells, autoantibody production, complement activation, and immune-complex deposition, resulting in tissue damage. However, data on immunologic disturbances in SLE, particularly regarding flares, are scarce. *Methods*: We investigated 35 patients with SLE: 12 (34.3%) with disease exacerbation (SLE disease activity index [SLEDAI] $\geq$ 5 points) and 23 (65.7%) in remission (SLEDAI < 5 points). All patients met the 2019 EULAR/ACR SLE criteria. Flow cytometry was used to identify B cell subsets, including memory B cells. *Results*: In the whole patient group, SLEDAI was positively related to the percentage of transitional/regulatory B cells (r = 0.38, p = 0.034). Some lymphocyte subsets correlated with complement levels, e.g., the percentage of naïve and memory B cells showed associations with C3c complement (r = 0.43, p = 0.018 and r = −0.45, p = 0.016, respectively). Furthermore, regarding inflammatory markers, we found associations between C-reactive protein and the percentage of plasmablasts (r = 0.40, p = 0.026) and plasmocytes (r = 0.44, p = 0.017). Finally, the percentage of plasmablasts correlated with SLE duration (r = 0.42, p = 0.016). In the follow-up analysis, during a median observation of 5 years, 5 out of the initially 23 inactive SLE patients developed a disease flare. They were characterized by longer disease duration stated in the beginning compared to patients who remained in remission (p = 0.019). *Conclusions*: Our study highlights significant associations between various B cell subsets and SLE disease activity. A more personalized approach to indicate patients with SLE at a higher risk of lupus flares is crucial for better management.

Keywords: systemic lupus erythematosus; lupus nephritis; lymphocytes; CD19+ cells; B cells

1. Introduction

Systemic lupus erythematosus (SLE) is a multifaceted autoimmune disease characterized by the dysregulation of the immune system, leading to widespread inflammation and tissue damage across various organs [1]. This condition predominantly affects women, particularly those of childbearing age, and presents with a broad spectrum of clinical manifestations, ranging from mild symptoms such as fatigue and joint pain to severe organ involvement, including nephritis and central nervous system disorders [2,3]. The complexity of SLE stems from its underlying pathophysiology, which involves an aberrant activation of innate and adaptive immune responses [4]. Interestingly, a hallmark of SLE is the presence of autoantibodies that target a variety of nuclear and cytoplasmic antigens, resulting in the formation of immune complexes [5]. These complexes can deposit in tissues, activating the complement system and leading to inflammatory cascades that cause organ damage [6]. Central to the pathogenesis of SLE are autoreactive T and B cells, which play crucial roles in the sustained autoimmune response and production of pathogenic autoantibodies [7]. Despite significant advances in understanding the immunological disturbances in SLE, there are still gaps in knowledge regarding the specific immune profiles and biomarkers associated with disease flares [8]. Indeed, flares in SLE are episodes of increased disease activity that can significantly impact a patient's quality of life and may lead to permanent organ damage if not adequately managed [9]. Identifying biomarkers and immune cell subsets that correlate with disease activity could enhance our ability to predict, monitor, and treat exacerbations effectively.

Emerging data indicate that B cell subsets may be essential for SLE pathophysiology, including exacerbation rate [10]. Plasmablasts and plasmocytes are involved in producing autoantibodies and regulating immune responses [11,12]. In turn, the B cell memory compartment in lupus nephritis (LN) is deficient in non-switched memory (NSM) cells. Next, during active disease, it becomes further skewed by the expansion of switched memory (SM) and exhausted memory phenotypes, most likely due to chronic antigenic stimulation [13]. In this context, regulatory B cells (B-regs) play a crucial role in modulating immune responses and maintaining tolerance. This is especially important in LN, where excessive immune activation can damage kidneys [14]. While interleukin (IL)-10 production is the most well-studied mechanism of B cell immune regulation, other IL-10-independent mechanisms have also been suggested [15]. Understanding how these lymphocyte subsets fluctuate during remission and exacerbation can provide valuable insights into the disease mechanism and potential therapeutic targets.

Evidence on immunologic disturbances in SLE regarding flares is still scarce. Therefore, in this study, we elucidated the changes within circulating B lymphocyte subsets in patients with SLE, particularly focusing on those experiencing disease exacerbation. Repeated flares can contribute to cumulative tissue damage over time, increasing the risk of long-term complications like chronic kidney disease and cardiovascular events [16]. By comparing the immune profiles of patients in remission and during flares, we hope to identify potentially useful immunologic biomarkers that correlate with disease activity and could serve as indicators for monitoring and managing SLE.

2. Patients and Methods

2.1. Characteristics of the Patients

This observational longitudinal study included 35 patients with SLE diagnosed according to the European League Against Rheumatism and the American College of Rheumatology (EULAR/ACR) criteria from 2019 [17]. We collected data about sex, present age, age at SLE onset, and disease duration. Blood samples were collected from all patients for B cell subset analysis.

The evaluation of LN was extended with a histologic type of nephropathy, classified according to the International Society of Nephrology/Renal Pathology Society (ISN/RPS) system (if kidney biopsy was performed) and numbers of LN exacerbations [18,19]. Renal biopsies were performed in 9 cases, representing 56.3% of LN patients. In 7 patients, renal biopsy was not performed due to lack of patient consent and/or medical contraindications. Patients with SLE were not previously treated with biological agents targeting B cells (e.g., rituximab, belimumab, and anifrolumab). We registered the current systemic glucocorticosteroids (GCS) dose and the cumulative cyclophosphamide (CTX) dose based on the clinical record. Importantly, patients were not treated with CTX 6 months preceding lymphocyte phenotyping. Disease activity was evaluated by the SLE disease activity index (SLEDAI) with renal SLEDAI (rSLEDAI) [20,21].

The Bioethics Committee of the Jagiellonian University Medical College approved the research (No: 1072.6120.34.2018, on 23 February 2018). All procedures adhered to the ethical principles outlined in the Declaration of Helsinki. Additionally, every individual received detailed information about the study's methods and safety procedures and provided written informed consent to participate in the research.

2.2. Laboratory Analysis

We collected laboratory data, including hematological, renal, and immunological parameters. Complete blood count (CBC), C-reactive protein, creatinine with estimated glomerular filtration rate (eGFR, using Modification of Diet in Renal Disease formula) [22], 24 h urine protein excretion, and urinary sediment analysis were measured using routine laboratory techniques. Anti-nuclear antibodies (ANAs) were evaluated by indirect immunofluorescence (IIF). Anti-double-stranded DNA (anti-dsDNA) antibodies were assayed by IIF on *Critidia luciliae* and by enzyme-linked immunosorbent assay (ELISA, EUROIMMUN, Lübeck, Germany). Serum complement levels (C3c and C4) were assessed using laser nephelometry.

2.3. Flow Cytometry

Aliquots of EDTA anticoagulated blood were stained with a mixture of monoclonal antibodies (all from BD Biosciences, Franklin Lakes, NJ, USA) for the detection of CD19+ B cells (anti-CD45, CD3, CD19, CD24, CD27, CD38, CD138, IgD; gating strategy shown in Figure 1). The samples were fixed with FACS lysing solution (BD Biosciences), washed, and analyzed in a FACS Canto II flow cytometer (BD Biosciences). Based on the differential expression of surface markers, the following B cell (CD19+) subsets were identified: transitional/regulatory (CD24+ CD38+) (B-trans/reg), naïve (IgD+ CD27−), non-switched memory (NSM, CD27+ IgD+), switched memory (SM, IgD− CD27+ CD38low), plasmablasts (CD38++ CD27++ CD24− CD138−), plasmocytes (CD38++ CD27++ CD24− CD138+), and double-negative B cells (IgD− CD27−) [13,23–26].

2.4. Statistical Elaboration

The results were analyzed using STATISTICA Tibco 13.3 software (StatSoft Inc., Tulsa, OK, USA). Categorical variables were presented as frequencies (number of cases) with relative frequencies (percentages) and compared using the Chi^2 test or the exact Fisher test, as appropriate. The normality of data distribution was evaluated by the Shapiro–Wilk test. All continuous variables were non-normally distributed and, thus, were presented as medians with Q1–Q3 ranges and compared using the Mann–Whitney test. A Pearson correlation coefficient or a Spearman rank correlation test was used to analyze the associations between continuous variables. The level of statistical significance was $\alpha < 0.05$.

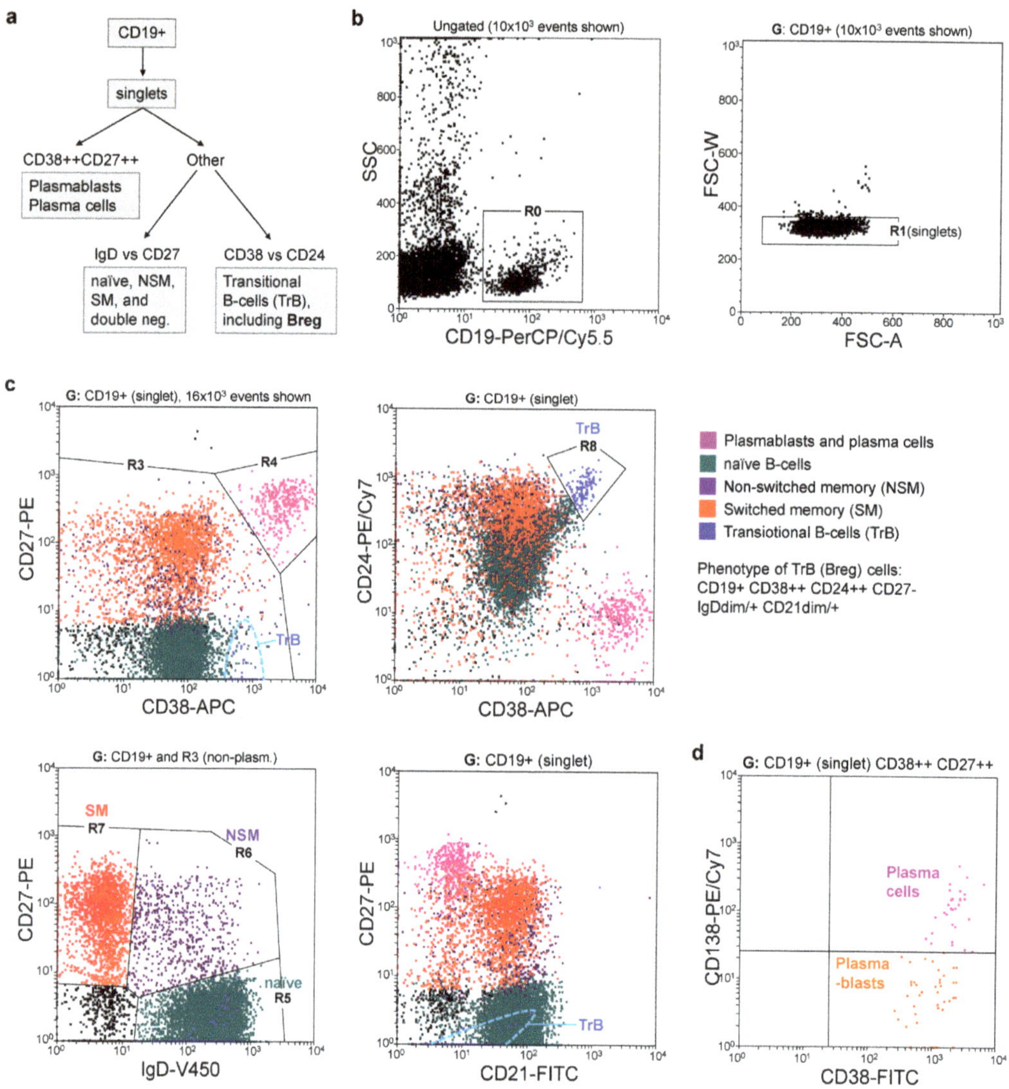

Figure 1. Flow cytometry staining of B cell subsets. (**a**) Schematic diagram showing the flow cytometry (FC) gating strategy used to identify major B cell subsets. Samples of peripheral blood mononuclear cells (PMBCs) were stained with pre-mixed antibodies (CD19-PerCP/Cy5.5, CD38-APC, CD27-PE, CD24-PE/Cy7, IgD-V450, CD21-FITC), and analyzed in FC (>10^3 events in B cell gate recorded). (**b**,**c**) Representative dot plots showing gates and analysis flowchart. (**b**) CD19+ singlets (R0 + R1, only FSC-A/W gate shown) were first analyzed to distinguish the CD38++ CD27++ subset of plasma cells and plasmablasts (R4 region). (**c**) The remaining non-plasma cells were gated (R3) to identify naïve B- B cells, non-switched memory (NSM) B cells, and switched-memory (SM) B cells. Transitional B cells (TrB)/regulatory B cells (Breg) were identified as CD38++ CD24++ using an oblique gate (R8). TrB cells showed the following phenotype: CD19+ CD38++ CD24++ CD27− IgD(low/+) CD21(low/+). (**d**) An additional sample (stained with CD19-PerCP/Cy5.5, CD38-FITC, CD27-PE, CD138-PE/Cy7, IgD-V450, and IgM-APC) was used to distinguish between plasmablasts (CD138−) and plasma cells (CD138+). These two subsets were CD27++ and were negative for membrane IgD and IgM.

3. Results

3.1. Clinical Characteristics

This study included 12 (34.3%) patients with SLE with disease exacerbation (SLEDAI ≥ 5 points) and 23 (65.7%) patients with SLE in remission (SLEDAI < 5 points). There was no difference in age, sex, age of disease onset, and duration between active and inactive SLE patients (Table 1).

Table 1. Demographic and clinical characteristics of active and inactive systemic lupus erythematosus patients.

Parameter	Active SLE Patients n = 12	Inactive SLE Patients n = 23	*p*-Value
Demographic characteristics			
Age at study enrolment, years	46.0 (36.5–50.5)	59.0 (41.0–65.0)	0.07
Sex, female, n (%)	11 (91.7%)	18 (78.3%)	0.64
Age at the SLE onset, years	24.0 (18.3–34.8)	31.0 (22.0–39.0)	0.26
SLE duration, years	16.5 (6.0–25.8)	20.0 (15.0–26.0)	0.26
Symptoms ever stated			
Skin, n (%)	9 (75.0%)	18 (78.3%)	1.00
Oral or nasopharyngeal ulcerations, n (%)	1 (8.3%)	4 (17.3%)	0.64
Photosensitivity, n (%)	7 (58.3%)	9 (39.1%)	0.28
Joints, n (%)	10 (83.3%)	20 (87.0%)	1.00
Serositis, n (%)	3 (25.0%)	2 (8.7%)	0.31
Renal, n (%)	6 (50.0%)	10 (43.5%)	0.71
Neurologic, n (%)	0 (0.0%)	3 (13.0%)	0.54
Hematologic, n (%)	11 (91.7%)	21 (91.3%)	1.00
Symptoms at the study enrolment			
Skin, n (%)	5 (41.7%)	2 (8.7%)	**0.033**
Joints, n (%)	6 (50.0%)	0 (0.0%)	**<0.001**
Serositis, n (%)	1 (8.3%)	0 (0.0%)	0.34
Renal, n (%)	5 (41.7%)	0 (0.0%)	**0.002**
Neurologic, n (%)	0 (0.0%)	0 (0.0%)	NA
Hematologic, n (%)	6 (50.0%)	4 (17.3%)	0.06
Clinical characteristics			
SLEDAI, score	12.0 (8.5–15.5)	2.0 (0.0–2.0)	**<0.001**
rSLEDAI, score	2.0 (0.0–12.0)	0.0 (0.0–0.0)	**0.016**
ANAs, titer	1:20,480 (1:2560–1:20,480)	1:2560 (1:160–1:20,480)	**0.002**
Anti-dsDNA antibodies, titer	1:80 (<1:10–1:5120)	<1:10 (<1:10–1:320)	**0.037**
Proteinuria, g/day	0.41 (0.10–1.66)	0.11 (0.08–0.14)	**0.007**
Creatinine, µmol/L	58.5 (51.0–89.0)	61.0 (56.0–83.0)	0.69
eGFR, mL/min/1.73 m^2	103.5 (65.3–121.5)	97.0 (82.0–107.0)	0.42
C3c, mg/dL	0.77 (0.51–1.01)	0.96 (0.82–1.20)	**0.013**
C4, mg/dL	0.08 (0.07–0.16)	0.17 (0.13–0.21)	**0.003**
C-reactive protein, mg/L	3.0 (1.4–16.0)	1.2 (1.0–3.3)	0.06

Table 1. *Cont.*

Parameter	Active SLE Patients n = 12	Inactive SLE Patients n = 23	*p*-Value
White blood cells, $10^3/\mu L$	4.9 (3.2–6.9)	5.5 (3.6–8.8)	0.29
Lymphocytes, $10^3/\mu L$	1.0 (0.5–1.6)	1.2 (0.9–1.7)	0.23
Neutrophils, $10^3/\mu L$	3.3 (1.9–5.3)	4.1 (2.3–6.6)	0.46
Platelets, $10^3/\mu L$	241 (145–280)	246 (214–296)	0.40
Current systemic GCS, mg/day	0.0 (0.0–5.5)	0.0 (0.0–4.0)	0.55
Cumulative CTX dose, g	4.0 (0.0–26.5)	0.0 (0.0–9.0)	0.38

Categorical variables are presented as numbers with percentages. Continuous variables as median with Q1–Q3 ranges (medians with min-max ranges in case of ANAs and anti-dsDNA titers). Statistically significant differences are marked in bold. Abbreviations: ANAs—anti-nuclear antibodies, C3c—complement component 3c, C4—complement component 4, CTX—cyclophosphamide, eGFR—estimated Glomerular Filtration Rate, GCS—glucocorticosteroids (recounted for methylprednisolone), NA—not applicable, n—number, rSLEDAI—renal SLEDAI, SLE—systemic lupus erythematosus, SLEDAI—SLE disease activity index.

Overall, the most frequent clinical SLE manifestations included hematological signs (n = 32, 91.4%), joint inflammation (n = 30, 85.7%), skin changes (n = 27, 77.1%), and photosensitivity (n = 16, 45.71%). In turn, serositis (n = 5, 14.3%), oral or nasopharyngeal ulcerations (n = 5, 14.3%), and nervous system involvement (n = 3, 8.6%) were much less common. Furthermore, all recruited patients had ANA titer ≥ 1:160, with anti-dsDNA antibodies being the most prevalent (n = 27, 77.1%). Regarding clinical parameters, we noticed higher SLEDAI and rSLEDAI scores with elevated ANA titer in the group of active SLE patients. Also, the active SLE patients had decreased concentrations of C3c and C4 complement components. Interestingly, at enrolment, we noticed more frequent renal manifestations and skin and joint involvement in the active group (Table 1).

LN was confirmed in 16 (45.1%) patients with SLE, of which in 5 (31.3%) cases, renal flare was diagnosed at the time of enrolment into the study. Overall, in LN patients, the most common histological type according to the ISN/RPS classification was class III, identified in 4 cases (44.4%), followed by classes IV (n = 3, 33.3%) and V (n = 2, 22.2%).

Only one patient was taking methylprednisolone > 8 mg/day (16 mg/day). Fourteen patients with SLE were previously (>6 months before blood sample) treated with CTX with a mean summary dose of 8.61 g. With the exception of hydroxychloroquine, none of the patients were taking other immunosuppressive drugs at the time of enrolment.

3.2. B Lymphocyte Subset Analysis in Active and Inactive Systemic Lupus Erythematosus Patients

Surprisingly, the analysis of B cell subset numbers and percentages revealed no significant differences between the active and inactive SLE groups (Table 2). In particular, the numbers and percentages of B-trans/reg cells were comparable between the analyzed subgroups ($p > 0.05$, both).

Table 2. B lymphocyte subset analysis in active and inactive systemic lupus erythematosus patients.

Parameter	Active SLE Patients n = 12	Inactive SLE Patients n = 23	*p*-Value
CD19+, % of lymphocytes	7.9 (5.6–17.5)	5.6 (3.6–10.0)	0.09
Naive, % of B lymphocytes	60.5 (45.1–77.3)	72.7 (53.9–84.7)	0.37
SM, % of B lymphocytes	14.1 (6.2–31.4)	13.4 (5.9–24.6)	0.87
NSM, % of B lymphocytes	8.7 (3.3–10.4)	7.1 (3.4–10.5)	0.87
DN, % of B lymphocytes	5.0 (1.4–9.6)	2.7 (1.4–5.3)	0.46
Plasmocytes, % of B lymphocytes	0.6 (0.1–1.7)	0.4 (0.2–0.7)	0.70

Table 2. *Cont.*

Parameter	Active SLE Patients n = 12	Inactive SLE Patients n = 23	*p*-Value
Plasmablasts, % of B lymphocytes	1.3 (0.5–3.7)	1.2 (0.5–3.3)	0.73
B-trans/reg, % of B lymphocytes	3.8 (2.1–5.0)	2.2 (0.7–3.6)	0.10
B cells per μL			
CD19+, cells/μL	91.6 (35.9–176.4)	88.5 (41.6–145.0)	0.87
Naive, cells/μL	39.9 (14.6–126.4)	53.2 (17.3–120.3)	0.79
SM, cells/μL	11.7 (7.4–26.9)	11.6 (5.2–18.2)	0.71
NSM, cells/μL	6.1 (3.0–8.3)	5.7 (1.8–9.3)	0.68
DN, cells/μL	3.5 (1.6–4.8)	2.2 (0.8–3.7)	0.24
Plasmocytes, cells/μL	0.5 (0.2–0.8)	0.2 (0.1–0.6)	0.29
Plasmablasts, cells/μL	1.3 (0.4–2.0)	0.7 (0.4–2.0)	0.55
B-trans/reg, cells/μL	3.8 (0.9–5.2)	1.7 (0.3–4.9)	0.40

Continuous variables are presented as medians with Q1–Q3 ranges. Abbreviations: B trans/reg—transitional/regulatory B cells, CD—cluster of differentiation, DN—double negative, n—number, NSM—non-switched memory, SLE—systemic lupus erythematosus, SM—switched memory.

3.3. Detailed Characteristics of Active Systemic Lupus Erythematosus Patients

We divided active SLE patients into two subgroups, with renal flare (n = 5) and other than renal flare (n = 7), and compared them using clinical and laboratory parameters (Table 3). Demographic characteristics were similar in both subgroups. As expected, we noticed a higher prevalence of renal symptoms with higher SLEDAI and rSLEDAI scores in the renal flare subgroup. Nevertheless, there were no differences in the numbers and percentages of B lymphocyte subsets between the analyzed subgroups (Supplementary Table S1).

Table 3. Demographic and clinical characteristics of active systemic lupus erythematosus patients with renal flare and other than renal flare.

Parameter	Active SLE Patients with Renal Flare n = 5	Active SLE Patients Other Than Renal Flare n = 7	*p*-Value
Demographic characteristics			
Age, years	42.0 (30.0–50.0)	48.0 (36.0–59.0)	0.53
Sex, female, n (%)	5 (100.0%)	6 (85.7%)	1.00
Age at the SLE onset, years	26.0 (19.5–32.5)	22.0 (18.0–44.0)	0.88
SLE duration, years	17.0 (6.0–21.5)	16.0 (5.0–36.0)	0.76
Symptoms ever stated			
Skin, n (%)	3 (60.0%)	6 (85.7%)	0.52
Oral or nasopharyngeal ulcerations, n (%)	0 (0.0%)	1 (14.3%)	1.00
Photosensitivity, n (%)	3 (60.0%)	4 (57.1%)	1.00
Joints, n (%)	3 (60.0%)	7 (100.0%)	0.15
Serositis, n (%)	2 (40.0%)	1 (14.3%)	0.52
Renal, n (%)	5 (100.0%)	1 (14.3%)	**0.015**
Neurologic, n (%)	0 (0.0%)	0 (0.0%)	NA
Hematologic, n (%)	4 (80.0%)	7 (100.0%)	0.42

Table 3. *Cont.*

Parameter	Active SLE Patients with Renal Flare n = 5	Active SLE Patients Other Than Renal Flare n = 7	*p*-Value
	Symptoms at the study enrolment		
Skin, n (%)	1 (20.0%)	4 (57.1%)	0.29
Joints, n (%)	1 (20.0%)	5 (71.4%)	0.24
Serositis, n (%)	1 (20.0%)	0 (0.0%)	0.42
Renal, n (%)	5 (100.0%)	0 (0.0%)	**0.001**
Neurologic, n (%)	0 (0.0%)	0 (0.0%)	NA
Hematologic, n (%)	4 (80.0%)	2 (28.6%)	0.24
	Clinical characteristics		
SLEDAI, score	16.0 (12.5–22.5)	10.0 (6.0–12.0)	**0.010**
rSLEDAI, score	12.0 (10.0–14.0)	0.0 (0.0–0.0)	**0.003**
ANAs, titer	1:5120 (1:2560–1:20,480)	1:20,480 (1:2560–1:20,480)	0.11
Anti-dsDNA antibodies, titer	1:1280 (<1:10–1:5120)	1:20 (<1:10–1:5120)	0.43
Proteinuria, g/day	1.79 (1.10–7.32)	0.14 (0.08–0.34)	**0.003**
Creatinine, μmol/L	93.0 (47.5–206.5)	57.0 (54.0–72.0)	0.43
eGFR, mL/min/1.73 m^2	59.0 (26.0–134.5)	105.0 (100.0–111.0)	0.53
C3c, mg/dL	0.80 (0.42–1.02)	0.74 (0.50–1.06)	0.88
C4, mg/dL	0.11 (0.06–0.17)	0.08 (0.07–0.17)	0.88
C-reactive protein, mg/L	2.1 (1.1–26.1)	5.2 (2.2–18.8)	0.53
White blood cells, $10^3/\mu L$	4.7 (2.6–7.9)	5.0 (4.4–6.3)	0.76
Lymphocytes, $10^3/\mu L$	0.9 (0.6–2.1)	1.0 (0.4–1.6)	0.88
Neutrophils, $10^3/\mu l$	3.1 (1.4–5.8)	3.4 (2.3–5.3)	0.53
Platelets, $10^3/\mu L$	242 (193–297)	204 (129–260)	0.43
Current systemic GCS, mg/day	0.0 (0.0–2.0)	4.0 (0.0–8.0)	0.20
Cumulative CTX dose, g	10.0 (0.0–35.8)	0.0 (0.0–10.0)	0.43

Categorical variables are presented as numbers with percentages. Continuous variables as medians with Q1–Q3 ranges (medians with min-max ranges in ANAs and anti-dsDNA titers). Statistically significant differences are marked in bold. Abbreviations: ANAs—anti-nuclear antibodies, C3c—complement component 3c, C4—complement component 4, CTX—cyclophosphamide, eGFR—estimated Glomerular Filtration Rate, GCS—glucocorticosteroids (recounted for methylprednisolone), NA—not applicable, n—number, rSLEDAI—renal SLEDAI, SLE—systemic lupus erythematosus, SLEDAI—SLE disease activity index.

3.4. *Detailed Characteristics of Non-Active Systemic Lupus Erythematosus Patients*

Next, we divided remissive SLE patients into two subgroups: patients with renal remission (n = 10) and patients in remission with never-diagnosed LN (n = 13) and also compared clinical and laboratory parameters (Table 4). SLEDAI and rSLEDAI scores were comparable between both groups. Inactive systemic lupus erythematosus patients with remission and LN versus remission without LN also did not differ in numbers and percentages of B lymphocyte subsets (Supplementary Table S2).

Table 4. Demographic and clinical characteristics of inactive systemic lupus erythematosus patients with remission and lupus nephritis versus remission without lupus nephritis.

Parameter	Inactive SLE Patients with Remission and Lupus Nephritis n = 10	Inactive SLE Patients with Remission Without Lupus Nephritis n = 13	*p*-Value
	Demographic characteristics		
Age, years	44.5 (36.8–66.0)	61.0 (49.5–66.0)	0.19
Sex, female, n (%)	7 (70.0%)	11 (84.6%)	0.62
Age at the SLE onset, years	24.5 (20.0–32.5)	36.0 (22.5–42.0)	0.26
SLE duration, years	16.5 (9.3–28.0)	23.0 (18.0–33.0)	0.23
	Symptoms ever stated		
Skin, n (%)	7 (70.0%)	11 (84.6%)	0.62
Oral or nasopharyngeal ulcerations, n (%)	2 (20.0%)	2 (15.4%)	1.00
Photosensitivity, n (%)	4 (40.0%)	5 (38.3%)	1.00
Joints. n (%)	9 (90.0%)	11 (84.6%)	1.00
Serositis, n (%)	1 (10.0%)	1 (7.7%)	1.00
Renal, n (%)	10 (100.0%)	0 (0.0%)	**<0.001**
Neurologic, n (%)	2 (20.0%)	1 (7.7%)	0.56
Hematologic, n (%)	10 (100.0%)	11 (84.6%)	0.49
	Symptoms at the study enrolment		
Skin, n (%)	1 (10.0%)	1 (7.7%)	1.00
Joints, n (%)	0 (0.0%)	0 (0.0%)	NA
Serositis, n (%)	0 (0.0%)	0 (0.0%)	NA
Renal, n (%)	0 (0.0%)	0 (0.0%)	NA
Neurologic, n (%)	0 (0.0%)	0 (0.0%)	NA
Hematologic, n (%)	1 (10.0%)	3 (23.1%)	0.60
	Clinical characteristics		
SLEDAI, score	1.0 (0.0–2.5)	2.0 (1.0–3.0)	0.38
rSLEDAI, score	0.0 (0.0–0.0)	0.0 (0.0–0.0)	1.00
ANAs, titer	1:1280 (1:160–1:10,240)	1:5120 (1:320–1:20,480)	**0.042**
Anti-dsDNA antibodies, titer	<1:10 (<1:10–1:320)	<1:10 (<1:10–1:160)	0.93
Proteinuria, g/day	0.13 (0.08–0.18)	0.10 (0.08–0.12)	0.26
Creatinine, μmol/L	70.0 (58.3–91.8)	59.0 (53.5–72.0)	0.10
eGFR, mL/min/1.73 m^2	82.5 (71.3–103.0)	99.0 (86.0–108.5)	0.21
C3c, mg/dL	1.09 (0.89–1.36)	0.90 (0.81–1.12)	0.17
C4, mg/dL	0.19 (0.14–0.22)	0.17 (0.11–0.21)	0.34
C-reactive protein, mg/L	2.6 (1.2–4.7)	1.0 (1.0–2.4)	0.11
White blood cells, $10^3/\mu L$	7.7 (4.8–9.5)	4.6 (3.4–8.0)	**0.042**
Lymphocytes, $10^3/\mu L$	1.7 (1.4–2.0)	1.0 (0.7–1.2)	**0.003**

Table 4. *Cont.*

Parameter	Inactive SLE Patients with Remission and Lupus Nephritis n = 10	Inactive SLE Patients with Remission Without Lupus Nephritis n = 13	*p*-Value
Neutrophils, $10^3/\mu L$	4.1 (2.5–6.8)	3.8 (2.1–6.0)	0.28
Platelets, $10^3/\mu L$	280 (180–336)	243 (220–264)	0.38
Current systemic GCS, mg/day	0.0 (0.0–4.0)	0.0 (0.0–3.0)	0.83
Cumulative CTX dose, g	7.5 (0.0–33.2)	0.0 (0.0–0.0)	**0.010**

Categorical variables are presented as numbers with percentages. Continuous variables as medians with Q1–Q3 ranges (medians with min-max ranges in ANAs and anti-dsDNA titers). Statistically significant differences are marked in bold. Abbreviations: ANAs—anti-nuclear antibodies, C3c—complement component 3c, C4—complement component 4, CTX—cyclophosphamide, GCS—glucocorticosteroids (recounted for methylprednisolone), eGFR—estimated Glomerular Filtration Rate, NA—not applicable, n—number, rSLEDAI—renal SLEDAI, SLE—systemic lupus erythematosus, SLEDAI—SLE disease activity index.

3.5. B Cell Subsets Correlate with Systemic Lupus Erythematosus Activity

Interestingly, we observed several correlations between B cell subsets and selected SLE parameters. The percentage of trans/reg B cells showed a positive correlation with SLEDAI, ANAs titers, and C-reactive protein (CRP) levels (r = 0.38, r = 0.38, and r = 0.41, respectively; $p < 0.05$ for all). The percentage of naïve B cells was positively associated only with complement C3c component levels (r = 0.43, $p = 0.018$). Furthermore, the frequency of SM B cells correlated positively with the duration of SLE (r = 0.41, $p = 0.028$) and negatively with complement C3c concentrations (r = −0.45, $p = 0.016$). Plasmablast percentage was linked to SLE duration and CRP levels (r = 0.42 and r = 0.40, respectively; $p < 0.05$ for both). Similarly, the percentage of plasmocytes correlated with CRP levels (r = 0.44, $p = 0.017$). The proportion of DN B cells was associated with anti-dsDNA titers (r = 0.44, $p = 0.02$). Interestingly, the percentage of NSM B cells did not relate to the classical disease activity parameters. Detailed data are presented in below in Table 5.

Table 5. Association of B cell subsets with clinical and laboratory parameters of systemic lupus erythematosus.

Parameter	CD19+, Cells/µL	Transitional/ Regulatory, % of B Lymphocytes	Naïve, % of B Lymphocytes	NSM, % of B Lymphocytes	SM, % of B Lymphocytes	Plasmablasts, % of B Lymphocytes	Plasmocytes, % of B Lymphocytes	DN, % of B Lymphocytes
SLEDAI, points	r = 0.19, *p* = 0.28	**r = 0.38, *p* = 0.034**	r = −0.12, *p* = 0.51	r = 0.13, *p* = 0.51	r = 0.02, *p* = 0.93	r = 0.10, *p* = 0.59	r = 0.11, *p* = 0.56	r = 0.19, *p* = 0.35
rSLEDAI, points	r = 0.24, *p* = 0.17	r = 0.28, *p* = 0.12	r = −0.14, *p* = 0.43	r = 0.22, *p* = 0.27	r = 0.10, *p* = 0.60	r = −0.12, *p* = 0.52	r = 0.09, *p* = 0.64	r = 0.06, *p* = 0.75
Anti-dsDNA, titer	r = −0.05, *p* = 0.77	r = 0.33, *p* = 0.07	r = −0.02, *p* = 0.92	r = −0.11, *p* = 0.58	r = −0.19, *p* = 0.33	r = 0.15, *p* = 0.41	r = 0.14, *p* = 0.46	**r = 0.44, *p* = 0.020**
ANAs, titer	r = 0.03, *p* = 0.85	**r = 0.38, *p* = 0.035**	r = 0.10, *p* = 0.59	r = 0.14, *p* = 0.50	r = −0.06, *p* = 0.75	r = 0.13, *p* = 0.47	r = 0.25, *p* = 0.19	r = 0.37, *p* = 0.06
C-reactive protein, mg/L	r = −0.19, *p* = 0.28	**r = 0.41, *p* = 0.023**	r = 0.00, *p* = 0.98	r = −0.21, *p* = 0.29	r = −0.08, *p* = 0.70	**r = 0.40, *p* = 0.026**	**r = 0.44, *p* = 0.017**	r = 0.13, *p* = 0.53

Table 5. *Cont.*

Parameter	CD19+, Cells/μL	Transitional/ Regulatory, % of B Lymphocytes	Naïve, % of B Lymphocytes	NSM, % of B Lymphocytes	SM, % of B Lymphocytes	Plasmablasts, % of B Lymphocytes	Plasmocytes, % of B Lymphocytes	DN, % of B Lymphocytes
Creatinine, μmol/L	r = 0.16, p = 0.36	r = −0.14, p = 0.44	r = −0.15, p = 0.41	r = −0.21, p = 0.29	r = −0.11, p = 0.58	r = −0.17, p = 0.37	r = −0.16, p = 0.40	r = −0.26, p = 0.18
eGFR, mL/min/1.73 m^2	r = −0.10, p = 0.58	r = 0.10, p = 0.58	r = 0.08, p = 0.66	r = 0.34, p = 0.08	r = 0.09, p = 0.66	r = 0.21, p = 0.25	r = 0.23, p = 0.23	r = 0.26, p = 0.20
C3c, mg/dL	r = 0.22, p = 0.21	r = −0.19, p = 0.30	**r = 0.43, *p* = 0.018**	r = −0.33, p = 0.09	**r = −0.45, *p* = 0.016**	r = −0.05, p = 0.79	r = −0.31, p = 0.09	r = −0.28, p = 0.15
C4, mg/dL	r = 0.16, p = 0.35	r = −0.19, p = 0.30	r = 0.28, p = 0.12	r = −0.25, p = 0.19	r = −0.30, p = 0.12	r = −0.02, p = 0.90	r = 0.11, p = 0.55	r = −0.18, p = 0.36
SLE duration, years	**r = −0.38, *p* = 0.026**	r = 0.17, p = 0.35	r = −0.12, p = 0.51	r = 0.25, p = 0.21	**r = 0.41, *p* = 0.028**	**r = 0.42, *p* = 0.016**	r = 0.31, p = 0.09	r = 0.17, p = 0.38
Proteinuria, g/day	**r = 0.43, *p* = 0.011**	r = 0.15, p = 0.42	r = −0.08, p = 0.67	r = 0.18, p = 0.37	r = −0.18, p = 0.35	r = −0.09, p = 0.64	r = −0.02, p = 0.91	r = 0.21, p = 0.28
Cumulative CTX dose, g	r = 0.01, p = 0.97	r = −0.07, p = 0.71	r = −0.11, p = 0.56	r = −0.16, p = 0.42	r = 0.18, p = 0.36	r = −0.05, p = 0.79	r = −0.13, p = 0.48	r = 0.23, p = 0.24

Correlation matrix showing significant associations between the main subsets of B cells and selected markers of active systemic lupus erythematosus (in the whole SLE group). Statistically significant differences are marked in bold. Abbreviations: ANAs—antinuclear antibodies, B trans/reg—transitional/regulatory B cells, C3c—complement component 3c, C4—complement component 4, CD—cluster of differentiation, CTX—cyclophosphamide (cumulative dose), eGFR—estimated Glomerular Filtration Rate, DN—double negative, n—number, NSM—non-switched memory, SLE—systemic lupus erythematosus, SM—switched memory, rSLEDAI—renal SLEDAI, SLE—systemic lupus erythematosus, SLEDAI—SLE disease activity index.

3.6. Follow-Up Analysis of Inactive Systemic Lupus Erythematosus Patients

In the follow-up analysis, we carefully examined flares in inactive SLE patients from the enrolment over the median observation of 5 years. During this time, five patients developed a disease flare (Table 6). We also compared groups of inactive SLE patients with a flare and without a flare over this period to look for potential biomarkers. They had longer disease duration, and no differences in B cell subsets analyzed at the enrolment (Supplementary Table S3).

Table 6. Demographic and clinical characteristics of inactive systemic lupus erythematosus patients with a flare and without a flare in the follow-up analysis.

Parameter	Inactive SLE Patients with a Flare in the Follow-Up n = 5	Inactive SLE Patients Without a Flare in the Follow-Up n = 18	*p*-Value
	Demographic characteristics		
Age, years	63.0 (52.0–69.0)	52.5 (38.5–65.0)	0.20
Sex, female, n (%)	4 (80.0%)	14 (77.8%)	1.00
Age at the SLE onset, years	23.0 (22.5–37.5)	31.0 (20.0–41.5)	0.80
SLE duration, years	25.0 (22.0–46.5)	18.0 (11.0–23.8)	**0.019**

Table 6. *Cont.*

Parameter	Inactive SLE Patients with a Flare in the Follow-Up n = 5	Inactive SLE Patients Without a Flare in the Follow-Up n = 18	*p*-Value
Symptoms ever stated			
Skin, n (%)	4 (80.0%)	14 (77.8%)	1.00
Oral or nasopharyngeal ulcerations, n (%)	2 (40.0%)	2 (11.1%)	0.19
Photosensitivity, n (%)	3 (60.0%)	6 (33.3%)	0.34
Joints, n (%)	5 (100.0%)	15 (83.3%)	1.00
Serositis, n (%)	0 (0.0%)	2 (11.1%)	1.00
Renal, n (%)	2 (40.0%)	8 (44.4%)	1.00
Neurologic, n (%)	1 (20.0%)	2 (11.1%)	0.54
Hematologic, n (%)	5 (100.0%)	16 (88.9%)	1.00
Symptoms at the study enrolment			
Skin, n (%)	0 (0.0%)	2 (11.1%)	1.00
Joints, n (%)	0 (0.0%)	0 (0.0%)	NA
Serositis, n (%)	0 (0.0%)	0 (0.0%)	NA
Renal, n (%)	0 (0.0%)	0 (0.0%)	NA
Neurologic, n (%)	0 (0.0%)	0 (0.0%)	NA
Hematologic, n (%)	0 (0.0%)	4 (22.2%)	0.54
Clinical characteristics			
SLEDAI, score	2.0 (1.0–2.0)	2.0 (0.0–4.0)	0.91
rSLEDAI, score	0.0 (0.0–0.0)	0.0 (0.0–0.0)	1.00
ANAs, titer	1:10,240 (1:1280–1:20,480)	1:1280 (1:160–1:20,480)	0.08
Anti-dsDNA antibodies, titer	<1:10 (<1:10–1:80)	<1:10 (<1:10–1:320)	0.36
Proteinuria, g/day	0.11 (0.05–0.16)	0.11 (0.08–0.14)	0.86
Creatinine, μmol/L	65.0 (59.0–92.0)	60.5 (52.5–80.8)	0.36
eGFR, mL/min/1.73 m^2	83.0 (66.0–99.0)	97.5 (82.0–111.0)	0.26
C3c, mg/dL	0.86 (0.66–1.16)	0.99 (0.82–1.32)	0.49
C4, mg/dL	0.17 (0.11–0.23)	0.18 (0.13–0.22)	0.86
C-reactive protein, mg/L	2.6 (1.3–3.1)	1.0 (1.0–3.7)	0.40
White blood cells, $10^3/\mu L$	3.6 (3.0–7.3)	6.4 (4.4–8.9)	0.23
Lymphocytes, $10^3/\mu L$	0.9 (0.7–2.5)	1.3 (1.0–1.7)	0.23
Neutrophils, $10^3/\mu L$	2.8 (1.7–4.1)	4.6 (2.3–6.7)	0.20
Platelets, $10^3/\mu L$	262 (162–312)	245 (217–273)	1.00
Current systemic GCS, mg/day	0.0 (0.0–4.0)	0.0 (0.0–2.5)	0.86
Cumulative CTX dose, g	0.0 (0.0–22.1)	0.0 (0.0–5.5)	0.91

Categorical variables are presented as numbers with percentages. Continuous variables as medians with Q1–Q3 ranges (medians with a min-max range in case of ANAs and anti-dsDNA titers). Statistically significant differences are marked in bold. Abbreviations: ANAs—anti-nuclear antibodies, C3c—complement component C3c, C4—complement component 4, CTX—cyclophosphamide, eGFR—estimated Glomerular Filtration Rate, GCS—glucocorticosteroids (recounted for methylprednisolone), NA—not applicable, n—number, rSLEDAI—renal SLEDAI, SLE—systemic lupus erythematosus, SLEDAI—SLE disease activity index.

4. Discussion

This study explored the immunological profile of patients with SLE, particularly focusing on those experiencing disease exacerbations. Surprisingly, no significant differences were observed in the numbers or percentages of B cell subsets between patients with active and inactive SLE. However, correlations were identified regarding specific B cell subsets and disease activity parameters, providing valuable insights into the pathophysiology of SLE flares and highlighting potential immune-related markers for monitoring disease activity.

Importantly, the demographic profile of our cohort mirrored typical SLE populations, with a predominance of females (n = 29, 82.9%) [27]. There were no differences in age at study enrolment, age of SLE diagnosis, or disease duration between analyzed active and inactive SLE patients. However, despite similar demographics, distinct clinical and laboratory features emerged, underscoring the multifaceted nature of the disease. As expected, active SLE patients showed elevated levels of anti-dsDNA antibodies, more severe proteinuria, lower complement component levels (C3c and C4), and higher C-reactive protein levels than inactive SLE patients. These differences, similar to discrepancies in clinical symptoms, are typical of exacerbated SLE [28,29].

We did not find any significant differences in the numbers or percentages of B cell subsets in active and inactive SLE. This contrasts with our previous findings in lupus nephritis (LN) patients, where we observed an increased percentage of immature/early-transitional B cells ($CD27^-IgD^+CD21^-$), a higher frequency of activated SM ($CD27^+IgD^-CD21^-$) and exhausted memory B cells ($CD27^-IgD^-$), and a decrease in NSM ($CD27^+IgD^+$) B cells [13]. Our findings also differ from those presented by Rodríguez-Bayona et al. [30], who demonstrated a deficiency in SM B cells and an increased proportion of naive B cells in active SLE cases. The discrepancy between our results and existing data may be due to the small sample sizes of both studied groups.

On the other hand, in the entire cohort of 35 patients, disease activity, as measured by the SLEDAI, was positively associated with the percentage of trans/reg B cells, suggesting their engagement in the immunologic response of disease flare [31] and highlighting the significant role of the immune system in the progression of SLE.

Next, we also observed that specific B subsets were correlated with complement component levels. Complement components are clinically useful as they serve as biomarkers in SLE activity and are used in some SLE disease scores, such as SLEDAI [32]. Our observation suggests additional interplay between complement activation and lymphocyte dynamics in SLE. Indeed, the percentage of naïve and memory B cells was linked with C3c complement levels. C3, a central component of the complement system, plays a critical role in immune complex clearance and inflammatory responses [33]. Next, elevated levels of complement split products, such as C3dg, iC3b, C4d, and cell-bound complement activation products, can serve as diagnostic biomarkers and indicate disease activity, as well as predict adverse outcomes, including in antiphospholipid syndrome [33]. Dysfunctions in the complement system are pivotal in the pathogenesis of SLE, both during the initiation of autoimmunity and the inflammatory phase [32–34]. Complement deficiencies, such as C1q, are among the strongest genetic risk factors for SLE [32]. Complement activation on immune complexes and autoantibodies drives chronic inflammation, promoting the activation and expansion of autoreactive T and B cells. While complement receptor signaling on B cells typically helps regulate their activation, reduced receptor expression (e.g., CR2) in autoimmune diseases may impair this mechanism. Thus, targeting the inhibitory CR1 and CR2 in autoreactive B cells could serve as a novel scenario for therapeutic options in autoimmune diseases [34]. However, further investigation is needed to delineate which specific B cell subsets are primarily involved in this correlation and how they influence complement dynamics.

Another interesting finding of our study is a positive correlation between an unspecific marker of inflammation CRP and the percentage of plasmablasts and plasmocytes, underscoring the role of these cells in the SLE flares. Plasmablasts and plasmocytes produce autoantibodies, which form immune complexes that deposit in tissues and activate the complement system, perpetuating the cycle of inflammation [35], especially in the kidneys, skin, and joints [36]. In turn, elevated CRP points to the active inflammation [37]. Thus, the association presented here reinforces these cells as central to the humoral immune response and simultaneously to the acute inflammatory response in SLE. Notably, the percentage of plasmablasts also showed a significant correlation with the duration of SLE, which may reflect the chronic activation and differentiation of B cells over the disease course.

One of the crucial aspects of SLE management is the presence of LN [38]. However, there are no reliable early non-invasive biomarkers for ongoing kidney damage [39]. For example, Kitagori et al. [40] proposed a urine osteopontin N-half concentration as a novel biomarker related to kidney inflammation; however, more extensive clinical studies are needed to confirm its suitability in LN prediction. Furthermore, previously, it was documented that some B cell compartments were deficient in those cases [13]. We did not find such an association; only a positive correlation was noted between CD19+ cells and proteinuria. The lack of significant correlations between CD19+ cells and other kidney function markers, such as creatinine or eGFR, suggests proteinuria, a hallmark feature of lupus nephritis [41], might be a more sensitive marker of immune-mediated kidney damage in SLE. Importantly, ongoing proteinuria is a risk factor for LN flares in patients discontinuing immunosuppressive therapy [42]. Therefore, monitoring CD19+ B cell levels, together with proteinuria, might serve as a specific marker for assessing the risk and severity of renal involvement in patients with SLE. This could be especially valuable in clinical settings where early detection of kidney involvement is crucial for preventing progression to more severe renal damage and chronic kidney disease. Additionally, targeting B cells with therapies such as B cell depletion (e.g., rituximab) might be particularly effective for patients with SLE with significant renal involvement, as it directly addresses a key component of the pathogenic mechanism leading to proteinuria [43]. Furthermore, similar to others [44–46], we showed that specific immunological profiles could be linked with disease activity referring to the SLEDAI score.

A novelty of our study was the long-term follow-up of inactive SLE patients to identify immunological markers of pre-active or smoldering disease. However, a few of those with exacerbations (n = 5, 21.7% out of 23 inactive SLE patients) do not allow us to draw reliable conclusions. In contrast, other researchers underscore that specific B cell subpopulations may be valuable biomarkers for flare prediction [47].

5. Limitations of the Study

Despite its valuable findings, this study has several limitations. Firstly, the relatively small sample size limits the statistical power and may affect the reliability of the conclusions. Secondly, the single-center design introduces the possibility of selection bias, which may reduce the generalizability of the findings to broader populations. Furthermore, the cross-sectional nature of the study restricts the ability to establish causal relationships, particularly in exploring predictive factors for relapses or disease progression. Additionally, while informative, the study overlooks other potential aspects of disease mechanisms. Future approaches will focus on cytokine profiles, genetic markers, and activation markers on B cells to better understand disease mechanisms and identify potential therapeutic targets.

6. Conclusions

Our study highlights significant associations between various B cell subsets and SLE disease activity. Some B lymphocyte subsets correlated with complement levels support its role as a biomarker for identifying and tracking exacerbations in patients with SLE. These findings contribute to a better understanding of disease variability and could inform clinical management strategies for patients with SLE, especially those with renal manifestations. Future studies with larger, multicenter cohorts and prospective designs are needed to validate our findings and elucidate the long-term impact of identified markers on clinical outcomes in SLE. A more personalized approach to indicate patients with SLE at a higher risk of lupus flares is crucial for better management.

Supplementary Materials: The following supporting information can be downloaded at https://www.mdpi.com/article/10.3390/medicina60121994/s1. Table S1: B cell subset analysis in active systemic lupus erythematosus patients with renal flare and other than renal flare; Table S2: B cell subset analysis in active systemic lupus erythematosus patients with remission and lupus nephritis versus remission without lupus nephritis; Table S3: B cell subset analysis in inactive systemic lupus erythematosus patients with a flare and without a flare in the follow-up analysis.

Author Contributions: Conceptualization, J.K.-W., B.J., M.S., J.M., S.B.-S. and M.K.; methods, J.K.-W., B.J., S.B.-S. and M.K.; software, J.K.-W., S.B.-S. and M.K.; validation, J.K.-W., B.J., R.D., S.B.-S. and M.K.; formal analysis, J.K.-W., R.D. and L.Z.; investigation, J.K.-W., M.M., A.S.-K. and S.B.-S.; resources, J.K.-W.; data curation, J.K.-W., R.D. and L.Z.; writing—original draft preparation, J.K.-W., B.J. and R.D.; writing—review and editing, M.M., A.S.-K., L.Z., S.B.-S., M.S., J.M. and M.K.; visualization, J.K.-W., B.J. and R.D.; supervision, M.S., J.M., S.B.-S. and M.K.; project administration, J.K.-W. All authors have read and agreed to the published version of the manuscript.

Funding: This work was supported by a research grant from the National Science Center in Poland, No. 2017/25/N/NZ5/02595 (to J.K.-W.).

Institutional Review Board Statement: The study was conducted in accordance with the guidelines of the Declaration of Helsinki and was approved by the Bioethical Committee of Jagiellonian University (Kraków, Poland) (Approval No: 1072.6120.34.2018, on 23 February 2018).

Informed Consent Statement: Informed consent was obtained from all subjects involved in the study.

Data Availability Statement: The data presented in this study are available upon reasonable request from the corresponding author.

Acknowledgments: The results of this study were presented at the 13th Annual Meeting of the Lupus Academy on 6–8 September 2024 (Amsterdam, The Netherlands).

Conflicts of Interest: The authors declare no conflicts of interest.

References

1. Hoi, A.; Igel, T.; Mok, C.C.; Arnaud, L. Systemic Lupus Erythematosus. *Lancet* **2024**, *403*, 2326–2338. [CrossRef] [PubMed]
2. Lisnevskaia, L.; Murphy, G.; Isenberg, D. Systemic Lupus Erythematosus. *Lancet* **2014**, *384*, 1878–1888. [CrossRef] [PubMed]
3. Piga, M.; Tselios, K.; Viveiros, L.; Chessa, E.; Neves, A.; Urowitz, M.B.; Isenberg, D. Clinical Patterns of Disease: From Early Systemic Lupus Erythematosus to Late-Onset Disease. *Best Pract. Res. Clin. Rheumatol.* **2024**, *37*, 101938. [CrossRef] [PubMed]
4. Hisada, R.; Kono, M. Potential Therapies Targeting Metabolic Pathways in Systemic Lupus Erythematosus. *Clin. Immunol.* **2024**, *263*, 110224. [CrossRef] [PubMed]
5. Dema, B.; Charles, N. Autoantibodies in SLE: Specificities, Isotypes and Receptors. *Antibodies* **2016**, *5*, 2. [CrossRef]
6. Accapezzato, D.; Caccavale, R.; Paroli, M.P.; Gioia, C.; Nguyen, B.L.; Spadea, L.; Paroli, M. Advances in the Pathogenesis and Treatment of Systemic Lupus Erythematosus. *Int. J. Mol. Sci.* **2023**, *24*, 6578. [CrossRef]
7. D'Cruz, D.P.; Khamashta, M.A.; Hughes, G.R. Systemic Lupus Erythematosus. *Lancet* **2007**, *369*, 587–596. [CrossRef]
8. Yu, H.; Nagafuchi, Y.; Fujio, K. Clinical and Immunological Biomarkers for Systemic Lupus Erythematosus. *Biomolecules* **2021**, *11*, 928. [CrossRef]
9. Moysidou, G.-S.; Mastrogiorgakis, D.; Boumpas, D.; Bertsias, G. Management of Systemic Lupus Erythematosus: A New Scenario. *Best Pract. Res. Clin. Rheumatol.* **2023**, *37*, 101895. [CrossRef]
10. Morand, E.F.; Fernandez-Ruiz, R.; Blazer, A.; Niewold, T.B. Advances in the Management of Systemic Lupus Erythematosus. *BMJ* **2023**, *383*, e073980. [CrossRef]
11. Fujio, K.; Okamura, T.; Sumitomo, S.; Yamamoto, K. Regulatory Cell Subsets in the Control of Autoantibody Production Related to Systemic Autoimmunity. *Ann. Rheum. Dis.* **2013**, *72*, ii85–ii89. [CrossRef] [PubMed]
12. Nutt, S.L.; Hodgkin, P.D.; Tarlinton, D.M.; Corcoran, L.M. The Generation of Antibody-Secreting Plasma Cells. *Nat. Rev. Immunol.* **2015**, *15*, 160–171. [CrossRef] [PubMed]
13. Kosalka, J.; Jakiela, B.; Musial, J. Changes of Memory B- and T-Cell Subsets in Lupus Nephritis Patients. *Folia Histochem. Cytobiol.* **2016**, *54*, 32–41. [CrossRef] [PubMed]
14. Bilate, A.M.; Lafaille, J.J. Induced $CD4^{+}Foxp3^{+}$ Regulatory T Cells in Immune Tolerance. *Annu. Rev. Immunol.* **2012**, *30*, 733–758. [CrossRef] [PubMed]
15. Ray, A.; Wang, L.; Dittel, B.N. IL-10-Independent Regulatory B-Cell Subsets and Mechanisms of Action. *Int. Immunol.* **2015**, *27*, 531–536. [CrossRef]
16. Lam, N.-C.V.; Brown, J.A.; Sharma, R. Systemic Lupus Erythematosus: Diagnosis and Treatment. *Am. Fam. Physician* **2023**, *107*, 383–395.
17. Aringer, M. EULAR/ACR Classification Criteria for SLE. *Semin. Arthritis Rheum.* **2019**, *49*, S14–S17. [CrossRef]

18. Kaczmarczyk, K.; Kosalka, J.; Soja, J.; Kuzniewski, M.; Musial, J.; Okon, K. Renal Interstitial Mast Cell Counts Differ across Classes of Proliferative Lupus Nephritis. *Folia Histochem. Cytobiol.* **2014**, *52*, 218–224. [CrossRef]
19. Szymanik-Grzelak, H.; Barabasz, M.; Wikiera-Magott, I.; Banaszak, B.; Wieczorkiewicz-Płaza, A.; Bieniaś, B.; Drożynska-Duklas, M.; Tkaczyk, M.; Pańczyk-Tomaszewska, M. Retrospective Analysis of Clinical and Pathomorphological Features of Lupus Nephritis in Children. *Adv. Med. Sci.* **2021**, *66*, 128–137. [CrossRef]
20. Jakiela, B.; Kosałka, J.; Plutecka, H.; Węgrzyn, A.S.; Bazan-Socha, S.; Sanak, M.; Musiał, J. Urinary Cytokines and mRNA Expression as Biomarkers of Disease Activity in Lupus Nephritis. *Lupus* **2018**, *27*, 1259–1270. [CrossRef]
21. Aljaberi, N.; Wenderfer, S.E.; Mathur, A.; Qiu, T.; Jose, S.; Merritt, A.; Rose, J.; Devarajan, P.; Huang, B.; Brunner, H. Clinical Measurement of Lupus Nephritis Activity Is Inferior to Biomarker-Based Activity Assessment Using the Renal Activity Index for Lupus Nephritis in Childhood-Onset Systemic Lupus Erythematosus. *Lupus Sci. Med.* **2022**, *9*, e000631. [CrossRef] [PubMed]
22. Levey, A.S.; Titan, S.M.; Powe, N.R.; Coresh, J.; Inker, L.A. Kidney Disease, Race, and GFR Estimation. *CJASN* **2020**, *15*, 1203–1212. [CrossRef] [PubMed]
23. Żabińska, M.; Kościelska-Kasprzak, K.; Krajewska, J.; Bartoszek, D.; Augustyniak-Bartosik, H.; Krajewska, M. Immune Cells Profiling in ANCA-Associated Vasculitis Patients—Relation to Disease Activity. *Cells* **2021**, *10*, 1773. [CrossRef] [PubMed]
24. Chung, M.K.Y.; Gong, L.; Kwong, D.L.; Lee, V.H.; Lee, A.W.; Guan, X.; Kam, N.; Dai, W. Functions of Double-negative B Cells in Autoimmune Diseases, Infections, and Cancers. *EMBO Mol. Med.* **2023**, *15*, e17341. [CrossRef] [PubMed]
25. Lebel, E.; Nachmias, B.; Pick, M.; Gross Even-Zohar, N.; Gatt, M.E. Understanding the Bioactivity and Prognostic Implication of Commonly Used Surface Antigens in Multiple Myeloma. *J. Clin. Med.* **2022**, *11*, 1809. [CrossRef]
26. Agarbati, S.; Benfaremo, D.; Viola, N.; Paolini, C.; Svegliati Baroni, S.; Funaro, A.; Moroncini, G.; Malavasi, F.; Gabrielli, A. Increased Expression of the Ectoenzyme CD38 in Peripheral Blood Plasmablasts and Plasma Cells of Patients with Systemic Sclerosis. *Front. Immunol.* **2022**, *13*, 1072462. [CrossRef]
27. Siegel, C.H.; Sammaritano, L.R. Systemic Lupus Erythematosus: A Review. *JAMA* **2024**, *331*, 1480–1491. [CrossRef] [PubMed]
28. Adamichou, C.; Bertsias, G. Flares in Systemic Lupus Erythematosus: Diagnosis, Risk Factors and Preventive Strategies. *Mediterr. J. Rheumatol.* **2017**, *28*, 4–12. [CrossRef] [PubMed]
29. Thong, B.; Olsen, N.J. Systemic Lupus Erythematosus Diagnosis and Management. *Rheumatology* **2016**, *56*, i3–i13. [CrossRef]
30. Rodríguez-Bayona, B.; Ramos-Amaya, A.; Pérez-Venegas, J.J.; Rodríguez, C.; Brieva, J.A. Decreased Frequency and Activated Phenotype of Blood CD27 IgD IgM B Lymphocytes Is a Permanent Abnormality in Systemic Lupus Erythematosus Patients. *Arthritis Res. Ther.* **2010**, *12*, R108. [CrossRef]
31. Cruciani, C.; Zen, M.; Gatto, M.; Morand, E.; Doria, A. Assessment of Disease Activity and Damage in SLE: Are We There Yet? *Best Pract. Res. Clin. Rheumatol.* **2023**, *37*, 101896. [CrossRef] [PubMed]
32. Leffler, J.; Bengtsson, A.A.; Blom, A.M. The Complement System in Systemic Lupus Erythematosus: An Update. *Ann. Rheum. Dis.* **2014**, *73*, 1601–1606. [CrossRef] [PubMed]
33. Weinstein, A.; Alexander, R.V.; Zack, D.J. A Review of Complement Activation in SLE. *Curr. Rheumatol. Rep.* **2021**, *23*, 16. [CrossRef] [PubMed]
34. Erdei, A.; Kovács, K.G.; Nagy-Baló, Z.; Lukácsi, S.; Mácsik-Valent, B.; Kurucz, I.; Bajtay, Z. New Aspects in the Regulation of Human B Cell Functions by Complement Receptors CR1, CR2, CR3 and CR4. *Immunol. Lett.* **2021**, *237*, 42–57. [CrossRef] [PubMed]
35. Parodis, I.; Gatto, M.; Sjöwall, C. B Cells in Systemic Lupus Erythematosus: Targets of New Therapies and Surveillance Tools. *Front. Med.* **2022**, *9*, 952304. [CrossRef]
36. Ceccarelli, F.; Natalucci, F.; Olivieri, G.; Perricone, C.; Pirone, C.; Spinelli, F.R.; Alessandri, C.; Conti, F. Erosive Arthritis in Systemic Lupus Erythematosus: Not Only Rhupus. *Lupus* **2021**, *30*, 2029–2041. [CrossRef]
37. Enocsson, H.; Karlsson, J.; Li, H.-Y.; Wu, Y.; Kushner, I.; Wetterö, J.; Sjöwall, C. The Complex Role of C-Reactive Protein in Systemic Lupus Erythematosus. *J. Clin. Med.* **2021**, *10*, 5837. [CrossRef]
38. Kostopoulou, M.; Mukhtyar, C.B.; Bertsias, G.; Boumpas, D.T.; Fanouriakis, A. Management of Systemic Lupus Erythematosus: A Systematic Literature Review Informing the 2023 Update of the EULAR Recommendations. *Ann. Rheum. Dis.* **2024**, *83*, 1489–1501. [CrossRef]
39. Alduraibi, F.K.; Tsokos, G.C. Lupus Nephritis Biomarkers: A Critical Review. *Int. J. Mol. Sci.* **2024**, *25*, 805. [CrossRef]
40. Kitagori, K.; Yoshifuji, H.; Oku, T.; Sasaki, C.; Miyata, H.; Mori, K.P.; Nakajima, T.; Ohmura, K.; Kawabata, D.; Yukawa, N.; et al. Cleaved Form of Osteopontin in Urine as a Clinical Marker of Lupus Nephritis. *PLoS ONE* **2016**, *11*, e0167141. [CrossRef]
41. Omer, M.H.; Shafqat, A.; Ahmad, O.; Nadri, J.; AlKattan, K.; Yaqinuddin, A. Urinary Biomarkers for Lupus Nephritis: A Systems Biology Approach. *J. Clin. Med.* **2024**, *13*, 2339. [CrossRef] [PubMed]
42. Alenzi, F.; Ateka-Barrutia, O.; Ken Cheah, C.; Khamashta, M.; Sangle, S.R.; D'Cruz, D.P. Lupus Nephritis Outcomes after Stopping Immunosuppression. *J. Clin. Med.* **2024**, *13*, 2211. [CrossRef] [PubMed]
43. Imran, T.F.; Yick, F.; Verma, S.; Estiverne, C.; Ogbonnaya-Odor, C.; Thiruvarudsothy, S.; Reddi, A.S.; Kothari, N. Lupus Nephritis: An Update. *Clin. Exp. Nephrol.* **2016**, *20*, 1–13. [CrossRef] [PubMed]
44. Szabó, E.; Faragó, A.; Bodor, G.; Gémes, N.; Puskás, L.G.; Kovács, L.; Szebeni, G.J. Identification of Immune Subsets with Distinct Lectin Binding Signatures Using Multi-Parameter Flow Cytometry: Correlations with Disease Activity in Systemic Lupus Erythematosus. *Front. Immunol.* **2024**, *15*, 1380481. [CrossRef]

45. Xiong, H.; Tang, Z.; Xu, Y.; Shi, Z.; Guo, Z.; Liu, X.; Tan, G.; Ai, X.; Guo, Q. CD19+CD24highCD27+ B Cell and Interleukin 35 as Potential Biomarkers of Disease Activity in Systemic Lupus Erythematosus Patients. *Adv. Rheumatol.* **2022**, *62*, 48. [CrossRef]
46. Zhou, H.; Li, B.; Li, J.; Wu, T.; Jin, X.; Yuan, R.; Shi, P.; Zhou, Y.; Li, L.; Yu, F. Dysregulated T Cell Activation and Aberrant Cytokine Expression Profile in Systemic Lupus Erythematosus. *Mediat. Inflamm.* **2019**, *2019*, 8450947. [CrossRef]
47. Loeser, R.F.; Arbeeva, L.; Kelley, K.; Fodor, A.A.; Sun, S.; Ulici, V.; Longobardi, L.; Cui, Y.; Stewart, D.A.; Sumner, S.J.; et al. Association of Increased Serum Lipopolysaccharide, But Not Microbial Dysbiosis, With Obesity-Related Osteoarthritis. *Arthritis Rheumatol.* **2022**, *74*, 227–236. [CrossRef]

medicina

MDPI

Article

Parents' Satisfaction with Juvenile Idiopathic Arthritis Care: Findings from a Cohort of Italian Children Using the JAMAR Questionnaire

Federica Romano [1], Precia Mombasi [1], Franco Garofalo [2], Nima Namarvari [3], Francesco Franco [3], Patrizia Defabianis [1] and Giovanni Nicolao Berta [3,*]

[1] Department of Surgical Sciences, C.I.R. Dental School, University of Turin, Via Nizza 230, 10126 Turin, Italy; federica.romano@unito.it (F.R.); mompasi20@gmail.com (P.M.); patrizia.defabianis@unito.it (P.D.)
[2] Paediatric Rheumatology Unit, Paediatric Department, Rivoli Hospital, Via Rivalta 29, 10098 Rivoli, Italy; franco.garofalo37@gmail.com
[3] Department of Clinical and Biological Sciences, Section of Translational Pharmacology, University of Turin, Regione Gonzole 10, 10043 Orbassano, Italy; nima.namarvari@unito.it (N.N.); francesco.franco@unito.it (F.F.)
* Correspondence: giovanni.berta@unito.it

Abstract: *Background and Objectives*: Despite recent advancements in treatment, children with juvenile idiopathic arthritis (JIA) continue to experience poor health-related quality of life, and data on patient and parent satisfaction with disease management remain limited. Thus, this cross-sectional study aimed to explore the factors influencing parental satisfaction with their child's JIA care, using the juvenile arthritis parent acceptable symptom state (JA-PASS). *Materials and Methods*: Parents of 63 children (43 females and 20 males; mean age 12.2 $\pm$ 3.7 years) diagnosed with JIA completed the Juvenile Arthritis Multidimensional Assessment Report (JAMAR). The study analyzed JAMAR responses, along with demographic data, disease duration and activity, and current medication use, to identify clinical factors that influence JA-PASS. *Results*: According to the JAMAR, 55.6% of parents expressed satisfaction with their child's current condition. In a multiple regression analysis, significant factors influencing JA-PASS included medication side effects ($p = 0.033$), current disease activity ($p = 0.009$), and the psychosocial well-being rating in the JAMAR questionnaire ($p = 0.048$). *Conclusions*: JA-PASS should be integrated into patient assessment protocols, as it provides valuable insight into parents' perceptions of disease progression and effectiveness of therapeutic interventions.

Keywords: juvenile idiopathic arthritis; quality of life; patient-reported outcomes; pediatric rheumatology

1. Introduction

Juvenile idiopathic arthritis (JIA) is a clinically heterogeneous group of chronic diseases characterized by joint inflammation of unknown etiology, with symptoms persisting for at least six weeks and an onset before the age of 16 years [1]. It is the most common rheumatic disorder in children, affecting approximately 16 to 50 children per 100,000 in high-income countries [2]. In Italy, around 10,000 children are affected by the disease [3].

The International League of Associations for Rheumatology (ILAR) classifies JIA into seven subtypes: systemic, polyarticular (rheumatoid factor [RF] negative or positive), oligoarticular, enthesitis-related (ERA), psoriatic, or undifferentiated [4]. Despite variations in disease course, all JIA subtypes share the hallmark of persistent synovial inflammation, leading to joint stiffness, swelling, and pain. These symptoms significantly impair daily activities and productivity compared to healthy peers [5]. In severe cases, this inflammatory process may result in permanent damage to articular cartilage and bone, leading to substantial physical disability [5].

The primary goal in managing JIA is to achieve and sustain disease remission, or at least minimal disease activity [6]. However, this remains challenging despite significant advances in drug therapy, especially with the introduction of advanced disease-modifying antirheumatic drugs (DMARDs) that target specific immune system pathways [7,8]. Consequently, the disease's symptoms and activity can greatly impact the health-related quality of life (HRQoL) of affected children [9,10]. Furthermore, medication side effects can contribute to additional pain and stress, further deteriorating the patient's overall well-being [11].

In this context, parent-/child-reported outcomes (PCROs) provide valuable insights into the disease's course and the perceived benefits of therapeutic interventions, aiding medical decision-making and improving patient care [12]. Among the available tools, the Juvenile Arthritis Multidimensional Assessment Report (JAMAR) questionnaire captures key PCROs in JIA, including overall well-being, functional status, HRQoL, and pain intensity [13,14]. It also assesses satisfaction with the current state of the illness through a binary final question [15,16]. The concept of patient acceptable symptom state (PASS) is particularly relevant, as it reflects the symptom threshold beyond which health status is considered satisfactory by children with JIA and their parents (JA-CASS and JA-PASS, respectively) [17].

PASS is a relatively recent concept that captures the patient's perception of being well [18], and it has been increasingly adopted across various medical disciplines, including orthopedics and rheumatology [19,20]. Its ease of use and strong association with healthcare outcomes make it a a valuable tool for evaluating treatment response on an individual level. As such, PASS should be considered a meaningful treatment target when balancing the benefits and risks of different therapeutic interventions [17]. However, PASS estimates may vary across different populations, even among individuals with the same condition [20].

While the impact of JIA on HRQoL and physical function has been extensively studied [6,21,22], there is limited research in the literature on patient and parent satisfaction [23]. Therefore, the objective of this cross-sectional study was to identify the clinical variables associated with JA-PASS using the JAMAR questionnaire in a specialized center in northern Italy.

2. Materials and Methods

2.1. Study Design and Patient Selection

Consecutive children diagnosed with JIA were recruited from those under follow-up at the Rheumatology Unit of Rivoli Hospital (Italy) between January 2020 and July 2022. Eligible patients were under 16 years of age, of both sexes, and diagnosed with any JIA subtype according to the ILAR criteria [4]. Patients with cognitive impairment and chronic conditions that could affect HRQoL or pain perception were excluded. They were also excluded if their parents lacked sufficient fluency in Italian to understand and complete the JAMAR questionnaire. Written informed consent was provided by parents/guardians prior to enrollment, and assent was obtained from participants as appropriate for their age. The study was conducted in accordance to the principles of the Helsinki Declaration, as revised in 2013, and was approved by the Institutional Ethics Committee. Reporting complied with the STROBE guidelines for cross-sectional studies.

2.2. Instrument

A parent (mother or father) or legal guardian of each enrolled patient was asked to complete the cross-culturally adapted and validated Italian parent version of the JAMAR questionnaire prior to a clinical visit [24]. The JAMAR is a multidimensional assessment tool consisting of 15 sections. For the purposes of this study, in addition to the question on the degree of satisfaction with the present child's disease status (with yes or no response), corresponding to the JA-PASS, data from 7 of the 15 original domains were utilized. They included the following: (1) physical function measured through the 15-item Juvenile Arthritis Functionality Scale (JAFS) [25], which rates the child's ability to perform daily tasks on a Likert scale (from 0 = without difficulty to 3 = unable to do), with total score ranging from 0 to 45; (2) HRQoL assessment using the 10-item Pediatric Rheumatology Quality of Life Scale (PRQL) questionnaire [26], organized into two subdimensions [physical health (PhH) and psychosocial health (PsH)]. Each consists of 5 items, with a scoring total from 0 to 15, with higher scores indicating worse HRQoL; (3) pain intensity graded using a visual analog scale (VAS), with scores ranging from 0 (no pain) to 10 (worst scenario) [27]; (4) degree and duration of morning stiffness; (5) perception of disease activity graduated from 0 (no activity) to 10 (maximum activity) on a VAS scale; (6) assessment of well-being on the VAS (from 0 = very well to 10 = very bad); and (7) degree of school difficulties caused by the disease, including difficulty attending school, inability to sit for extended periods, disagreement with teachers, or problems performing well.

2.3. Additional Information

The following information was collected from the patient's medical records: demographic characteristics, disease-related variables such as JIA category, positivity for antinuclear antibody (ANA), RF, presence of human leukocyte antigen (HLA) B27 (HLA-B27) and B51 (HLA-B51), age at disease onset, age at visit, disease duration, and disease-activity parameters including the number of active and limited joints as assessed by the physician. Disease status (remission, continued activity, or flare) and current use of medication (type of medication, treatment adhesion, side effects) were also recorded. The involvement of the temporomandibular joint was assessed by an experienced dentist.

2.4. Data Analysis

The primary outcome of the study was satisfaction with child's disease status. Thus, parents/caregivers were divided in two groups based on positive/negative JA-PASS according to the JAMAR questionnaire.

Data were all anonymously collected, analyzed, and published as aggregates. Quantitative data were reported using the mean value and standard deviation or the median and interquartile range (IQR). Categorical data were summarized using absolute and relative frequencies. The normality of continuous variables was verified with the Shapiro–Wilk test. For the comparison of quantitative variables between the two groups, the Student's *t*-test for independent samples or the non-parametric Mann–Whitney test were applied according to their normal/non-normal distribution. Categorical variables were analyzed using the chi-square test or Fisher's exact test, as appropriate.

A multiple logistic regression model was built to identify predictors of positive JA-PASS using a stepwise backward selection procedure. All potential explanatory variables that were significantly associated with the outcome in univariate models were entered in the multivariate logistic regression analysis. The results were presented as odds ratio (OR) with 95% confidence interval (CI). Finally, the area under the receiver operating characteristic curve (AUC) of the best-fitting model was used as an indicator of its predictive ability.

A p-value of 5% was set for statistical significance. All statistical tests were 2-sided and were performed using SPSS statistical package version 28 (IBM, Chicago, IL, USA).

3. Results

3.1. Patient Characteristics

Sixty-three consecutive children with JIA, with a mean age of 12.2 ± 3.7 years, were enrolled in the study. Of these, 43 (68.3%) were girls. A parent of each patient, consisting of 44 mothers and 19 fathers, completed the JAMAR questionnaire. As reported in Figure 1, the majority of children (57.1%) had oligoarticular JIA, followed by polyarticular (12.7%) and psoriatic disease subtypes (7.9%).

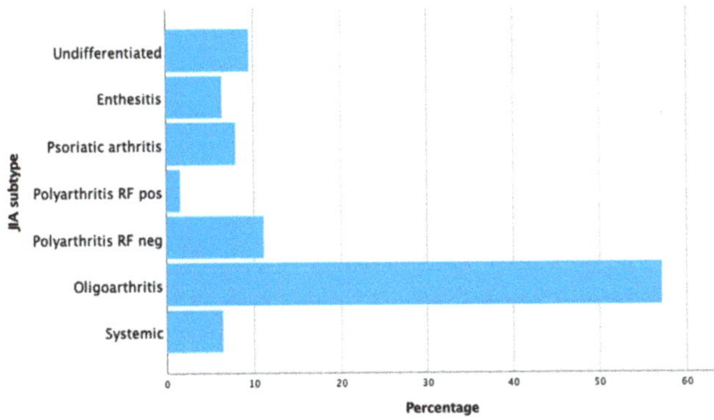

Figure 1. Frequency distribution by juvenile idiopathic arthritis subtype.

The child's demographic and clinical characteristics, along with disease-related measures and JAMAR domain scores, are presented in Table 1. The mean disease duration was 6.0 ± 3.8 years. The presence of ANA was found in 46% (n = 29) of individuals, while 6.3% (n = 4) tested positive for HLA-B27. The median active joint count was 0 (IQR 0–2). Fever and skin rashes were observed in only two children.

Table 1. Demographic and disease severity characteristics of children with JIA at enrolment.

Variables	N = 63
Patient's characteristics	
Sex female, n (%)	43 (68.3)
JIA subtypes, n (%)	
Oligoarthritis	36 (57.1)
Polyarthritis, RF positive	1 (1.6)
Polyarthritis, RF negative	7 (11.1)
Psoriatic arthritis	5 (7.9)
Enthesitis-related arthritis	4 (6.3)
Systemic arthritis	4 (6.3)
Undifferentiated arthritis	6 (9.6)
ANA positive, n (%)	29 (46.0)
HLA-B27 positive, n (%)	4 (6.3)
HLA-B51 positive, n (%)	1 (1.6)
Age at disease onset, mean (SD), years	6.0 (3.8)
Disease duration, mean (SD), years	6.1 (3.3)
Drug therapy	
Medication intake, n (%)	40 (63.5)

Table 1. *Cont.*

Variables	N = 63
Type of medication, n (%)	
NSAIDS	6 (9.5)
Glucocorticoids	4 (6.3)
bDMARDS (TNFi)	10 (15.9)
MTX	21 (33.3)
MTX + TNFi	6 (9.5)
bDMARDS (non-TNFi)	2 (3.2)
None	23 (36.5)
Side effects, n (%)	27 (47.9)
Active joints, median (IQR)	0 (0–2)
TMJ pain, n (%)	25 (39.7)
TMJ stiffness, n (%)	24 (38.1)
Morning stiffness over the past week by JAMAR report, n (%)	19 (30.2)
JAFS, median (IQR)	2.0 (0.0–3.0)
PhH, median (IQR)	1.0 (0.0–2.0)
PsH, median (IQR)	2.0 (0.0–4.0)
VAS pain, median (IQR)	1.5 (0.0–4.3)
VAS disease activity, median (IQR)	1.0 (0.0–5.0)
VAS well-being, median (IQR)	2.0 (1.0–3.6)
School difficulties, n (%)	17 (27.0)

JIA: juvenile idiopathic arthritis; ANA: antinuclear antibody; RF: rheumatoid factor; NSAIDS: non-steroidal inflammatory drugs; MTX: methotrexate; bDMARDS: biological disease-modifying antirheumatic drugs; TNFi: tumor necrosis factor inhibitor; SD: standard deviation; IQR: interquartile range; TMJ: temporomandibular joint; JAFS: Juvenile Arthritis Functionality Scale; PhH: physical health; PsH: psychological health; VAS: visual analog scale.

Methotrexate and tumor necrosis factor inhibitor agents were the most commonly used drugs, either as monotherapy or in combination. Nearly half of the patients experienced side effects, with nausea, gastritis, and vomiting being the most frequently reported. However, all parents declared children adhering to their prescribed medication regimen.

3.2. Assessment of JA-PASS Status

The majority of the parents (55.6%) were satisfied with their child's current disease condition according to the JA-PASS. Demographic and disease-related characteristics of positive/negative JA-PASS are separately shown in Table 2.

Table 2. Demographic and disease severity characteristics stratified by JA-PASS.

Variables	JA-PASS Positive (n = 35)	JA-PASS Negative (n = 28)	*p* Value
Father, n (%)	15 (42.9)	4 (14.3)	0.026
Patient's characteristics			
Sex female, n (%)	21 (60.0)	22 (78.6)	0.173
JIA subtypes, n (%)			0.004
Oligoarthritis	27 (77.1)	9 (32.2)	
Poliarthritis	2 (5.7)	6 (21.4)	
Systemic arthritis—ERA	2 (5.7)	6 (21.4)	
Others	4 (11.5)	7 (25.0)	
Age at visit, mean (SD), years	11.7 (3.5)	12.6 (4.0)	0.321
Age at disease onset, mean (SD), years	5.3 (3.4)	6.9 (4.1)	0.090
Disease duration, mean (SD), years	5.7 (3.7)	6.3 (3.0)	0.436
Drug therapy			
Medication intake, n (%)	17 (48.6)	23 (82.1)	0.015
Side effects, n (%)	3 (8.6)	24 (85.7)	<0.001
Disease severity			
Current disease state, n (%)			<0.001
Disease activity	2 (5.7)	19 (67.9)	

Table 2. *Cont.*

Variables	JA-PASS Positive (n = 35)	JA-PASS Negative (n = 28)	*p* Value
Relapse	0 (0.0)	4 (14.3)	
Remission	33 (94.3)	5 (17.9)	
Active joints, median (IQR)	0.0 (0.0–0.0)	1.0 (0.0–2.0)	<0.001
TMJ pain, n (%)	9 (25.7)	16 (57.1)	0.011
TMJ stiffness, n (%)	5 (14.3)	19 (67.9)	<0.001
Morning stiffness by JAMAR report, n (%)	10 (28.6)	9 (32.1)	0.756
JAFS, median (IQR)	0.0 (0.0–1.5)	3.0 (2.0–4.0)	<0.001
PhH, median (IQR)	0.0 (0.0–1.0)	2.0 (2.0–3.0)	<0.001
PsH, median (IQR)	0.0 (0.0–1.3)	4.0 (3.3–5.8)	<0.001
VAS pain, median (IQR)	0.0 (0.0–1.0)	4.0 (1.6–6.0)	<0.001
VAS disease activity, median (IQR)	0.0 (0.0–0.0)	5.0 (2.1–7.0)	<0.001
VAS well-being, median (IQR)	3.0 (2.0–5.0)	1.0 (0.0–2.0)	<0.001
School difficulties, n (%)	3 (8.6)	14 (50.0)	0.001

JIA: juvenile idiopathic arthritis; SD: standard deviation; IQR: interquartile range; TMJ: temporomandibular joint; JAFS: Juvenile Arthritis Functionality Scale; PhH: physical health; PsH: psychological health; VAS: visual analog scale.

A negative JA-PASS was significantly associated with specific JIA types, with a higher prevalence of ERA, systemic arthritis, and polyarticular arthritis ($p = 0.004$). However, no associations were found between the JA-PASS and patients' demographic characteristics, although a higher proportion of fathers reported satisfaction than mothers ($p = 0.026$). The duration of the disease or age at diagnosis appeared to have no impact.

Conversely, active disease state, current medication intake, and drug side effects were reported more frequently among participants whose parents expressed dissatisfaction with the child's JIA condition. Regarding the JAMAR domains, as displayed in Figure 2, statistically significant differences were found between parents with positive and negative JA-PASS in terms of functional ability, physical and psychosocial health, pain level, and child's current well-being. Parents of children with a negative JA-PASS reported worse scores across all these items (all $p < 0.001$).

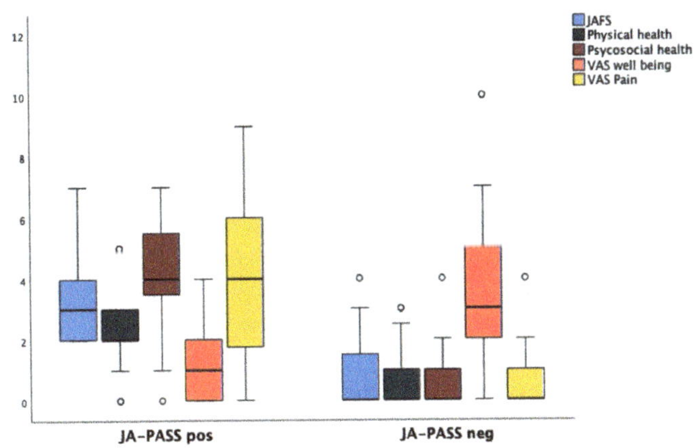

Figure 2. Parents' score in the JAMAR domains grouped by positive or negative JA-PASS (box and whisker plots).

With the exception of four cases, all parents in the positive JA-PASS group rated the severity of disease activity as 0, whereas none of the parents in the negative JA-PASS group reported a severity score of 0 ($p < 0.001$).

3.3. Variables Associated with JA-PASS

In the stepwise logistic regression model (Table 3), the child's current illness status (OR = 0.024, $p = 0.009$), the presence of at least one medication side effect (OR = 0.054, $p = 0.033$), and a higher psychosocial well-being rating on the JAMAR questionnaire (OR = 0.443, $p = 0.048$) were identified as the most significant independent variables associated with a negative JA-PASS. Other predictors that were statistically significant in the univariate analysis were no longer significant contributors to the model. The AUC value for the final regression model was 0.97 (95% CI 0.95–0.99).

Table 3. Multiple logistic regression model with a positive JA-PASS status as dependent variable ($R^2 = 0.897$).

Variables	Odds Ratio (95% CI)	p Value
Intercept	124.399	
Current disease state (activity or relapse vs. remission)	0.024 (0.001–0.389)	0.009
Psychosocial well-being, points	0.443 (0.199–0.984)	0.048
Presence of drug side effects (yes vs. no)	0.054 (0.004–0.785)	0.033

4. Discussion

Juvenile idiopathic arthritis is a clinically heterogeneous disease, characterized by wide variability in presentation and disease course, often leading to significant impairment in quality of life [1]. Its impact is influenced not only by physical symptoms but also by parents' perceptions of disease progression and treatment effectiveness [5]. This cross-sectional study aimed to identify factors influencing parental satisfaction with the treatment of JIA in a cohort of pre-adolescent children. Key contributors to parental satisfaction included the child's current disease activity, medication side effects, and psychosocial well-being, as measured by the JAMAR questionnaire. A stepwise logistic regression model identified these variables as significant predictors, yielding an AUC of 0.97.

Assessing overall quality of life in children with JIA requires consideration of multiple complex and interrelated factors. The JAMAR is regarded as a gold-standard tool for evaluating these complexities, as it allows for a comprehensive assessment of the child's symptoms, addressing both physical and psychosocial domains [15]. Additionally, the JA-PASS score, which is a component of the broader JAMAR tool, assesses parental perspectives on treatment effectiveness and whether they perceive their child's current health status as acceptable [17]. Although it consists of a global dichotomized simple question, it has a good construct/discriminative validity, yielding a positive association with disease activity and severity [17,23,28]. Nevertheless, aspects such as emotional burden, coping mechanisms, or dissatisfaction with specific elements of care may not be fully addressed by the current structure of the questionnaire. These limitations should be taken into account in future research efforts aimed at improving the JAMAR questionnaire.

This study, conducted on 63 children in Italy, predominantly female, found oligoarticular JIA to be the most common disease subtype. A median active joint count of zero, along with a high proportion of children in remission at the time of evaluation, indicates a relatively low overall disease burden. These findings suggest that the study population is well-positioned to achieve and sustain an optimal HRQoL.

In line with previous studies [17,23], more than half of the parents (55.6%) expressed satisfaction with their child's disease condition, despite significant side effects associated with standard medications such as methotrexate and tumor necrosis factor inhibitors [1,9]. Nevertheless, adherence to prescribed treatments remained high, even in the presence of common adverse effects such as nausea, gastritis, and vomiting. This highlights the substantial burden of managing treatment-related side effects, which adds to the challenges faced by families coping with JIA. While parents acknowledge that no treatment is without risk and appreciate the importance of therapy, their dissatisfaction often arises from adverse reactions that are perceived as intolerable. Addressing these concerns through a more individualized approach to JIA management, which carefully balances the benefits of treatment with its potential adverse effects, may enable healthcare providers to improve the overall treatment framework.

A key finding in this study is the strong influence of disease activity on parental satisfaction. Dissatisfaction was significantly associated with more severe disease presentations, particularly among patients with ERA, systemic arthritis, and polyarticular JIA. These subtypes are often linked to higher disease activity and greater functional impairment, which likely contribute to increased parental concern [1]. Consequently, a reduction in disease activity is strongly correlated with improved parental perceptions of treatment effectiveness and their child's overall well-being. Notably, when children with JIA achieve disease remission, parents report higher satisfaction with care and enhanced quality of life for their children [20]. These findings underscore the importance of achieving and sustaining disease remission as the central goal in JIA treatment [21].

Furthermore, the present study further highlights the significant role of psychosocial well-being in shaping parental satisfaction. Parents of children who reported better psychosocial scores on the JAMAR questionnaire were more likely to express satisfaction with treatments. Although often underrecognized, the psychosocial impact of JIA emerges as a critical factor influencing the perceptions of both children and their families. Importantly, psychosocial stress is not only a consequence, but also a potential contributor to worse disease outcomes through mechanisms involving poor treatment adherence or amplifying symptoms' perception. Thus, effective management strategies should address not only physical symptoms, but also promote psychosocial well-being, as this is essential for the child's overall health and also for improving parental satisfaction with care.

The reliability of the assessment tools is supported by the finding that patients' demographic characteristics did not influence JA-PASS outcomes, suggesting that the tool is not biased by such factors. Interestingly, a higher proportion of fathers reported satisfaction compared to mothers ($p = 0.026$), highlighting the potential need for a parent-specific approach in future research. Previous studies have identified gender differences with respect to caregiving roles and illness perception. Mothers usually assume the role of primary caregivers and report significantly higher levels of parenting stress and depressive symptoms compared with fathers when caring children with chronic or rare diseases [29–31]. Moreover, mothers tend to focus more on the negative aspects of their children's chronic illnesses, whereas fathers are generally more accepting of their child's disease conditions [29,32]. Thus, developing a tailored questionnaire that independently captures the perspectives of both mothers and fathers could provide a more nuanced and comprehensive understanding of parental experience with JIA care.

While this study provides valuable insights into the factors influencing parental satisfaction with JIA care, some limitations should be acknowledged. First, the study was conducted on a relatively small, single-center, cohort of Italian children, all receiving care at the same hospital. Larger, multicenter studies are needed to validate these findings and to explore potential country variations. Additionally, longitudinal studies that follow patients over time would provide a deeper understanding of how parental satisfaction evolves in relation to changes in disease activity and treatment plans.

Furthermore, this analysis was limited to the items included in the JAMAR, excluding factors such as fatigue, which is a common and burdensome issue not captured by the tool. Future research should also explore the influence of additional factors, such as socioeconomic status and healthcare access, on parental satisfaction. These variables may affect families' ability to manage the disease, adhere to treatment protocols, and impact the quality of life for both children and parents [33]. Finally, exploring interventions aimed at improving psychosocial well-being and mitigating treatment-related side effects could help identify strategies that enhance overall treatment outcomes and satisfaction.

5. Conclusions

The present study shows that the JA-PASS provides valuable insight into parents' perceptions of disease progression and effectiveness of therapeutic interventions. Thus, it should be incorporated into patient assessment protocols in both routine clinical practice and clinical trials.

Despite the improvement in functional outcomes achieved in the last few years, about 44% of parents are still unsatisfied with the current state of their child's disease. The factors most strongly associated with parental dissatisfaction are child's current disease activity, psychosocial well-being, and medication side effects. These areas highlight key opportunities for improving medical management. If left unaddressed, parental dissatisfaction may contribute to therapy nonadherence and increased distress in patients. Thus, incorporating the questionnaire into medical decision-making could play a significant role in enhancing the quality of care for children with JIA. Although pain was not significantly associated with parents' dissatisfaction in the regression logistic model, the high VAS scores for pain perception suggest that there is also a need for improvement in children's pain control.

Author Contributions: Conceptualization, G.N.B. and F.R.; methodology, P.D. and F.R.; validation, G.N.B. and N.N.; formal analysis, F.F. and F.R.; investigation, P.M. and F.G.; data curation, F.F. and N.N.; writing—original draft preparation, F.F., N.N. and F.R.; writing—review and editing, G.N.B. and F.R.; supervision, G.N.B. All authors have read and agreed to the published version of the manuscript.

Funding: This research received no external funding.

Institutional Review Board Statement: The study was conducted in accordance with the Declaration of Helsinki, and approved by the Institutional Review Board of AOU Città della Salute e della Scienza of Turin (protocol n. 0038521, date of approval: 9 April 2019).

Informed Consent Statement: Informed consent was obtained from all parents/caregivers of all children involved in the study.

Data Availability Statement: The data presented in this study are available on request from the corresponding author due to ethical restriction.

Conflicts of Interest: The authors declare no conflicts of interest.

Abbreviations

The following abbreviations are used in this manuscript:

JIA	Juvenile idiopathic arthritis
ANA	Antinuclear antibody
RF	Rheumatoid factor
ERA	Enthesitis-related arthritis
NSAIDS	Non-steroidal inflammatory drugs
MTX	Methotrexate
bDMARDS	Biological disease-modifying antirheumatic drugs
TNFi	Tumoral necrosis factor inhibitor
SD	Standard deviation
IQR	Interquartile range

OR	Odds ratio
CI	Confidence interval
TMJ	Temporomandibular joint
JAFS	Juvenile Arthritis Functionality Scale
PhH	Physical health
PsH	Psychological health
VAS	Visual analog scale

References

1. Zaripova, L.N.; Midgley, A.; Christmas, S.E.; Beresford, M.W.; Baildam, E.M.; Oldershaw, R.A. Juvenile idiopathic arthritis: From etiopathogenesis to therapeutic approaches. *Pediatr. Rheumatol.* **2021**, *19*, 135. [CrossRef]
2. Thierry, S.; Fautrel, B.; Lemelle, I.; Guillemin, F. Prevalence and incidence of juvenile idiopathic arthritis: A systematic review. *Jt. Bone Spine* **2014**, *81*, 112–117. [CrossRef] [PubMed]
3. Marini, F.; Falcini, F.; Stagi, S.; Fabbri, S.; Ciuffi, S.; Rigante, D.; Matucci Cerinic, M.; Brandi, M.L. Study of vitamin D status and vitamin D receptor polymorphisms in a cohort of Italian patients with juvenile idiopathic arthritis. *Sci. Rep.* **2020**, *10*, 17550. [CrossRef] [PubMed]
4. Petty, R.; Southwood, T.R.; Manners, P.; Baum, J.; Glass, D.N.; Goldenberg, J.; He, X.; Maldonado-Cocco, J.; Orozco-Alcala, J.; Prieur, A.-M.; et al. International League of Associations for Rheumatology classification of juvenile idiopathic arthritis: Second revision, Edmonton, 2001. *J. Rheumatol.* **2004**, *31*, 390–392. [PubMed]
5. Onel, K.; Rumsey, D.G.; Shenoi, S. Juvenile idiopathic arthritis treatment updates. *Rheum. Dis. Clin. N. Am.* **2021**, *47*, 545–563. [CrossRef]
6. Martini, A. Are there new targets for juvenile idiopathic arthritis? *Semin. Arthritis Rheum.* **2019**, *49*, S1–S54. [CrossRef]
7. Welzel, T.; Winskill, C.; Zhang, N.; Woerner, A.; Pfister, M. Biologic disease modifying antirheumatic drugs and Janus kinase inhibitors in pediatric rheumatology—What we know and what we do not know from randomized controlled trials. *Pediatr. Rheumatol. Online J.* **2021**, *19*, 46. [CrossRef]
8. Selvaag, A.M.; Aulie, H.A.; Lilleby, V.; Flato, B. Disease progression into adulthood and predictors of long-term active disease in juvenile idiopathic arthritis. *Ann. Rheum. Dis.* **2016**, *75*, 190–195. [CrossRef]
9. Doeleman, M.J.H.; de Roock, S.; Buijsse, N.; Klein, M.; Bonsel, G.J.; Seyfert-Margolis, V.; Swart, J.F.; Wulffraat, N.M. Monitoring patients with juvenile idiopathic arthritis using health-related quality of life. *Pediatr. Rheumatol.* **2021**, *19*, 40. [CrossRef]
10. Chédeville, G.; McGuire, K.; Cabral, D.A.; Shiff, N.J.; Rumsey, D.G.; Proulx-Gauthier, J.P.; Schmeling, H.; Berard, R.A.; Batthish, M.; Soon, G.; et al. Parent-reported medication side effects and their impact on health-related quality of life in children with juvenile idiopathic arthritis. *Arthritis Care Res.* **2022**, *74*, 1567–1574. [CrossRef]
11. Hassan, S.; Wamithi, S.; Riang'a, R.M.; Migowa, A. Experiences among parents caring for children with juvenile idiopathic arthritis at a tertiary referral hospital in Kenya. *Front. Pediatr.* **2025**, *13*, 1443529. [CrossRef]
12. Lavallee, D.C.; Chenok, K.E.; Love, R.M.; Petersen, C.; Holve, E.; Segal, C.D.; Franklin, P.D. Incorporating patient-reported outcomes into health care to engage patients and enhance care. *Health Aff.* **2016**, *35*, 575–582. [CrossRef] [PubMed]
13. Taxter, A.J.; Wileyto, E.P.; Behrens, E.M.; Weiss, P.F. Patient-reported outcomes across categories of juvenile idiopathic arthritis. *J. Rheumatol.* **2015**, *42*, 1914–1921. [CrossRef] [PubMed]
14. Esi, M.M.; Carle, A.C. Measures of health status and quality of life in juvenile idiopathic arthritis. *Arthritis Care Res.* **2020**, *72* (Suppl. S10), 565–576. [CrossRef]
15. Filocamo, G.; Consolaro, A.; Schiappapietra, B.; Dalprà, S.; Lattanzi, B.; Magni-Manzoni, S.; Ruperto, N.; Pistorio, A.; Pederzoli, S.; Civino, A.; et al. A new approach to clinical care of juvenile idiopathic arthritis: The Juvenile Arthritis Multidimensional Assessment Report. *J. Rheumatol.* **2011**, *38*, 938–953. [CrossRef]
16. Bovis, F.; Consolaro, A.; Pistorio, A.; Garrone, M.; Scala, S.; Patrone, E.; Rinaldi, M.; Villa, L.; Martini, A.; Ravelli, A.; et al. Cross-cultural adaptation and psychometric evaluation of the Juvenile Arthritis Multi-Dimensional Assessment Report (JAMAR) in 54 languages across 52 countries: Review of the general methodology. *Rheumatol. Int.* **2018**, *38*, 5–17. [CrossRef]
17. Filocamo, G.; Consolaro, A.; Schiappapietra, B.; Ruperto, N.; Pistorio, A.; Solari, N.; Pederzoli, S.; Verazza, S.; Martini, A.; Ravelli, A. Parent and child acceptable symptom state in juvenile idiopathic arthritis. *J. Rheumatol.* **2012**, *39*, 856–863. [CrossRef]
18. Tubach, F.; Dougados, M.; Falissard, B.; Baron, G.; Logeart, I.; Ravaud, P. Feeling good rather than feeling better matters more to patients. *Arthr. Rheum.* **2006**, *55*, 526–530. [CrossRef]
19. De Wolff, L.; Vissink, A.; van Nimwegen, J.F.; van Zuiden, G.; Mossel, E.; Olie, L.; Stel, A.J.; Delli, K.; Verstappen, G.M.; Kroese, F.G.M.; et al. Patient Acceptable Symptom State (PASS) in patients with primary Sjögren's syndrome in daily clinical practice. *Clin. Exp. Rheumatol.* **2022**, *40*, 2303–2309. [CrossRef]

20. Daste, C.; Abdoul, H.; Foissac, F.; Lefèvre-Colau, M.M.; Poiraudeau, S.; Rannou, F.; Nguyen, C. Patient acceptable symptom state for patient-reported outcomes in people with non-specific chronic low back pain. *Ann. Phys. Rehabil. Med.* **2022**, *65*, 101451. [CrossRef]
21. Vanoni, F.; Suris, J.C.; Scheven-gete, A.V.; Fonjallaz, B.; Hofer, M. The difference of disease perception by juvenile idiopathic arthritis patients and their parents: Analysis of the JAMAR questionnaire. *Pediatr. Rheumatol.* **2016**, *14*, 2–5. [CrossRef]
22. Consolaro, A.; Ruperto, N.; Filocamo, G.; Lanni, S.; Bracciolini, G.; Garrone, M.; Scala, S.; Villa, L.; Silvestri, G.; Tani, D.; et al. Pediatric Rheumatology International Trials Organization (PRINTO). Seeking insights into the EPidemiology, treatment and Outcome of Childhood Arthritis through a multinational collaborative effort: Introduction of the EPOCA study. *Pediatr. Rheumatol.* **2012**, *10*, 39. [CrossRef] [PubMed]
23. Del Giudice, E.; de Roock, S.; Vastert, S.J.; Wulffraat, N.M.; Swart, J.F.; van Dijkhuizen, E.H.P. Patients' and parents' satisfaction to improve patient care in JIA: Factors determining acceptable symptom state measured with JAMAR. *Rheumatology* **2023**, *62*, 1920–1925. [CrossRef] [PubMed]
24. Consolaro, A.; Bovis, F.; Pistorio, A.; Cimaz, R.; De Benedetti, F.; Miniaci, A.; Corona, F.; Gerloni, V.; Martino, S.; Pastore, S.; et al. The Italian version of the Juvenile Arthritis Multidimensional Assessment Report (JAMAR). *Rheumatol. Int.* **2018**, *38* (Suppl. S1), S251–S258. [CrossRef] [PubMed]
25. Balay-Dustrude, E.; Shenoi, S. Current validated clinical and patient reported disease outcome measures in juvenile idiopathic arthritis. *Open Access Rheumatol.* **2023**, *15*, 189–200. [CrossRef]
26. Ford, J.P.; Soriano, E.R.; Andreu, M. Evaluation of the psychometric properties of the Functional Ability Scale in children with juvenile idiopathic arthritis. *Reumatol. Clin. (Engl. Ed.)* **2025**, *21*, 101802. [CrossRef]
27. Filocamo, G.; Davi, S.; Pistorio, A.; Bertamino, M.; Ruperto, N.; Lattanzi, B.; Consolaro, A.; Magni-Manzoni, S.; Galasso, R.; Varnier, G.C.; et al. Evaluation of 21-numbered circle and 10-centimeter horizontal line visual analog scales for physician and parent subjective ratings in juvenile idiopathic arthritis. *J. Rheumatol.* **2010**, *37*, 1534–1541. [CrossRef]
28. Salaffi, F.; Carotti, M.; Gutierrez, M.; Di Carlo, M.; De Angelis, R. Patient acceptable symptom state in self-report questionnaires and composite clinical disease index for assessing rheumatoid arthritis activity: Identification of cut-off points for routine care. *BioMed Res. Int.* **2015**, *2015*, 930756. [CrossRef]
29. Cardinali, P.; Migliorini, L.; Rania, N. The caregiving experiences of fathers and mothers of children with rare diseases in Italy: Challenges and social support perceptions. *Front. Psychol.* **2019**, *10*, 1780. [CrossRef]
30. Chu, S.-Y.; Wen, C.-C.; Weng, C.-Y. Gender differences in caring for children with genetic or rare diseases: A mixed-methods study. *Children* **2022**, *9*, 627. [CrossRef]
31. Matthews, A.; Lenz, K.R.; Peugh, J.; Copps, E.C.; Peterson, C.M. Caregiver burden and illness perceptions in caregivers of medically hospitalized youth with anorexia nervosa. *Eat. Behav.* **2018**, *29*, 14–18. [CrossRef] [PubMed]
32. Knafl, K.; Zoeller, L. Childhood chronic illness: A comparison of mothers' and fathers' experiences. *J. Fam. Nurs.* **2000**, *6*, 287–302. [CrossRef]
33. Kraft, P.; Kraft, B. Explaining socioeconomic disparities in health behaviors: A review of biopsychological pathways involving stress and inflammation. *Neurosci. Biobehav. Rev.* **2021**, *127*, 689–708. [CrossRef] [PubMed]

medicina MDPI

Review

Dietary Principles, Interventions and Oxidative Stress in Psoriasis Management: Current and Future Perspectives

Oana-Georgiana Vaduva [1], Aristodemos-Theodoros Periferakis [1,2,*], Roxana Elena Doncu [1], Vlad Mihai Voiculescu [1,3,*] and Calin Giurcaneanu [1,3]

1 Faculty of Medicine, "Carol Davila" University of Medicine and Pharmacy, 050474 Bucharest, Romania
2 Elkyda, Research & Education Centre of Charismatheia, 17675 Athens, Greece
3 Dermatology Department, Elias Emergency University Hospital, 011461 Bucharest, Romania
* Correspondence: theodoros.periferakis0920@stud.umfcd.ro (A.-T.P.); vlad.voiculescu@umfcd.ro (V.M.V.)

Abstract

Psoriasis is a chronic inflammatory autoimmune disease that causes significant deterioration of the quality of life, and due to its multifactorial causes, it is often difficult to manage. Apart from genetic and environmental components, an important part of its pathophysiology comprises an oxidative stress induction that the standard antioxidative mechanisms of the human body cannot compensate for. Moreover, in many psoriatic patients, there is a documented imbalance between antioxidant and pro-oxidative factors. Usually, psoriasis is evaluated using the Psoriasis Area and Severity Index (PASI) score. It has been demonstrated that dietary choices can lead to significant modification of PASI scores. Hypocaloric diets that are rich in antioxidants are highly effective in this regard, especially when focusing on vegetables and restricting consumption of animal-derived protein. Specific dietary regimens, namely the Mediterranean diet and potentially the ketogenic diet, are very beneficial, in the former case owing in large part to the omega-three fatty acids it provides and its ability to alter gut microbiome, a factor which seems to play a notable role in the pathogenesis of the disease. Another option is the topical application of vitamin D and its analogues, combined with corticosteroids, which can ameliorate the manifestations of psoriasis at the level of the skin. Finally, oral vitamin D supplementation has a positive impact on psoriatic arthritis and can mitigate the risk of associated comorbidities.

Keywords: psoriasis; nutrition; diet; oxidative stress; vitamin D; supplements

1. Introduction

In recent years there has been an increased incidence of autoimmune pathologies, and this has led to an heightened awareness of the associated morbidity as well as psychological and mental challenges. One of the most well-known autoimmune diseases is psoriasis, a complex chronic immune-mediated disease presenting with a variety of manifestations, of which the most prominent are usually the cutaneous ones, although other locations and systems may be affected as well [1–4].

Currently, it is estimated that psoriasis affects over 120 million people at a worldwide level, with incidence and prevalence showing great geographical variations [5]. Notably, it seems that higher-income countries and people of Caucasian ancestry are at higher risk of developing psoriasis [6]. The average prevalence is around 8% in the adult population [6], while, based on recent research results, the actual burden of disease is higher due to underdiagnosis of psoriasis-related morbidities like psoriatic arthritis [7]. The systemic inflammatory nature of the disease means that patients usually exhibit numerous comorbidities [8,9], which in turn decrease their quality of life [10–12]. The most common signs of the disease are red and scaly plaques, which usually cause some degree of itching and discomfort [13]; other comorbidities, of varying degrees of severity, are also associated with psoriasis [14].

While there is a genetic component in psoriasis, not all patients carrying the implicated genes will develop the disease. Perhaps the most prominent genetic associations at the moment are genes of the HLA complex [15]. It becomes therefore apparent that since genetic determinism alone cannot justify on its own the pathogenetic model, the onset of the disease must be related to environmental factors as well. It is also well established that the course and severity of the disease are influenced predominantly by environmental rather than intrinsic factors [16,17]. Another important contributing factor, based on recent research, is an increased amount of oxidative stress, which leads to the activation of a number of proinflammatory signalling pathways [18] (Figure 1).

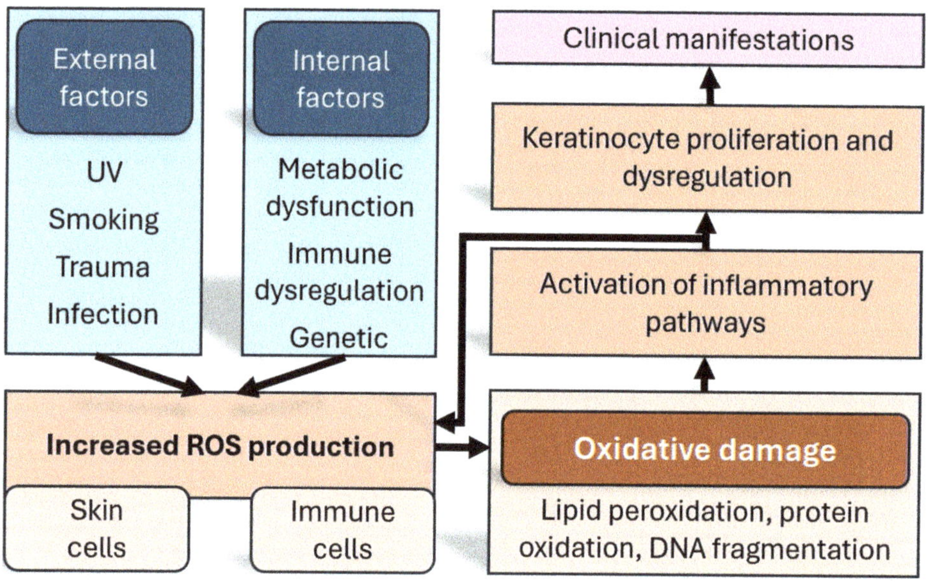

Figure 1. Schematic representation of the how oxidative stress affects inflammation, and the manifestations of psoriasis. ROS = reactive oxygen species. DNA = deoxyribonucleic acid.

One of the distinguishing features of psoriasis is the exaggerated production of reactive oxygen species (ROS) inside keratinocytes and immune cells [19]. The generated redox imbalance aggravates the inflammation via signalling pathways such as MAPK, STAT3, and NF-κB and contributes not only to local skin lesions but also to systemic comorbidities [20,21]. Cutaneous oxidative stress is generated in response to inflammatory cytokines such as IL-17 and TNF-α, leading to lipid peroxidation, protein oxidation, and DNA fragmentation; in contrast, systemic oxidative stress appears as an extension of the chronic inflammatory process beyond the skin, and the increased pro-inflammatory cytokine levels can negatively affect endothelial cells, leading to dysfunction [22,23].

Aside from medical interventions, the environmental factors implicated are psychological stress, substance and tobacco use and abuse, and diet. By themselves, these factors have been studied for decades by numerous researchers trying to establish causal relationships between diseases and risk factors. Indeed, physiological and psychological stress is now seen as being associated with both mortality and morbidity [24–26]. Smoking and excessive alcohol consumption have a host of research data demonstrating their importance as risk factors [27–32], while the role of diet in health maintenance and disease prevention has come into focus in the 21st century [33–38].

In the specific case of psoriasis, it seems that the principal associated comorbidity is obesity [39–43]. Obesity increases the risk of psoriasis incidence, while the cytokine profile in patients with metabolic syndrome and obesity and psoriatic patients is similar [44,45]. Obesity is more likely to develop in people following a sedentary lifestyle [46,47] and with high-fat diets [48,49]; dietary factors, both in the context of obesity and on their own, can modify disease progression and severity in the case of psoriasis.

In the last decades medical innovations have led to the development of novel therapeutic strategies [50]. Given the recent focus on the influence of nutrition and oxidative stress in psoriatic patients, the focus of this review will be the presentation of how diet, both from a quantitative and a qualitative perspective, influences the onset and severity of psoriasis, and via which mechanisms such influences are exerted.

2. Materials and Methods

In endeavoring to gather a complete and representative sample of research on psoriasis and nutrition, we have performed a thorough search in the most complete and widely used medical databases, namely PubMed, Scopus, Science Direct, and Medline. The search strategy relied on the terms "psoriasis", "diet", "obesity", "oxidative", "oxidants", "antioxidants", and "inflammation" in different combinations so as to cover as much probable relevant research material as possible, using the appropriate Boolean operators. For a paper to be considered as appropriate, the search terms should have to be included either in the title or abstract, preferably both. We tried different combinations of these keywords to ensure, as much as possible, the inclusion of all possible relevant papers, and we subsequently removed from our selection papers that did not exclusively deal with psoriasis but with oxidative stress in the context of autoimmune diseases. We have further excluded papers published in languages other than English, manuscripts not published in peer-reviewed journals, and those with a research question or patient population that were not relevant for our study.

Even though psoriasis was first described in modern medical terminology in the 18th century [51], the role of diet in its evolution and management began to be assessed after the 1950s, and research has only specifically focused on this aspect after 2010. Therefore, we have elected to confine our search to papers published between 2014 and 2024; the starting year has been selected specifically due to the relevant WHO resolution [52], which raised awareness of psoriasis and served as an impetus for intensifying research efforts. We have chosen to include, wherever possible, reviews that delve into mechanisms and associations, but where original papers reported essential or novel information, we have included them as well.

3. The Interplay Between Psoriasis and Nutrition

The profound influence of diet on human health and disease [53] has begun to be understood in the last decades [38,54]. At the same time, a notable majority of adults in the Western world suffer from at least one chronic disease, whose evolution and even risk of incidence may be associated with dietary factors [55,56].

At the same time, several different diet patterns have been implicated in the management of different diseases. For example, ketogenic diets may be useful in the management of neurological conditions [57]. Furthermore, nutritional supplementation may have potential in inflammatory biomarker control [58], and certain nutritional products may be useful in managing macular degeneration [59,60]. Other authors have focused on the role of gut microbiota in disease [61,62]. All these and other factors have been implicated in the incidence and management of psoriasis. As such, in this section, we will explore the role of oxidative stress, of diet and nutritional choices, of other supplements in general, and of vitamin D supplementation in particular.

3.1. The Role of Oxidative Stress in the Pathogenesis of Psoriasis

Oxidative stress can be defined as an imbalance manifesting as a temporary or chronic increase in the levels of free oxygen/nitrogen radicals resulting either from an increased production or a decrease in the ability of antioxidant systems to eliminate them [63], contributing to the pathogenesis of psoriasis.

Oxidative stress levels are measured by markers such as malondialdehyde (MDA), total oxidative stress (TOS), oxidative stress index (OSI), catalase (CAT), myeloperoxidase (MPO), ferroxidase (FOX), ischemia-modified albumin (IMA), paraoxonase-1 (PON-1), total antioxidant status (TAS), and 8-hydroxy 2′-deoxyguanosine (8H2D) [18,64]. Other useful markers include adipokines, namely adiponectin, leptin, visfatin, and resistin, due to their immunomodulating action [63,65], as well as urinary biopyrins [63,66]. There exist correlations between these markers and the severity of psoriasis, as measured by the Psoriasis Area and Severity Index (PASI) [18,63,66]; higher oxidative stress levels were associated with increased PASI scores. Out of all of them, the strongest correlation was found to exist between MDA levels and PASI, highlighting its potential as a biomarker for assessing psoriasis severity [67]. Thus, these findings support the theory that oxidative stress plays a crucial role in the development and complications of psoriasis.

Antioxidant enzymes, such as superoxide dismutase (SOD) and CAT, play a crucial role in reducing ROS levels, which are implicated in the pathogenesis of psoriasis [68–70]. A deficiency in these enzymes can lead to oxidative stress, contributing to inflammation and hyperproliferation of keratinocytes [43]. Therefore, maintaining or restoring the activity of these enzymes may offer therapeutic benefits in managing psoriasis symptoms [18].

In patients with active psoriasis, the levels of antioxidant enzyme levels, particularly SOD and CAT, are often reduced, indicating an impaired antioxidant defense system [18]. This deficiency can lead to increased oxidative stress, exacerbating inflammation and skin lesions associated with psoriasis. Consequently, monitoring and potentially restoring antioxidant enzyme levels may have therapeutic implications, offering a strategy to mitigate oxidative damage and improve disease management [18].

Another study emphasizes systemic inflammation through redox mechanisms, showing that oxidative stress associated with the development of psoriasis leads to oxidative protein changes, including a wide range of lipid peroxidation products [71]; the authors demonstrate that psoriasis-associated diseases can be effectively treated by inhibiting the formation of lipid peroxidation product–protein adducts and adjusting their concentrations during psoriasis therapy [71].

3.2. The Role of Diet in the Management of Psoriasis

Most studies agree that dietary patterns play a significant role in the management of psoriasis [40,70,72–80], as various skin diseases and conditions can be prevented or improved through changes in diet. Various dietary interventions, as well as single nutrients, can positively impact the clinical presentation, severity, and course of the disease [81]. Hypocaloric diets as well as antioxidant-rich diets can promote weight loss, reduce oxidative stress, and improve both the severity and the response of the condition to systemic treatments [40,73,76,82].

Since reducing caloric intake was found to alleviate symptoms [80,81], some forms of fasting, such as intermittent circadian fasting [74,83,84] and TRE (time-restricted eating) [78], may be promising in terms of their potential for symptom amelioration. This is in line with findings that suggest that intermittent fasting is associated with beneficial effects on autoimmune pathologies [74,83,84].

Generally, specialized diets, such as protein-restricted and vegetarian diets, may suppress systemic inflammation and inhibit angiogenesis [73], creating a less favorable environment for psoriasis. Diets rich in vegetables, with low or even zero animal protein intake, when combined with appropriate nutritional supplementation, seem to be associated with symptom amelioration in some patients, presumably due to their high fiber content and low saturated fat intake [73]. Although they may be wrongly characterized as risky for skin health due to nutritional deficiencies, such as lack of riboflavin (B2) and vitamin A, well-devised vegan diets can nevertheless meet nutritional needs and benefit inflammatory skin conditions like psoriasis, acne, and atopic dermatitis [85].

Elimination diets (e.g., gluten-free diet) may work for some patients, who report improvement by eliminating specific foods that may trigger flare-ups [82,86–88]. Common triggers include gluten-containing grains for those with gluten sensitivity or intolerance, dairy products, refined carbohydrates, nightshade vegetables (like tomatoes and potatoes), high-sugar foods, and processed foods [88]. However, these effects are individualistic; what triggers one person's condition may not affect another. Consequently, when it comes to the totality of psoriatic patients, the benefits of a gluten-free diet are indeterminate [81].

The Mediterranean diet, which is rich in fruits and vegetables, provides polyphenols and antioxidants that help combat oxidative stress. Antioxidants such as flavonoids, vitamins A, C, and E, and β-carotene, along with oligo-elements like copper, manganese, zinc, and selenium, may offer protective effects against intrinsic skin damage [89]. Interestingly, it has been suggested that this diet's beneficial effects can also be tied to changes in the gut microbiota [90]. Overall, greater adherence to the Mediterranean diet is linked to less severe forms of psoriasis and improved quality of life for patients [73,76,78,82,89,91,92]. The Mediterranean-like model tested by Castaldo et al. [93] on obese, drug-naïve patients in particular, consisting of a protein-sparing, very-low caloric ketogenic diet, resulted in notable alterations of PASI scores. While the Mediterranean diet sensu stricto may be considered culturally specific to the Mediterranean region, its basic tenets and principles may be applicable in a wide range of populations, irrespective of their nationality or residential region. The effectiveness of the Mediterranean diet, but also of the ketogenic diet, in affecting psoriatic activity and the associated inflammatory markers is also corroborated by Lambadiari et al. [94] and Katsimbri et al. [95]. It is worth mentioning, however, that the ketogenic diet has been reported to have both ameliorating and exacerbating effects on psoriasis [96]. Apart from the presence of ambiguous data on this matter, it should also be mentioned that ketogenic diets have a number of potential adverse effects, including nutrient deficiency, fatigue, increased LDL cholesterol, or other chronic diseases [97,98]; therefore, a careful risk-benefit assessment should be undertaken on a patient-by-patient basis.

At the opposite end of the spectrum, there are the high-fat diets, like the Western diet, which may exacerbate the cutaneous manifestations, particularly through the action of saturated fatty acids (SFAs), such as palmitic acid, due to enhancement of skin inflammation via immune activation, independent of obesity [78,99].

Thus, this kind of fatty acid should be avoided in order to reduce psoriasis-related inflammatory lesions at the level of the skin [72]. The opposite is true of unsaturated fatty acids, namely monounsaturated (MUFA) and polyunsaturated (PUFA) fatty acids, which have been found to be able to decrease the risk of immunometabolic diseases. MUFAs, such as oleic acid, which are found in extra-virgin olive oil, safeguard lipoproteins and cell membranes from detrimental oxidative damage. PUFAs are divided into omega-3 and omega-6 fatty acids. Patients should be encouraged to increase their intake of omega-3 fatty acids (found in fish, flaxseed, and walnuts) since they can reduce inflammation [67,76,89]. Conversely, omega-6 fatty acids (commonly found in processed foods and vegetable oils) are promoters of inflammation, and consumption of the associated food sources should be restricted [43]. A cross-sectional study focusing on patterns of food consumption in psoriasis patients illustrates this point by assessing Pattern 1, consisting mostly of processed foods, and Pattern 2, being made up predominantly of fresh foods. Compliance with Pattern 2 was linked to normal serum lipids and blood pressure, a lower waist-to-hip ratio, and decreased psoriasis (skin) activity [100]. In the same vein, Clark et al. [101] conclude that the supplementation of omega-3 fatty acids leads to improvement of PASI score, as well as of the erythema and scaling, though it remains uncertain whether they can help with other signs and symptoms, like desquamation and itching. The beneficial nature of omega-3 fatty acids is also supported by the fact that the Mediterranean diet, the effectiveness of which was described previously, has a favorable omega-3 to omega-6 ratio [40].

As far as specific dietary instructions are concerned, according to the United States National Institutes of Health Panel [102], the ideal ratio of omega-3 to omega-6 fatty acids should be approximately 1:1.80, though other reports place it at a range of 1:30 to 1:50 [103–105].

Natural antioxidants can be used to treat inflammatory diseases, including psoriasis. Because of its anti-inflammatory and antioxidant properties, it has been discovered that the natural phytocannabinoid oil has been suggested as a treatment for psoriasis [106].

Similarly, it has been discovered that cannabidiol (CBD) can provide considerable protection from UV-induced oxidative stress to skin cells [107,108], as, after applying CBD to psoriatic skin, there was a decrease in proinflammatory mediators and relevant proteins [107], and it induces metabolic alterations in keratinocytes [109]; other authors report a decrease in keratinocyte proliferation [103,108]. Furthermore, psoriatic arthritis patients report less pain when using CBD [75,108]. Although there is insufficient evidence to confirm this, other antioxidant and anti-inflammatory substances, such as the lipid extract of microalgae [69], are proposed as possible anti-psoriatic factors, their actions being based on preventing lipid peroxidation products from interacting with proteins. Regarding CBD, it must be stressed that this is not a risk-free substance, and a host of adverse effects have been reported [110]; at the same time, more clinical trials on its use in psoriasis patients must be designed, with the aim of elucidating the full spectrum of its therapeutical value and its benefit-to-adverse-effect ratio. We must note that the aforementioned CBD applications are mostly researched at a cellular level in vitro; however, based on these encouraging results, several authors have explored its possible use as a supplement [111,112].

Anti-inflammatory effects can be exerted by adhering to diets that include foods such as fruits, vegetables, whole grains, fatty fish (rich in omega-3 fatty acids), nuts, and seeds [85,87,89]. This is made possible due to their ability to assist in lowering oxidative stress and modulating immune responses, having been associated with lower levels of inflammation markers, such as C-reactive protein (CRP) [87].

As mentioned before, obesity is a known risk factor for psoriasis. This is because adipose tissue produces adipokines, the proinflammatory action of which is implicated in the pathophysiology of the condition, being able to bring about exacerbations [79]; hence, this is why they are useful as markers [63,65]. As such, it can be said that adipokines play a crucial role in the relationship between obesity, psoriasis, and nonalcoholic fatty liver disease (NAFLD); adiponectin, a hormone that promotes insulin sensitivity and fatty acid oxidation, is closely associated with both psoriasis and NAFLD [113]. Therefore, weight loss or weight management through any of the aforementioned balanced diet patterns can lead to a decrease in blood serum inflammatory factors and consequently to significant improvements in psoriatic symptoms [40,42,70,75,78,87]. Since high alcohol consumption and smoking are associated with increased severity of psoriasis [105,114], studies also show that reducing or excluding these substances can lead to improvements in skin health and overall well-being [80,87].

3.3. The Role of Vitamin D in the Management of Psoriasis

Vitamins play a significant role in the treatment of mild to moderate psoriasis. Currently, various vitamins and their analogues are employed to manage these forms of psoriasis, either administered individually or in combination with other medications [68]. Vitamins are essential in psoriasis treatment, with two primary therapeutic vitamins and their derivatives being vitamin A and vitamin D [68].

Vitamin D, also called the sunshine vitamin, is mainly produced by the skin upon exposure to UVB radiation [115]. It is then hydroxylated in the liver to form 25-hydroxyvitamin D, or 25(OH)D3, an inactive form of the vitamin, and undergoes further hydroxylation in the kidneys to produce the biologically active form of vitamin D, calcitriol, or 1,25(OH)D3. In order to ensure the required amount of vitamin D, it is necessary to expose the forearm for 15–20 min to UV sunrays. A major problem is advanced technology, which induces people to spend more and more time indoors, and this leads to a significant decrease in vitamin D levels [116,117].

There are two main forms of this vitamin, ergocalciferol (vitamin D2) and cholecalciferol (vitamin D3); only vitamin D3 is the bioactive form [118]. Few foods naturally contain vitamin D, and they are primarily of animal origin [118]. Vitamin D2 is produced by plants, but fruits and vegetables in the human diet contain only minimal amounts. The best sources of vitamin D2 are nuts, whole cereals, and vegetables. Mushrooms provide variable amounts of vitamin D2, which can be enhanced through ultraviolet light exposure under controlled conditions [119]. In contrast, vitamin D3 is naturally found in certain animal foods, particularly meat, egg yolk, butter, pork liver, and fatty fish such as salmon, herring, and mackerel, as well as in fish oils [118].

Additionally, vitamin D3 is available through dietary supplements and is the form present in vitamin D-fortified foods such as milk, orange juice, and cereals [118]. Fortification with vitamin D is considered a promising and impactful strategy [120]. The recommended daily dose of vitamin D3 for adults between 19 and 50 is 600 UI/day, while for adults over 60, the International Osteoporosis Foundation recommends 800–1000 UI per day [41].

Vitamin D's properties have been investigated for decades in the treatment of psoriasis [121], as it plays a crucial part in the maintenance of the homeostasis of the cutaneous barrier [118]. Various studies have explored the correlation between vitamin D-specific receptors and susceptibility to psoriasis [122,123]; it has been discovered that the A-1012G promoter polymorphism of the vitamin D receptor (VDR) gene is linked to an increased risk of psoriasis due to reduced expression of VDR mRNA, which may contribute to changes in the cutaneous barrier and the formation of psoriatic lesions [124]. Moreover, a reduced expression of VDR and decreased tight junction proteins are commonly observed on the skin of psoriatic patients [125,126]. Tight junctions are essential for regulating the adhesion and permeability of keratinocytes, polarizing cutaneous cell differentiation, and managing the extracellular calcium gradient. They interact with nuclear and cytoplasmic proteins and influence the regulation of specific genes involved in keratinocyte differentiation and proliferation [41]. Thus, maintaining the skin barrier homeostasis is essential for maintaining the tight junctions of epithelial and endothelial cells, which are under threat of being dysregulated due to psoriasis, and it reduces the pathological inflammatory response. As far as associated comorbidities are concerned, the study of Barrea et al. [41] suggests that vitamin D deficiency in psoriasis may be linked to both obesity and cardiovascular disease.

Topical vitamin D is commonly prescribed, either alone or with topical corticosteroids, for localized plaque psoriasis, showing good results [127]. Especially when combined with vitamin D analogues, corticosteroids are more effective and provide remission for longer periods of time when compared to monotherapy [94]. Those analogs are especially useful for sensitive areas like the face and do not lead to tolerance like corticosteroids do. They can be used indefinitely without serious side effects and are effective for both children and the elderly [41]. A recent analysis showed that topical vitamin D treatments have similar effectiveness to corticosteroids and even better results when combined with potent steroids, showing a "steroid-sparing" effect [118]. That being said, the findings of Ford et al. [81] suggest that oral vitamin D supplementation can help with psoriatic arthritis but not with the skin-related manifestations. In a similar vein, according to Formisano et al. [128], vitamin D supplementation does not affect PASI values in any notable way. Despite not affecting the PASI values, vitamin D deficiency is considered a risk factor for psoriasis [128], and, as mentioned earlier, while the cutaneous manifestations of psoriasis may be more concerning from the point of view of quality of life, other manifestations of the disease may benefit from such an intervention.

At any rate, in addition to its topical application, oral vitamin D supplementation serves as an important adjunctive treatment option for patients with psoriasis [118]. Secondly, vitamin D supplementation may play a crucial role in the prevention of psoriasis-related comorbidities, including hypertension [129] and metabolic syndrome [120], the latter being correlated with vitamin D deficiency [130]. Furthermore, its derivatives are capable of ameliorating the efficacy of phototherapy without causing any unwanted side effects [131].

3.4. The Role of Dietary Supplements in Psoriasis

Due to the potential side effects and benefits of simultaneous conventional and complementary and alternative medicine (CAM) practices, alternative or integrative therapies that may serve as substitutes or supplements to conventional treatment should be explored. The positive impact of macro- and micronutrient supplementation on improving psoriasis should be taken into account. The most frequently utilized oral dietary supplements among psoriasis patients are fish oil, selenium, and zinc [132]. Studies show that the evidence for zinc supplementation is controversial, yet supplements such as fish oil (omega-3 fatty acids) and selenium have been found beneficial for psoriasis patients. Results on the effectiveness of fish oil supplementation in psoriasis are ambivalent, with some reviews demonstrating a benefit [67] and some a lack of effectiveness [133]. The dosages varied, with the average being 4 g/day of eicosapentaenoic acid (EPA) and 2.6 g/day of docosahexaenoic acid (DHA). These supplements should be taken for an extended period (1–6 months) to achieve a noteworthy improvement in psoriasis. It was shown that consuming 6 ounces (170 g) of fatty fish daily improved psoriasis compared to the intake of white fish [67].

As for vitamin D, studies reveal that while topical vitamin D is effective [79,89] in counteracting inflammation at the skin level [79], oral supplementation is not recommended for psoriasis treatment in adults with normal vitamin D levels [73]. As mentioned before, vitamin D supplementation may be beneficial in selected cases, particularly in those with documented hypovitaminosis to prevent psoriasis-related comorbidities [76]. Topical application of phytoestrogens like genistein, present in soybeans, ameliorated the symptoms of psoriasiform dermatitis [99].

In addition, certain phytochemical compounds like *Dunaliella bardawil* (the richest known source of the antioxidant β-carotene), *Tripterygium wilfordii* (which contains bioactive triptolides and terpenoids), *Azadirachta indica* (the neem tree), and *Curcuma longa* (turmeric) are worth mentioning. Similarly, HESA-A is a compound produced in accordance with traditional Persian medicine, comprising mineral, herbal, and animal (marine shrimp) components, which has exhibited important benefits in clinical trials for improving psoriasis severity [73]. It is predominantly an herbal formulation, with all of its constituents being derived from the Apiaceae family; *Kelussia odoratissima* Mozaff. (wild celery) is paired with *Cuminum cyminum* L. (cumin), while *Apium graveolens* L. (cultivated celery) is paired with *Carum carvi* (*C. carvi*) L. (wild cumin) [73]. While more research is required in such traditional medical schemes, from the point of view of documenting their efficacy and their dosage and toxicity profiles, specifically in the case of HESA-A, there is a host of data documenting its use in certain pathological states [134,135].

Finally, prebiotics and probiotics may help by reducing lipopolysaccharide production and promoting a healthy gut microbiota, which can decrease inflammation [76,89,99,136–138].

4. Discussion

From all the aforementioned, it is evident that there exist numerous extrinsic factors that can be modified in the context of psoriasis management. Perhaps the most important aspect, from the point of view of pathophysiology and inflammation, is oxidative stress. Oxidative stress, which can be caused by numerous factors [139–142], is under research for its importance in several different pathologies [143]. Based on current evidence, in psoriatic patients there is an impairment of most antioxidant mechanisms [18], and the adjustment of lipid peroxidation may lead to improved outcomes [71]. Regarding the role of diet, there are several interventions that can contribute to more favorable outcomes, such as phytocannabinoid oil intake [106], reduced calorie intake, or elimination diets; specialized diets may be of benefit for some patients (Table 1).

Table 1. Dietary and nutritional interventions and supplements, and their effects on psoriatic patients, and some foods or dietary patterns that aggravating the disease are also presented.

Type of Intervention/Diet Scheme	Results	Year	Reference
General Diet and Weight Loss Interventions			
Weight loss via caloric restriction or surgery	Improvement of disease status in many patients in conjunction with standard medical treatment	2014	[42]
Weight loss via caloric restriction and increase in unsaturated fats and antioxidant intake	Improvement of disease status and general health condition of patients	2015	[114]
Weight loss via different diet patterns	Increase in drug pharmacokinetics and efficiency and general improvement of patient condition	2016	[40]
Weight loss via different diet patterns	Increase in treatment efficacy and improvement in the cardiovascular profile of the patients	2016	[113]
Weight loss via diet modifications and a healthy lifestyle	Improvement in PASI scores	2018	[73]
Weight loss via caloric restriction in overweight or obese patients	Probability of reduction in disease severity	2018	[81]
Gluten-free diet only in patients with a proven gluten sensitivity	Probably improvement in patient state		

Table 1. *Cont.*

Type of Intervention/Diet Scheme	Results	Year	Reference
Intermittent circadian fasting	Positive impact on psoriasis and psoriatic arthritis	2019	[74]
Adherence to a Mediterranean diet scheme	Decrease in a subjective and objective severity of psoriasis	2019	[91]
Predominance of fresh instead of processed foods in diet	Lower skin disease activity in many patients	2020	[100]
Weight loss and adoption of the Mediterranean diet patterns	Decrease of inflammation and improvement in patient state	2021	[95]
Adoption of the Mediterranean diet	Improvement in patient status in conjunction with standard medical treatment	2022	[76]
Adoption of the Mediterranean diet	Decreased severity of psoriasis and psoriatic arthritis	2023	[82]
Intermittent fasting patterns	Possible effects in psoriasis and other autoimmune disorders of inflammatory nature	2023	[84]
Adoption of the Mediterranean diet	Potential anti-inflammatory benefit	2024	[92]
Combination of ketogenic and Mediterranean diets	Reduction of inflammatory and disease markers	2024	[94]
Nutritional Supplementation			
Supplementation with Zn, Se, Ω3, HESA-A, and other botanical species	Various benefits in psoriatic patients (depending on the supplements, patient condition, etc.)	2018	[73]
Intake of proanthocyanidins (along with possible topical application)	Possible correction of Th17/Treg cell imbalances, keratinocyte overproliferation, and angiogenesis	2018	[87]
Ω3 supplementation	Improvement of disease parameters in psoriatic patients	2019	[101]
Supplementation with oral probiotics	Potential benefits in conjunction with standard medical therapy	2022	[76]
Vitamin D Supplementation			
Oral vitamin D supplementation in deficient patients	Prevention of psoriasis-related comorbidities	2018	[73]
Oral vitamin D supplementation in conjunction with weight loss	Possible benefits to patients status if used along with standard medical treatment	2018	[81]
Local In Vitro Cannabidiol Applications			
Cannabidiol application in irradiated keratinocytes	Reduction of oxidative stress in cells isolated from healthy individuals—possible protective effect	2020	[109]
Cannabidiol application in 3D-cultured keratinocytes	Protective effect of cannabidiol against irradiation	2021	[107]
Cannabidiol application in irradiated keratinocytes	Possible protective effect against irradiation	2021	[108]
Aggravation of Psoriasis			
Increased alcohol consumption	Increased severity of psoriasis manifestations	2017	[105]
Increased saturated fatty acid intake	Increase of skin inflammation	2018	[72]
Increased BMI	Increased chances of psoriasis incidence	2019	[83]
Western-style diet, rich in sugars and fats	Promotion of a pro-inflammatory state possibly due to gut microbiota dysregulation	2021	[75]
Western-style diet, rich in sugars and fats	Immune aberration in the production of pro-inflammatory cytokines	2021	[95]
Poor dietary habits and alcohol abuse	Increased chance of psoriasis incidence or increase in disease severity	2023	[80]

Probably the most important role may be that of substances, phytochemicals in particular, which have concurrent antioxidant and anti-inflammatory properties; some such compounds have already been explored as a potential management solution [73]. Other such phytochemicals may be tried in the management of psoriasis, like kaempferol [144,145], pinosylvin [146], compounds derived from black pepper [147,148], capsaicin [149,150], and thymol [151]. Other recent concepts concern the role of probiotics and of gut microbiota in inflammation and disease [75,137,152,153]; the modification of gut microbiota may be useful in the management of psoriasis [136,154–157] and surely represents an interesting avenue for future research. Intestinal microbial dysbiosis has already been documented in psoriatic patients [158,159], while the dysregulation of the skin microbiome has also been proposed as a contributing factor [160].

In the introduction we have mentioned the influence of certain risk factors such as smoking and stress on mortality and morbidity. Stress and obesity are interconnected in many cases [161,162], and smoking often coexists with higher body mass index (BMI) [163,164], even though this relationship is not causal. Therefore, it can be seen that there is, most likely, an interplay between all these factors, directly or indirectly [165]; stress leads to psoriasis exacerbation [166], in turn leading to more stress [167], in a vicious cycle scheme. Therefore, the need for multidisciplinary management [168], including psychological management, in such patients becomes apparent. Similar multidisciplinary approaches have already been successfully tried in psoriatic arthritis [169,170]. Apart from such factors, the multidisciplinary aspect should be focused on other aspects such as joint involvement in psoriasis [171]; advanced modern concepts such as 3D printing applications [172–175] can be considered in such cases.

A proper diet and exercise regimen will lead, in the absence of other metabolic pathologies, to weight loss and the maintenance of a healthy physique. This is important when considering the interplay between obesity and inflammation [176,177]. Even in psoriatic patients, where there is persistent systemic inflammation, it follows that weight loss will be correlated with an improvement of disease status. Finally, the role of hormonal imbalances and treatment in psoriasis must be considered. In particular, hormonal imbalances may alter the presentation and clinical course of psoriasis [178,179], while hormonal treatment may be effective. For example, somatostatin treatment has been tried in the past with mixed results [180,181]; perhaps the use of more modern somatostatin analogs [182,183] should be more eagerly investigated in the future.

Even though the pathophysiology of psoriasis is extremely complex [184,185], there exists a host of modifiable factors that can influence its development, severity, and impact on quality of life. Altering dietary habits can greatly enhance the quality of life for patients, benefiting both psoriatic lesions and decreasing the likelihood of other associated diseases. Though there are no national or international guidelines recommending a specific nutritional approach to the management of psoriasis, several approaches may be tried based on the data reported in this review, either as a general rule or on an individualized patient-by-patient basis.

In considering the clinical significance of all the data herein presented, we must, at first, emphasize that while the data on the reduction of oxidative stress using dietary interventions are promising, in most cases there are additional steps which that be taken in order to obtain statistically significant correlations in wide and diverse patient samples. On the other hand, the wealth of encouraging data enables us to suggest that, pending further research, the implementation of dietary interventions in a patient-by-patient case may be of use at the moment. However, in certain cases, for example, when implementing ketogenic diet schemes or administering herbal or traditional supplements, the medical personnel should be mindful of potential adverse effects or toxicity.

The improvement in patient quality of life may be further increased by stress management and the elimination or reduction of other risk factors, which have already been presented. Modifying such factors, especially based on patient decision, may lead to self-empowerment, which can lead to better treatment outcomes [186,187].

5. Conclusions

It can be concluded that the management and clinical course of psoriasis, while in part depending on genetic factors, is mostly attributable to extrinsic factors. An important aspect of such factors is nutrition; in the context of nutrition, there are various approaches that have been tried, ranging from adopting different diet patterns to altering caloric intake or administering supplements. Perhaps the most crucial implicated factors, which can be modified by said interventions, are oxidative stress and obesity. Both are linked to and influence inflammation, which is arguably the most prominent component in the majority of psoriasis cases. Future studies should aim to expand on quantifying the influence of such factors in the management and quality of life of such patients and on examining the potential beneficial effects of other antioxidants, namely phytochemicals, in oral or topical administration.

Author Contributions: Conceptualization, O.-G.V., V.M.V. and C.G.; methodology, O.-G.V., A.-T.P. and R.E.D.; validation, O.-G.V. and A.-T.P.; formal analysis, O.-G.V., A.-T.P. and R.E.D.; investigation, O.-G.V. and A.-T.P.; resources, R.E.D., V.M.V. and C.G.; writing—original draft preparation, O.-G.V., A.-T.P., R.E.D., V.M.V. and C.G.; writing—review and editing, O.-G.V., A.-T.P. and R.E.D.; visualization, R.E.D., V.M.V. and C.G.; supervision, V.M.V. and C.G. All authors have read and agreed to the published version of the manuscript.

Funding: This research received no external funding.

Institutional Review Board Statement: Not applicable.

Informed Consent Statement: Not applicable.

Data Availability Statement: Not applicable.

Conflicts of Interest: The authors declare no conflicts of interest.

Abbreviations

The following abbreviations are used in this manuscript:

25(OH)D3	25-hydroxyvitamin D
8H2D	8-hydroxy 2′-deoxyguanosine
CAM	Complementary and alternative medicine
CAT	Catalase
CBD	Cannabidiol
CRP	C-reactive protein
DHA	Docosahexaenoic acid
EPA	Eicosapentaenoic acid
FOX	Ferroxidase
HLA	Human leucocyte antigen
IMA	Ischemia-modified albumin
MDA	Malondialdehyde
MPO	Myeloperoxidase
MUFA	Monounsaturated fatty acids
NAFLD	Nonalcoholic fatty liver disease
OSI	Oxidative stress index
PASI	Psoriasis area and severity index
PON-1	Paraoxonase-1
PUFA	Polyunsaturated fatty acids

SFAs	Saturated fatty acids
SOD	Superoxide dismutase
TAS	Total antioxidant status
TOS	Total oxidative stress
VDR	Vitamin D receptor
WHO	World Health Organization

References

1. Greb, J.E.; Goldminz, A.M.; Elder, J.T.; Lebwohl, M.G.; Gladman, D.D.; Wu, J.J.; Mehta, N.N.; Finlay, A.Y.; Gottlieb, A.B. Psoriasis. *Nat. Rev. Dis. Primers* **2016**, *2*, 16082. [CrossRef] [PubMed]
2. Schett, G.; Lories, R.J.; D'Agostino, M.A.; Elewaut, D.; Kirkham, B.; Soriano, E.R.; McGonagle, D. Enthesitis: From pathophysiology to treatment. *Nat. Rev. Rheumatol.* **2017**, *13*, 731–741. [CrossRef] [PubMed]
3. Haneke, E. Nail psoriasis: Clinical features, pathogenesis, differential diagnoses, and management. *Psoriasis* **2017**, *7*, 51–63. [CrossRef] [PubMed]
4. McGonagle, D.; Tan, A.L.; Watad, A.; Helliwell, P. Pathophysiology, assessment and treatment of psoriatic dactylitis. *Nat. Rev. Rheumatol.* **2019**, *15*, 113–122. [CrossRef] [PubMed]
5. Nicolescu, A.C.; Bucur, Ș.; Giurcăneanu, C.; Gheucă-Solovăstru, L.; Constantin, T.; Furtunescu, F.; Ancuța, I.; Constantin, M.M. Prevalence and characteristics of psoriasis in Romania—First study in overall population. *J. Pers. Med.* **2021**, *11*, 523. [CrossRef] [PubMed]
6. Parisi, R.; Symmons, D.P.; Griffiths, C.E.; Ashcroft, D.M. Global epidemiology of psoriasis: A systematic review of incidence and prevalence. *J. Investig. Dermatol.* **2013**, *133*, 377–385. [CrossRef] [PubMed]
7. Haroon, M.; Kirby, B.; FitzGerald, O. High prevalence of psoriatic arthritis in patients with severe psoriasis with suboptimal performance of screening questionnaires. *Ann. Rheum. Dis.* **2013**, *72*, 736–740. [CrossRef]
8. Takeshita, J.; Grewal, S.; Langan, S.M.; Mehta, N.N.; Ogdie, A.; Van Voorhees, A.S.; Gelfand, J.M. Psoriasis and comorbid diseases: Epidemiology. *J. Am. Acad. Dermatol.* **2017**, *76*, 377–390. [CrossRef]
9. Morariu, S.H.; Cotoi, O.S.; Tiucă, O.M.; Baican, A.; Gheucă-Solovăstru, L.; Decean, H.; Brihan, I.; Silaghi, K.; Biro, V.; Șerban-Pescar, D.; et al. Blood-Count-Derived Inflammatory Markers as Predictors of Response to Biologics and Small-Molecule Inhibitors in Psoriasis: A Multicenter Study. *J. Clin. Med.* **2024**, *13*, 3229. [CrossRef] [PubMed]
10. Gonzalez, J.; Cunningham, K.; Perlmutter, J.; Gottlieb, A. Systematic Review of Health-Related Quality of Life in Adolescents with Psoriasis. *Dermatology* **2016**, *232*, 541–549. [CrossRef] [PubMed]
11. Koo, J.; Marangell, L.B.; Nakamura, M.; Armstrong, A.; Jeon, C.; Bhutani, T.; Wu, J.J. Depression and suicidality in psoriasis: Review of the literature including the cytokine theory of depression. *J. Eur. Acad. Dermatol. Venereol.* **2017**, *31*, 1999–2009. [CrossRef] [PubMed]
12. Strober, B.; Karki, C.; Mason, M.; Guo, N.; Holmgren, S.H.; Greenberg, J.D.; Lebwohl, M. Characterization of disease burden, comorbidities, and treatment use in a large, US-based cohort: Results from the Corrona Psoriasis Registry. *J. Am. Acad. Dermatol.* **2018**, *78*, 323–332. [CrossRef] [PubMed]
13. Gao, Y.; Xu, T.; Wang, Y.; Hu, Y.; Yin, S.; Qin, Z.; Yu, H. Pathophysiology and Treatment of Psoriasis: From Clinical Practice to Basic Research. *Pharmaceutics* **2025**, *17*, 56. [CrossRef] [PubMed]
14. Nowowiejska, J.; Baran, A.; Grabowska, P.; Lewoc, M.; Kamiński, T.W.; Flisiak, I. Assessment of life quality, stress and physical activity among patients with psoriasis. *Dermatol. Ther.* **2022**, *12*, 395–406. [CrossRef] [PubMed]
15. Capon, F. The Genetic Basis of Psoriasis. *Int. J. Mol. Sci.* **2017**, *18*, 2526. [CrossRef] [PubMed]
16. Balato, N.; Di Costanzo, L.; Patruno, C.; Patrì, A.; Ayala, F. Effect of weather and environmental factors on the clinical course of psoriasis. *Occup. Environ. Med.* **2013**, *70*, 600. [CrossRef] [PubMed]
17. Zeng, J.; Luo, S.; Huang, Y.; Lu, Q. Critical role of environmental factors in the pathogenesis of psoriasis. *J. Dermatol.* **2017**, *44*, 863–872. [CrossRef] [PubMed]
18. Pleńkowska, J.; Gabig-Cimińska, M.; Mozolewski, P. Oxidative Stress as an Important Contributor to the Pathogenesis of Psoriasis. *Int. J. Mol. Sci.* **2020**, *21*, 6206. [CrossRef] [PubMed]
19. Wroński, A.; Wójcik, P. Impact of ROS-Dependent Lipid Metabolism on Psoriasis Pathophysiology. *Int. J. Mol. Sci.* **2022**, *23*, 12137. [CrossRef] [PubMed]
20. Xu, F.; Xu, J.; Xiong, X.; Deng, Y. Salidroside inhibits MAPK, NF-κB, and STAT3 pathways in psoriasis-associated oxidative stress via SIRT1 activation. *Redox Rep.* **2019**, *24*, 70–74. [CrossRef] [PubMed]
21. Wójcik, P.; Gęgotek, A.; Žarković, N.; Skrzydlewska, E. Oxidative Stress and Lipid Mediators Modulate Immune Cell Functions in Autoimmune Diseases. *Int. J. Mol. Sci.* **2021**, *22*, 723. [CrossRef] [PubMed]

22. Schaller, T.; Ringen, J.; Fischer, B.; Bieler, T.; Perius, K.; Knopp, T.; Kommoss, K.S.; Korn, T.; Heikenwälder, M.; Oelze, M.; et al. Reactive oxygen species produced by myeloid cells in psoriasis as a potential biofactor contributing to the development of vascular inflammation. *BioFactors* **2023**, *49*, 861–874. [CrossRef] [PubMed]
23. Karbach, S.; Croxford, A.L.; Oelze, M.; Schüler, R.; Minwegen, D.; Wegner, J.; Koukes, L.; Yogev, N.; Nikolaev, A.; Reißig, S.; et al. Interleukin 17 drives vascular inflammation, endothelial dysfunction, and arterial hypertension in psoriasis-like skin disease. *Arter. Thromb. Vasc. Biol.* **2014**, *34*, 2658–2668. [CrossRef] [PubMed]
24. Martens, W.J.M. Climate change, thermal stress and mortality changes. *Soc. Sci. Med.* **1998**, *46*, 331–344. [CrossRef] [PubMed]
25. Puttonen, S.; Härmä, M.; Hublin, C. Shift work and cardiovascular disease—Pathways from circadian stress to morbidity. *Scand. J. Work Environ. Health* **2010**, *36*, 96–108. [CrossRef] [PubMed]
26. Poulin, M.J.; Brown, S.L.; Dillard, A.J.; Smith, D.M. Giving to others and the association between stress and mortality. *Am. J. Public Health* **2013**, *103*, 1649–1655. [CrossRef]
27. Hammond, E.C. Smoking in Relation to Mortality and Morbidity. Findings in First Thirty-Four Months of Follow-Up in a Prospective Study Started in 19592. *JNCI J. Natl. Cancer Inst.* **1964**, *32*, 1161–1188. [CrossRef] [PubMed]
28. Poikolainen, K. Alcohol and mortality: A review. *J. Clin. Epidemiol.* **1995**, *48*, 455–465. [CrossRef] [PubMed]
29. Rehm, J.; Gmel, G.; Sempos, C.T.; Trevisan, M. Alcohol-related morbidity and mortality. *Alcohol. Res. Health* **2003**, *27*, 39–51. [PubMed]
30. White, W.B. Smoking-Related Morbidity and Mortality in the Cardiovascular Setting. *Prev. Cardiol.* **2007**, *10*, 1–4. [CrossRef] [PubMed]
31. Hingson, R.W.; Zha, W.; Weitzman, E.R. Magnitude of and trends in alcohol-related mortality and morbidity among US college students ages 18–24, 1998–2005. *J. Stud. Alcohol Drugs Suppl.* **2009**, 12–20. [CrossRef] [PubMed]
32. Carter, B.D.; Abnet, C.C.; Feskanich, D.; Freedman, N.D.; Hartge, P.; Lewis, C.E.; Ockene, J.K.; Prentice, R.L.; Speizer, F.E.; Thun, M.J. Smoking and mortality—Beyond established causes. *N. Engl. J. Med.* **2015**, *372*, 631–640. [CrossRef] [PubMed]
33. Sofi, F.; Abbate, R.; Gensini, G.F.; Casini, A. Importance of diet on disease prevention. *Int. J. Med. Med. Sci.* **2013**, *5*, 55–59.
34. Sakurai, M.; Nakamura, K.; Miura, K.; Takamura, T.; Yoshita, K.; Nagasawa, S.Y.; Morikawa, Y.; Ishizaki, M.; Kido, T.; Naruse, Y.; et al. Dietary carbohydrate intake, presence of obesity and the incident risk of type 2 diabetes in Japanese men. *J. Diabetes Investig.* **2016**, *7*, 343–351. [CrossRef] [PubMed]
35. Rosa, R.; Ornella, R.; Maria, G.C.; Elisa, S.; Maria, N.; Chiara, M.; Antonio, N.; Tiziana, M.; Gian, L.d.A.; Francesco, D.M. The role of diet in the prevention and treatment of Inflammatory Bowel Diseases. *Acta Biomed. Atenei Parm.* **2018**, *89*, 60.
36. Requena, T.; Martínez-Cuesta, M.C.; Peláez, C. Diet and microbiota linked in health and disease. *Food Funct.* **2018**, *9*, 688–704. [CrossRef] [PubMed]
37. Neuhouser, M.L. The importance of healthy dietary patterns in chronic disease prevention. *Nutr. Res.* **2019**, *70*, 3–6. [CrossRef] [PubMed]
38. Cena, H.; Calder, P.C. Defining a Healthy Diet: Evidence for the Role of Contemporary Dietary Patterns in Health and Disease. *Nutrients* **2020**, *12*, 334. [CrossRef] [PubMed]
39. Armstrong, A.W.; Harskamp, C.T.; Armstrong, E.J. The association between psoriasis and obesity: A systematic review and meta-analysis of observational studies. *Nutr. Diabetes* **2012**, *2*, e54. [CrossRef] [PubMed]
40. Barrea, L.; Nappi, F.; Di Somma, C.; Savanelli, M.C.; Falco, A.; Balato, A.; Balato, N.; Savastano, S. Environmental Risk Factors in Psoriasis: The Point of View of the Nutritionist. *Int. J. Environ. Res. Public Health* **2016**, *13*, 743. [CrossRef] [PubMed]
41. Barrea, L.; Savanelli, M.C.; Di Somma, C.; Napolitano, M.; Megna, M.; Colao, A.; Savastano, S. Vitamin D and its role in psoriasis: An overview of the dermatologist and nutritionist. *Rev. Endocr. Metab. Disord.* **2017**, *18*, 195–205. [CrossRef] [PubMed]
42. Debbaneh, M.; Millsop, J.W.; Bhatia, B.K.; Koo, J.; Liao, W. Diet and psoriasis, part I: Impact of weight loss interventions. *J. Am. Acad. Dermatol.* **2014**, *71*, 133–140. [CrossRef] [PubMed]
43. Garbicz, J.; Całyniuk, B.; Górski, M.; Buczkowska, M.; Piecuch, M.; Kulik, A.; Rozentryt, P. Nutritional Therapy in Persons Suffering from Psoriasis. *Nutrients* **2021**, *14*, 119. [CrossRef] [PubMed]
44. Katta, R.; Desai, S.P. Diet and dermatology: The role of dietary intervention in skin disease. *J. Clin. Aesthet. Dermatol.* **2014**, *7*, 46–51. [PubMed]
45. Katta, R.; Kramer, M.J. Skin and Diet: An Update on the Role of Dietary Change as a Treatment Strategy for Skin Disease. *Ski. Ther. Lett.* **2018**, *23*, 1–5.
46. Martínez-González, M.A.; Martínez, J.A.; Hu, F.B.; Gibney, M.J.; Kearney, J. Physical inactivity, sedentary lifestyle and obesity in the European Union. *Int. J. Obes. Relat. Metab. Disord.* **1999**, *23*, 1192–1201. [CrossRef] [PubMed]
47. Silveira, E.A.; Mendonça, C.R.; Delpino, F.M.; Elias Souza, G.V.; Pereira de Souza Rosa, L.; de Oliveira, C.; Noll, M. Sedentary behavior, physical inactivity, abdominal obesity and obesity in adults and older adults: A systematic review and meta-analysis. *Clin. Nutr. ESPEN* **2022**, *50*, 63–73. [CrossRef] [PubMed]

48. Black, M.H.; Watanabe, R.M.; Trigo, E.; Takayanagi, M.; Lawrence, J.M.; Buchanan, T.A.; Xiang, A.H. High-fat diet is associated with obesity-mediated insulin resistance and β-cell dysfunction in Mexican Americans. *J. Nutr.* **2013**, *143*, 479–485. [CrossRef]
49. Wang, L.; Wang, H.; Zhang, B.; Popkin, B.M.; Du, S. Elevated Fat Intake Increases Body Weight and the Risk of Overweight and Obesity among Chinese Adults: 1991–2015 Trends. *Nutrients* **2020**, *12*, 3272. [CrossRef] [PubMed]
50. Periferakis, A.; Bolocan, A.; Ion, D. A review of innovation in medicine. *Technol. Innov. Life Sci.* **2022**, *1*, 42–48. [CrossRef]
51. Meenan, F.O. A note on the history of psoriasis. *Ir. J. Med. Sci.* **1955**, *30*, 141–142. [CrossRef] [PubMed]
52. Sommer, R.; Mrowietz, U.; Radtke, M.A.; Schäfer, I.; von Kiedrowski, R.; Strömer, K.; Enk, A.; Maul, J.-T.; Reich, K.; Zander, N.; et al. What is psoriasis?—Perception and assessment of psoriasis among the German population. *JDDG J. Dtsch. Dermatol. Ges.* **2018**, *16*, 703–710. [CrossRef] [PubMed]
53. Xiao, Y.-L.; Gong, Y.; Qi, Y.-J.; Shao, Z.-M.; Jiang, Y.-Z. Effects of dietary intervention on human diseases: Molecular mechanisms and therapeutic potential. *Signal Transduct. Target. Ther.* **2024**, *9*, 59. [CrossRef] [PubMed]
54. Kandel, S. An Evidence-based Look at the Effects of Diet on Health. *Cureus* **2019**, *11*, e4715. [CrossRef] [PubMed]
55. Kim, J.; Giovannucci, E. Healthful Plant-Based Diet and Incidence of Type 2 Diabetes in Asian Population. *Nutrients* **2022**, *14*, 3078. [CrossRef] [PubMed]
56. Giosuè, A.; Calabrese, I.; Vitale, M.; Riccardi, G.; Vaccaro, O. Consumption of Dairy Foods and Cardiovascular Disease: A Systematic Review. *Nutrients* **2022**, *14*, 831. [CrossRef] [PubMed]
57. Dyńka, D.; Kowalcze, K.; Paziewska, A. The Role of Ketogenic Diet in the Treatment of Neurological Diseases. *Nutrients* **2022**, *14*, 5003. [CrossRef] [PubMed]
58. Basiri, R.; Spicer, M.; Levenson, C.; Ledermann, T.; Akhavan, N.; Arjmandi, B. Improving Dietary Intake of Essential Nutrients Can Ameliorate Inflammation in Patients with Diabetic Foot Ulcers. *Nutrients* **2022**, *14*, 2393. [CrossRef] [PubMed]
59. Lewis Luján, L.M.; McCarty, M.F.; Di Nicolantonio, J.J.; Gálvez Ruiz, J.C.; Rosas-Burgos, E.C.; Plascencia-Jatomea, M.; Iloki Assanga, S.B. Nutraceuticals/Drugs Promoting Mitophagy and Mitochondrial Biogenesis May Combat the Mitochondrial Dysfunction Driving Progression of Dry Age-Related Macular Degeneration. *Nutrients* **2022**, *14*, 1985. [CrossRef]
60. Bartimoccia, S.; Cammisotto, V.; Nocella, C.; Del Ben, M.; D'Amico, A.; Castellani, V.; Baratta, F.; Pignatelli, P.; Loffredo, L.; Violi, F.; et al. Extra Virgin Olive Oil Reduces Gut Permeability and Metabolic Endotoxemia in Diabetic Patients. *Nutrients* **2022**, *14*, 2153. [CrossRef] [PubMed]
61. Araujo, R.; Borges-Canha, M.; Pimentel-Nunes, P. Microbiota Modulation in Patients with Metabolic Syndrome. *Nutrients* **2022**, *14*, 4490. [CrossRef] [PubMed]
62. Cozma, E.C.; Avram, I.; Voiculescu, V.M.; Mihai, M.M.; Găman, A.M. Correlations between Gut Microbiota and Hematological, Inflammatory, Biochemical and Oxidative Stress Parameters in Treatment-Naïve Psoriasis Patients. *Int. J. Mol. Sci.* **2024**, *25*, 6649. [CrossRef] [PubMed]
63. Dobrică, E.C.; Cozma, M.A.; Găman, M.A.; Voiculescu, V.M.; Găman, A.M. The Involvement of Oxidative Stress in Psoriasis: A Systematic Review. *Antioxidants* **2022**, *11*, 282. [CrossRef] [PubMed]
64. Cannavò, S.P.; Riso, G.; Casciaro, M.; Di Salvo, E.; Gangemi, S. Oxidative stress involvement in psoriasis: A systematic review. *Free Radic. Res.* **2019**, *53*, 829–840. [CrossRef] [PubMed]
65. Kiełbowski, K.; Bakinowska, E.; Ostrowski, P.; Pala, B.; Gromowska, E.; Gurazda, K.; Dec, P.; Modrzejewski, A.; Pawlik, A. The Role of Adipokines in the Pathogenesis of Psoriasis. *Int. J. Mol. Sci.* **2023**, *24*, 6390. [CrossRef] [PubMed]
66. Bakry, O.A.; El Hefnawy, S.; Mariee, A.H.; El Gendy, Y. Urinary Biopyrrins: A New Marker of Oxidative Stress in Psoriasis. *Indian J. Dermatol.* **2016**, *61*, 169–173. [CrossRef] [PubMed]
67. Millsop, J.W.; Bhatia, B.K.; Debbaneh, M.; Koo, J.; Liao, W. Diet and psoriasis, part III: Role of nutritional supplements. *J. Am. Acad. Dermatol.* **2014**, *71*, 561–569. [CrossRef] [PubMed]
68. Torsekar, R.; Gautam, M.M. Topical Therapies in Psoriasis. *Indian Dermatol. Online J.* **2017**, *8*, 235–245. [CrossRef] [PubMed]
69. Conde, T.; Lopes, D.; Łuczaj, W.; Neves, B.; Pinto, B.; Maurício, T.; Domingues, P.; Skrzydlewska, E.; Domingues, M.R. Algal Lipids as Modulators of Skin Disease: A Critical Review. *Metabolites* **2022**, *12*, 96. [CrossRef] [PubMed]
70. Bellinato, F.; Maurelli, M.; Geat, D.; Girolomoni, G.; Gisondi, P. Managing the Patient with Psoriasis and Metabolic Comorbidities. *Am. J. Clin. Dermatol.* **2024**, *25*, 527–540. [CrossRef] [PubMed]
71. Wroński, A.; Gęgotek, A.; Skrzydlewska, E. Protein adducts with lipid peroxidation products in patients with psoriasis. *Redox Biol.* **2023**, *63*, 102729. [CrossRef] [PubMed]
72. Herbert, D.; Franz, S.; Popkova, Y.; Anderegg, U.; Schiller, J.; Schwede, K.; Lorz, A.; Simon, J.C.; Saalbach, A. High-Fat Diet Exacerbates Early Psoriatic Skin Inflammation Independent of Obesity: Saturated Fatty Acids as Key Players. *J. Investig. Dermatol.* **2018**, *138*, 1999–2009. [CrossRef] [PubMed]
73. Zuccotti, E.; Oliveri, M.; Girometta, C.; Ratto, D.; Di Iorio, C.; Occhinegro, A.; Rossi, P. Nutritional strategies for psoriasis: Current scientific evidence in clinical trials. *Eur. Rev. Med. Pharmacol. Sci.* **2018**, *22*, 8537–8551. [CrossRef] [PubMed]

74. Adawi, M.; Damiani, G.; Bragazzi, N.L.; Bridgewood, C.; Pacifico, A.; Conic, R.R.Z.; Morrone, A.; Malagoli, P.; Pigatto, P.D.M.; Amital, H.; et al. The Impact of Intermittent Fasting (Ramadan Fasting) on Psoriatic Arthritis Disease Activity, Enthesitis, and Dactylitis: A Multicentre Study. *Nutrients* **2019**, *11*, 601. [CrossRef] [PubMed]
75. Nayak, R.R. Western Diet and Psoriatic-Like Skin and Joint Diseases: A Potential Role for the Gut Microbiota. *J. Investig. Dermatol.* **2021**, *141*, 1630–1632. [CrossRef] [PubMed]
76. Musumeci, M.L.; Nasca, M.R.; Boscaglia, S.; Micali, G. The role of lifestyle and nutrition in psoriasis: Current status of knowledge and interventions. *Dermatol. Ther.* **2022**, *35*, e15685. [CrossRef] [PubMed]
77. Ingkapairoj, K.; Chularojanamontri, L.; Chaiyabutr, C.; Silpa-Archa, N.; Wongpraparut, C.; Bunyaratavej, S. Dietary habits and perceptions of psoriatic patients: Mediterranean versus Asian diets. *J. Dermatol. Treat.* **2022**, *33*, 2290–2296. [CrossRef] [PubMed]
78. Zanesco, S.; Hall, W.; Gibson, R.; Griffiths, C.; Maruthappu, T. Approaches to nutrition intervention in plaque psoriasis, a multi-system inflammatory disease-The Diet and Psoriasis Project (DIEPP). *Nutr. Bull.* **2022**, *47*, 524–537. [CrossRef] [PubMed]
79. Cintoni, M.; Palombaro, M.; Maramao, F.S.; Raoul, P.; Egidi, G.; Leonardi, E.; Bianchi, L.; Campione, E.; Rinninella, E.; Gasbarrini, A.; et al. Metabolic Disorders and Psoriasis: Exploring the Role of Nutritional Interventions. *Nutrients* **2023**, *15*, 3876. [CrossRef] [PubMed]
80. Michalski, P.; Palazzo-Michalska, V.; Buda, P.; Michalska-Bańkowska, A.; Bańkowski, M.; Strojny, D.; Grabarek, B.O. A crossroads between dietary habits, alcohol consumption, and smoking in the clinical course of psoriasis: A narrative review. *Postep. Dermatol. Alergol.* **2023**, *40*, 599–605. [CrossRef] [PubMed]
81. Ford, A.R.; Siegel, M.; Bagel, J.; Cordoro, K.M.; Garg, A.; Gottlieb, A.; Green, L.J.; Gudjonsson, J.E.; Koo, J.; Lebwohl, M.; et al. Dietary Recommendations for Adults With Psoriasis or Psoriatic Arthritis From the Medical Board of the National Psoriasis Foundation: A Systematic Review. *JAMA Dermatol.* **2018**, *154*, 934–950. [CrossRef] [PubMed]
82. Berna-Rico, E.; Fernandez-Nieto, D.; Gonzalez-Cantero, A. RF—Role of the Mediterranean Diet in the Treatment of Psoriasis. *Actas Dermosifiliogr.* **2023**, *114*, 152–155. [CrossRef] [PubMed]
83. Budu-Aggrey, A.; Brumpton, B.; Tyrrell, J.; Watkins, S.; Modalsli, E.H.; Celis-Morales, C.; Ferguson, L.D.; Vie, G.; Palmer, T.; Fritsche, L.G.; et al. Evidence of a causal relationship between body mass index and psoriasis: A mendelian randomization study. *PLoS Med.* **2019**, *16*, e1002739. [CrossRef] [PubMed]
84. Barati, M.; Ghahremani, A.; Namdar Ahmadabad, H. Intermittent fasting: A promising dietary intervention for autoimmune diseases. *Autoimmun. Rev.* **2023**, *22*, 103408. [CrossRef] [PubMed]
85. Lee, H.; Sim, N.; Fotouhi, A.; Daveluy, S. Vegan Diet in Dermatology: A Review. *J. Clin. Med.* **2023**, *12*, 5800. [CrossRef] [PubMed]
86. Bhatia, B.K.; Millsop, J.W.; Debbaneh, M.; Koo, J.; Linos, E.; Liao, W. Diet and psoriasis, part II: Celiac disease and role of a gluten-free diet. *J. Am. Acad. Dermatol.* **2014**, *71*, 350–358. [CrossRef] [PubMed]
87. Lai, R.; Xian, D.; Xiong, X.; Yang, L.; Song, J.; Zhong, J. Proanthocyanidins: Novel treatment for psoriasis that reduces oxidative stress and modulates Th17 and Treg cells. *Redox Rep.* **2018**, *23*, 130–135. [CrossRef] [PubMed]
88. Passali, M.; Josefsen, K.; Frederiksen, J.L.; Antvorskov, J.C. Current Evidence on the Efficacy of Gluten-Free Diets in Multiple Sclerosis, Psoriasis, Type 1 Diabetes and Autoimmune Thyroid Diseases. *Nutrients* **2020**, *12*, 2316. [CrossRef] [PubMed]
89. Duchnik, E.; Kruk, J.; Tuchowska, A.; Marchlewicz, M. The Impact of Diet and Physical Activity on Psoriasis: A Narrative Review of the Current Evidence. *Nutrients* **2023**, *15*, 840. [CrossRef] [PubMed]
90. Kranyak, A.; Haran, K.; Smith, P.; Johnson, C.; Liao, W.; Bhutani, T. The Mediterranean Diet as a Potential Solution to the Gut Microbiome Dysbiosis in Psoriasis Patients. *J. Psoriasis Psoriatic Arthritis* **2024**, *9*, 69–81. [CrossRef] [PubMed]
91. Molina-Leyva, A.; Cuenca-Barrales, C.; Vega-Castillo, J.J.; Ruiz-Carrascosa, J.C.; Ruiz-Villaverde, R. Adherence to Mediterranean diet in Spanish patients with psoriasis: Cardiovascular benefits? *Dermatol. Ther.* **2019**, *32*, e12810. [CrossRef] [PubMed]
92. Aryanian, Z.; Asghari, M.; Zanousi, P.P.; Ghadimi, R.; Kebria, A.S.; Hatami, P. Adherence to the Mediterranean diet in patients with psoriasis and its relationship with the severity of the disease: A case-control study. *Health Sci. Rep.* **2024**, *7*, e70049. [CrossRef] [PubMed]
93. Castaldo, G.; Rastrelli, L.; Galdo, G.; Molettieri, P.; Rotondi Aufiero, F.; Cereda, E. Aggressive weight-loss program with a ketogenic induction phase for the treatment of chronic plaque psoriasis: A proof-of-concept, single-arm, open-label clinical trial. *Nutrition* **2020**, *74*, 110757. [CrossRef]
94. Lambadiari, V.; Katsimbri, P.; Kountouri, A.; Korakas, E.; Papathanasi, A.; Maratou, E.; Pavlidis, G.; Pliouta, L.; Ikonomidis, I.; Malisova, S.; et al. The Effect of a Ketogenic Diet versus Mediterranean Diet on Clinical and Biochemical Markers of Inflammation in Patients with Obesity and Psoriatic Arthritis: A Randomized Crossover Trial. *Int. J. Mol. Sci.* **2024**, *25*, 2475. [CrossRef] [PubMed]
95. Katsimbri, P.; Korakas, E.; Kountouri, A.; Ikonomidis, I.; Tsougos, E.; Vlachos, D.; Papadavid, E.; Raptis, A.; Lambadiari, V. The Effect of Antioxidant and Anti-Inflammatory Capacity of Diet on Psoriasis and Psoriatic Arthritis Phenotype: Nutrition as Therapeutic Tool? *Antioxidants* **2021**, *10*, 157. [CrossRef] [PubMed]

96. Sternberg, F.; Leitner, J.; Aminzadeh-Gohari, S.; Weber, D.D.; Sanio, P.; Koller, A.; Feichtinger, R.G.; Weiss, R.; Kofler, B.; Lang, R. The Influence of Ketogenic Diets on Psoriasiform-Like Skin Inflammation. *J. Investig. Dermatol.* **2020**, *140*, 707–710.e7. [CrossRef] [PubMed]
97. Hartman, A.L.; Vining, E.P.G. Clinical Aspects of the Ketogenic Diet. *Epilepsia* **2007**, *48*, 31–42. [CrossRef] [PubMed]
98. Batch, J.T.; Lamsal, S.P.; Adkins, M.; Sultan, S.; Ramirez, M.N. Advantages and Disadvantages of the Ketogenic Diet: A Review Article. *Cureus* **2020**, *12*, e9639. [CrossRef] [PubMed]
99. Kanda, N.; Hoashi, T.; Saeki, H. Nutrition and Psoriasis. *Int. J. Mol. Sci.* **2020**, *21*, 5405. [CrossRef] [PubMed]
100. Polo, T.C.F.; Corrente, J.E.; Miot, L.D.B.; Papini, S.J.; Miot, H.A. Dietary patterns of patients with psoriasis at a public healthcare institution in Brazil. *Bras. Dermatol.* **2020**, *95*, 452–458. [CrossRef] [PubMed]
101. Clark, C.C.T.; Taghizadeh, M.; Nahavandi, M.; Jafarnejad, S. Efficacy of ω-3 supplementation in patients with psoriasis: A me-ta-analysis of randomized controlled trials. *Clin. Rheumatol.* **2019**, *38*, 977–988. [CrossRef] [PubMed]
102. Owczarczyk-Saczonek, A.; Purzycka-Bohdan, D.; Nedoszytko, B.; Reich, A.; Szczerkowska-Dobosz, A.; Bartosińska, J.; Batycka-Baran, A.; Czajkowski, R.; Dobrucki, I.T.; Dobrucki, L.W.; et al. Pathogenesis of psoriasis in the "omic" era. Part III. Metabolic disorders, metabolomics, nutrigenomics in psoriasis. *Postep. Dermatol. Alergol.* **2020**, *37*, 452–467. [CrossRef] [PubMed]
103. Sicińska, P.; Pytel, E.; Kurowska, J.; Koter-Michalak, M. Supplementation with omega fatty acids in various diseases. *Postep. Hig. Med. Dosw.* **2015**, *69*, 838–852. [CrossRef] [PubMed]
104. Baran, A.; Kiluk, P.; Myśliwiec, H.; Flisiak, I. The role of lipids in psoriasis. *Dermatol. Rev./Przegląd Dermatol.* **2017**, *104*, 619–635. [CrossRef]
105. Antosik, K.; Krzęcio-Nieczyporuk, E.; Kurowska-Socha, B. Diet and nutrition in psoriasis treatment. *Hygeia Public Health* **2017**, *52*, 131–137.
106. Puaratanaarunkon, T.; Sittisaksomjai, S.; Sivapornpan, N.; Pongcharoen, P.; Chakkavittumrong, P.; Ingkaninan, K.; Temkitthawon, P.; Promgool, T.; Waranuch, N.; Asawanonda, P. Topical cannabidiol-based treatment for psoriasis: A dual-centre randomized placebo-controlled study. *J. Eur. Acad. Dermatol. Venereol.* **2022**, *36*, e718–e720. [CrossRef] [PubMed]
107. Gęgotek, A.; Atalay, S.; Rogowska-Wrzesińska, A.; Skrzydlewska, E. The Effect of Cannabidiol on UV-Induced Changes in Intracellular Signaling of 3D-Cultured Skin Keratinocytes. *Int. J. Mol. Sci.* **2021**, *22*, 1501. [CrossRef] [PubMed]
108. Atalay, S.; Gęgotek, A.; Skrzydlewska, E. Protective Effects of Cannabidiol on the Membrane Proteome of UVB-Irradiated Keratinocytes. *Antioxidants* **2021**, *10*, 402. [CrossRef] [PubMed]
109. Jarocka-Karpowicz, I.; Biernacki, M.; Wroński, A.; Gęgotek, A.; Skrzydlewska, E. Cannabidiol Effects on Phospholipid Metabolism in Keratinocytes from Patients with Psoriasis Vulgaris. *Biomolecules* **2020**, *10*, 367. [CrossRef] [PubMed]
110. Huestis, M.A.; Solimini, R.; Pichini, S.; Pacifici, R.; Carlier, J.; Busardò, F.P. Cannabidiol Adverse Effects and Toxicity. *Curr. Neuropharmacol.* **2019**, *17*, 974–989. [CrossRef] [PubMed]
111. Cerino, P.; Buonerba, C.; Cannazza, G.; D'Auria, J.; Ottoni, E.; Fulgione, A.; Di Stasio, A.; Pierri, B.; Gallo, A. A Review of Hemp as Food and Nutritional Supplement. *Cannabis Cannabinoid Res.* **2021**, *6*, 19–27. [CrossRef] [PubMed]
112. Engeli, B.E.; Lachenmeier, D.W.; Diel, P.; Guth, S.; Villar Fernandez, M.A.; Roth, A.; Lampen, A.; Cartus, A.T.; Wätjen, W.; Hengstler, J.G.; et al. Cannabidiol in Foods and Food Supplements: Evaluation of Health Risks and Health Claims. *Nutrients* **2025**, *17*, 489. [CrossRef] [PubMed]
113. Jensen, P.; Skov, L. Psoriasis and Obesity. *Dermatology* **2016**, *232*, 633–639. [CrossRef] [PubMed]
114. Trojacka, E.; Zaleska, M.; Galus, R. Influence of exogenous and endogenous factors on the course of psoriasis. *Pol. Merkur. Lek.* **2015**, *38*, 169–173.
115. Voiculescu, V.M.; Nelson Twakor, A.; Jerpelea, N.; Pantea Stoian, A. Vitamin D: Beyond Traditional Roles—Insights into Its Biochemical Pathways and Physiological Impacts. *Nutrients* **2025**, *17*, 803. [CrossRef] [PubMed]
116. Bârsan, M.; Chelaru, V.F.; Râjnoveanu, A.G.; Popa, Ș.L.; Socaciu, A.I.; Bădulescu, A.V. Difference in Levels of Vitamin D between Indoor and Outdoor Athletes: A Systematic Review and Meta-Analysis. *Int. J. Mol. Sci.* **2023**, *24*, 7584. [CrossRef] [PubMed]
117. Santana, K.V.d.S.d.; Oliver, S.L.; Mendes, M.M.; Lanham-New, S.; Charlton, K.E.; Ribeiro, H. Association between vitamin D status and lifestyle factors in Brazilian women: Implications of Sun Exposure Levels, Diet, and Health. *Eclinicalmedicine* **2022**, *47*, 101400. [CrossRef] [PubMed]
118. Mattozzi, C.; Paolino, G.; Richetta, A.G.; Calvieri, S. Psoriasis, vitamin D and the importance of the cutaneous barrier's integrity: An update. *J. Dermatol.* **2016**, *43*, 507–514. [CrossRef] [PubMed]
119. Cardwell, G.; Bornman, J.F.; James, A.P.; Black, L.J. A Review of Mushrooms as a Potential Source of Dietary Vitamin D. *Nutrients* **2018**, *10*, 1498. [CrossRef] [PubMed]
120. Orgaz-Molina, J.; Magro-Checa, C.; Arrabal-Polo, M.A.; Raya-Álvarez, E.; Naranjo, R.; Buendía-Eisman, A.; Arias-Santiago, S. Association of 25-hydroxyvitamin D with metabolic syndrome in patients with psoriasis: A case-control study. *Acta Derm. Venereol.* **2014**, *94*, 142–145. [CrossRef] [PubMed]

121. Pradhan, M.; Alexander, A.; Singh, M.R.; Singh, D.; Saraf, S.; Saraf, S.; Ajazuddin. Understanding the prospective of nanoformulations towards the treatment of psoriasis. *Biomed. Pharmacother.* **2018**, *107*, 447–463. [CrossRef] [PubMed]
122. Wadhwa, B.; Relhan, V.; Goel, K.; Kochhar, A.M.; Garg, V.K. Vitamin D and skin diseases: A review. *Indian J. Dermatol. Venereol. Leprol.* **2015**, *81*, 344–355. [CrossRef] [PubMed]
123. Soleymani, T.; Hung, T.; Soung, J. The role of vitamin D in psoriasis: A review. *Int. J. Dermatol.* **2015**, *54*, 383–392. [CrossRef] [PubMed]
124. Richetta, A.G.; Silvestri, V.; Giancristoforo, S.; Rizzolo, P.; D'Epiro, S.; Graziano, V.; Mattozzi, C.; Navazio, A.S.; Campoli, M.; D'Amico, C.; et al. A-1012G promoter polymorphism of vitamin D receptor gene is associated with psoriasis risk and lower allele-specific expression. *DNA Cell Biol.* **2014**, *33*, 102–109. [CrossRef] [PubMed]
125. Visconti, B.; Paolino, G.; Carotti, S.; Pendolino, A.L.; Morini, S.; Richetta, A.G.; Calvieri, S. Immunohistochemical expression of VDR is associated with reduced integrity of tight junction complex in psoriatic skin. *J. Eur. Acad. Dermatol. Venereol.* **2015**, *29*, 2038–2042. [CrossRef] [PubMed]
126. Almohanna, H.M.; Ahmed, A.A.; Tsatalis, J.P.; Tosti, A. The Role of Vitamins and Minerals in Hair Loss: A Review. *Dermatol. Ther.* **2019**, *9*, 51–70. [CrossRef] [PubMed]
127. Mostafa, W.Z.; Hegazy, R.A. Vitamin D and the skin: Focus on a complex relationship: A review. *J. Adv. Res.* **2015**, *6*, 793–804. [CrossRef] [PubMed]
128. Formisano, E.; Proietti, E.; Borgarelli, C.; Pisciotta, L. Psoriasis and Vitamin D: A Systematic Review and Meta-Analysis. *Nutrients* **2023**, *15*, 3387. [CrossRef] [PubMed]
129. Qi, D.; Nie, X.; Cai, J. The effect of vitamin D supplementation on hypertension in non-CKD populations: A systemic review and meta-analysis. *Int. J. Cardiol.* **2017**, *227*, 177–186. [CrossRef] [PubMed]
130. Melguizo-Rodríguez, L.; Costela-Ruiz, V.J.; García-Recio, E.; De Luna-Bertos, E.; Ruiz, C.; Illescas-Montes, R. Role of Vitamin D in the Metabolic Syndrome. *Nutrients* **2021**, *13*, 830. [CrossRef]
131. Brożyna, A.A.; Slominski, R.M.; Nedoszytko, B.; Zmijewski, M.A.; Slominski, A.T. Vitamin D Signaling in Psoriasis: Pathogenesis and Therapy. *Int. J. Mol. Sci.* **2022**, *23*, 8575. [CrossRef] [PubMed]
132. Talbott, W.; Duffy, N. Complementary and alternative medicine for psoriasis: What the dermatologist needs to know. *Am. J. Clin. Dermatol.* **2015**, *16*, 147–165. [CrossRef] [PubMed]
133. Yang, S.J.; Chi, C.C. Effects of fish oil supplement on psoriasis: A meta-analysis of randomized controlled trials. *BMC Complement. Altern. Med.* **2019**, *19*, 354. [CrossRef] [PubMed]
134. Ahmadi, A.; Barikbin, B.; Naseri, M.; Mohagheghi, M. The effect of HESA-A on psoriasis vulgaris. *J. Drugs Dermatol.* **2008**, *7*, 559–561. [PubMed]
135. Mousavi, S.R.; Moshiri, M.; Darchini-Maragheh, E.; Ghasempouri, S.K.; Dadpour, B.; Sardar Antighechi, F.; Balali-Mood, M. Therapeutic effects of HESA-A (a herbal-marine compound) in acute organophosphorus pesticide poisoning. *Avicenna J. Phytomed* **2020**, *10*, 235–242. [PubMed]
136. Navarro-López, V.; Martínez-Andrés, A.; Ramírez-Boscá, A.; Ruzafa-Costas, B.; Núñez-Delegido, E.; Carrión-Gutiérrez, M.A.; Prieto-Merino, D.; Codoñer-Cortés, F.; Ramón-Vidal, D.; Genovés-Martínez, S.; et al. Efficacy and Safety of Oral Administration of a Mixture of Probiotic Strains in Patients with Psoriasis: A Randomized Controlled Clinical Trial. *Acta Derm. Venereol.* **2019**, *99*, 1078–1084. [CrossRef] [PubMed]
137. Navarro-López, V.; Núñez-Delegido, E.; Ruzafa-Costas, B.; Sánchez-Pellicer, P.; Agüera-Santos, J.; Navarro-Moratalla, L. Probiotics in the Therapeutic Arsenal of Dermatologists. *Microorganisms* **2021**, *9*, 1513. [CrossRef] [PubMed]
138. Buhaș, M.C.; Candrea, R.; Gavrilaș, L.I.; Miere, D.; Tătaru, A.; Boca, A.; Cătinean, A. Transforming Psoriasis Care: Probiotics and Prebiotics as Novel Therapeutic Approaches. *Int. J. Mol. Sci.* **2023**, *24*, 11225. [CrossRef] [PubMed]
139. Pizzino, G.; Irrera, N.; Cucinotta, M.; Pallio, G.; Mannino, F.; Arcoraci, V.; Squadrito, F.; Altavilla, D.; Bitto, A. Oxidative Stress: Harms and Benefits for Human Health. *Oxid. Med. Cell Longev.* **2017**, *2017*, 8416763. [CrossRef] [PubMed]
140. Abdelazim, A.M.; and Abomughaid, M.M. Oxidative stress: An overview of past research and future insights. *All Life* **2024**, *17*, 2316092. [CrossRef]
141. Reddy, V.P. Oxidative Stress in Health and Disease. *Biomedicines* **2023**, *11*, 2925. [CrossRef] [PubMed]
142. Periferakis, A.; Caruntu, A.; Periferakis, A.-T.; Scheau, A.-E.; Badarau, I.A.; Caruntu, C.; Scheau, C. Availability, Toxicology and Medical Significance of Antimony. *Int. J. Environ. Res. Public Health* **2022**, *19*, 4669. [CrossRef] [PubMed]
143. Teleanu, D.M.; Niculescu, A.-G.; Lungu, I.I.; Radu, C.I.; Vladâcenco, O.; Roza, E.; Costăchescu, B.; Grumezescu, A.M.; Teleanu, R.I. An Overview of Oxidative Stress, Neuroinflammation, and Neurodegenerative Diseases. *Int. J. Mol. Sci.* **2022**, *23*, 5938. [CrossRef] [PubMed]

144. Periferakis, A.; Periferakis, K.; Badarau, I.A.; Petran, E.M.; Popa, D.C.; Caruntu, A.; Costache, R.S.; Scheau, C.; Caruntu, C.; Costache, D.O. Kaempferol: Antimicrobial Properties, Sources, Clinical, and Traditional Applications. *Int. J. Mol. Sci.* **2022**, *23*, 15054. [CrossRef] [PubMed]
145. Periferakis, A.; Periferakis, A.-T.; Troumpata, L.; Periferakis, K.; Scheau, A.-E.; Savulescu-Fiedler, I.; Caruntu, A.; Badarau, I.A.; Caruntu, C.; Scheau, C. Kaempferol: A Review of Current Evidence of Its Antiviral Potential. *Int. J. Mol. Sci.* **2023**, *24*, 16299. [CrossRef] [PubMed]
146. Periferakis, A.; Periferakis, A.-T.; Troumpata, L.; Periferakis, K.; Georgatos-Garcia, S.; Touriki, G.; Dragosloveanu, C.D.M.; Caruntu, A.; Savulescu-Fiedler, I.; Dragosloveanu, S.; et al. Pinosylvin: A Multifunctional Stilbenoid with Antimicrobial, Antioxidant, and Anti-Inflammatory Potential. *Curr. Issues Mol. Biol.* **2025**, *47*, 204. [CrossRef] [PubMed]
147. Kumar, S.; Malhotra, S.; Prasad, A.K.; Van der Eycken, E.V.; Bracke, M.E.; Stetler-Stevenson, W.G.; Parmar, V.S.; Ghosh, B. Anti-inflammatory and antioxidant properties of Piper species: A perspective from screening to molecular mechanisms. *Curr. Top. Med. Chem.* **2015**, *15*, 886–893. [CrossRef] [PubMed]
148. Periferakis, A.; Troumpata, L.; Periferakis, K.; Adalis, G.; Periferakis, A.; Georgatos-Garcia, S.; Maier, C.; Costache, A.; Garofil, D.; Costache, D. Traditional Ethnomedical and Ethnobotanical Applications and Uses of Piper Nigrum. *Rom. J. Mil. Med.* **2025**, *128*, 286–303. [CrossRef]
149. Periferakis, A.-T.; Periferakis, A.; Periferakis, K.; Caruntu, A.; Badarau, I.A.; Savulescu-Fiedler, I.; Scheau, C.; Caruntu, C. Antimicrobial Properties of Capsaicin: Available Data and Future Research Perspectives. *Nutrients* **2023**, *15*, 4097. [CrossRef] [PubMed]
150. Petran, E.M.; Periferakis, A.; Troumpata, L.; Periferakis, A.-T.; Scheau, A.-E.; Badarau, I.A.; Periferakis, K.; Caruntu, A.; Savulescu-Fiedler, I.; Sima, R.-M.; et al. Capsaicin: Emerging Pharmacological and Therapeutic Insights. *Curr. Issues Mol. Biol.* **2024**, *46*, 7895–7943. [CrossRef] [PubMed]
151. Gago, C.; Serralheiro, A.; Miguel, M.d.G. Anti-Inflammatory Activity of Thymol and Thymol-Rich Essential Oils: Mechanisms, Applications, and Recent Findings. *Molecules* **2025**, *30*, 2450. [CrossRef] [PubMed]
152. Teleanu, R.I.; Moldoveanu, E.-T.; Niculescu, A.-G.; Predescu, E.; Roza, E.; Tincu, I.F.; Grumezescu, A.M.; Teleanu, D.M. Liposomal and Lipid-Based Drug Delivery Systems: Bridging Gut Microbiota and Pediatric Disorder Treatments. *Pharmaceutics* **2025**, *17*, 707. [CrossRef] [PubMed]
153. Wu, D.; Lin, Q.; Hou, S.; Cui, X.; Shou, N.; Yuan, X.; Xu, W.; Fu, K.; Wang, Q.; Shi, Z. Gut Microbiota and Its Metabolite Taurine-β-Muricholic Acid Contribute to Antimony- and/or Copper-Induced Liver Inflammation. *Int. J. Mol. Sci.* **2025**, *26*, 3332. [CrossRef] [PubMed]
154. Benhadou, F.; Mintoff, D.; Schnebert, B.; Thio, H.B. Psoriasis and Microbiota: A Systematic Review. *Diseases* **2018**, *6*, 47. [CrossRef] [PubMed]
155. Polak, K.; Bergler-Czop, B.; Szczepanek, M.; Wojciechowska, K.; Frątczak, A.; Kiss, N. Psoriasis and Gut Microbiome-Current State of Art. *Int. J. Mol. Sci.* **2021**, *22*, 4529. [CrossRef] [PubMed]
156. Zhu, Q.; Wu, K.; Yang, Q.; Meng, B.; Niu, Y.; Zhao, F. Advances in psoriasis and gut microorganisms with co-metabolites. *Front. Microbiol.* **2023**, *14*, 1192543. [CrossRef] [PubMed]
157. Zou, X.; Zou, X.; Gao, L.; Zhao, H. Gut microbiota and psoriasis: Pathogenesis, targeted therapy, and future directions. *Front. Cell Infect. Microbiol.* **2024**, *14*, 1430586. [CrossRef] [PubMed]
158. Hidalgo-Cantabrana, C.; Gómez, J.; Delgado, S.; Requena-López, S.; Queiro-Silva, R.; Margolles, A.; Coto, E.; Sánchez, B.; Coto-Segura, P. Gut microbiota dysbiosis in a cohort of patients with psoriasis. *Br. J. Dermatol.* **2019**, *181*, 1287–1295. [CrossRef] [PubMed]
159. Zhang, X.; Shi, L.; Sun, T.; Guo, K.; Geng, S. Dysbiosis of gut microbiota and its correlation with dysregulation of cytokines in psoriasis patients. *BMC Microbiol.* **2021**, *21*, 78. [CrossRef] [PubMed]
160. Visser, M.J.E.; Kell, D.B.; Pretorius, E. Bacterial Dysbiosis and Translocation in Psoriasis Vulgaris. *Front. Cell Infect. Microbiol.* **2019**, *9*, 7. [CrossRef] [PubMed]
161. Kumar, R.; Rizvi, M.R.; Saraswat, S. Obesity and Stress: A Contingent Paralysis. *Int. J. Prev. Med.* **2022**, *13*, 95. [CrossRef] [PubMed]
162. Goens, D.; Virzi, N.E.; Jung, S.E.; Rutledge, T.R.; Zarrinpar, A. Obesity, Chronic Stress, and Stress Reduction. *Gastroenterol. Clin. N. Am.* **2023**, *52*, 347–362. [CrossRef] [PubMed]
163. Kaufman, A.; Augustson, E.M.; Patrick, H. Unraveling the Relationship between Smoking and Weight: The Role of Sedentary Behavior. *J. Obes.* **2012**, *2012*, 735465. [CrossRef] [PubMed]
164. Dare, S.; Mackay, D.F.; Pell, J.P. Relationship between smoking and obesity: A cross-sectional study of 499,504 middle-aged adults in the UK general population. *PLoS ONE* **2015**, *10*, e0123579. [CrossRef] [PubMed]
165. Voiculescu, V.M.; Popa, L.G.; Bumbacea, R.S.; Nitipir, C.; Giurcaneanu, C. Genetics of psoriasis susceptibility and treatment response. *Farmacia* **2016**, *64*, 313–322.
166. Snast, I.; Reiter, O.; Atzmony, L.; Leshem, Y.A.; Hodak, E.; Mimouni, D.; Pavlovsky, L. Psychological stress and psoriasis: A systematic review and meta-analysis. *Br. J. Dermatol.* **2018**, *178*, 1044–1055. [CrossRef] [PubMed]

167. Rigas, H.M.; Bucur, S.; Ciurduc, D.M.; Nita, I.E.; Constantin, M.M. Psychological Stress and Depression in Psoriasis Patients—A Dermatologist's Perspective. *Maedica* **2019**, *14*, 287–291. [CrossRef] [PubMed]
168. Urruticoechea-Arana, A.; Serra Torres, M.; Hergueta Diaz, M.; González Guerrero, M.E.; Fariñas Padron, L.; Navarro Martín, S.; Vargas Osorio, K.; Palacios Abufón, A.; García de Yébenes, M.J.; Loza, E. Experience and satisfaction with a multidisciplinary care unit for patients with psoriasis and psoriatic arthritis. *Reumatol. Clínica* **2019**, *15*, 237–241. [CrossRef] [PubMed]
169. Zheng, Y.X.; Zheng, M. A multidisciplinary team for the diagnosis and management of psoriatic arthritis. *Chin. Med. J.* **2021**, *134*, 1387–1389. [CrossRef]
170. Jadon, D.R.; Helliwell, P.S. The role of the multidisciplinary team in the management of psoriatic arthritis. *Musculoskelet. Care* **2022**, *20* (Suppl. S1), S32–S40. [CrossRef] [PubMed]
171. Holzmann, H.; Hoede, N.; Eißner, D.; Hahn, K.; Hülse, R. Joint involvement in psoriasis. *Arch. Für Dermatol. Forsch.* **1974**, *250*, 95–107. [CrossRef] [PubMed]
172. Periferakis, A.; Periferakis, A.-T.; Troumpata, L.; Dragosloveanu, S.; Timofticiuc, I.-A.; Georgatos-Garcia, S.; Scheau, A.-E.; Periferakis, K.; Caruntu, A.; Badarau, I.A.; et al. Use of Biomaterials in 3D Printing as a Solution to Microbial Infections in Arthroplasty and Osseous Reconstruction. *Biomimetics* **2024**, *9*, 154. [CrossRef] [PubMed]
173. Timofticiuc, I.-A.; Călinescu, O.; Iftime, A.; Dragosloveanu, S.; Caruntu, A.; Scheau, A.-E.; Badarau, I.A.; Didilescu, A.C.; Caruntu, C.; Scheau, C. Biomaterials Adapted to Vat Photopolymerization in 3D Printing: Characteristics and Medical Applications. *J. Funct. Biomater.* **2024**, *15*, 7. [CrossRef] [PubMed]
174. Timofticiuc, I.-A.; Dragosloveanu, S.; Caruntu, A.; Scheau, A.-E.; Badarau, I.A.; Garofil, N.D.; Didilescu, A.C.; Caruntu, C.; Scheau, C. 3D Bioprinting in Limb Salvage Surgery. *J. Funct. Biomater.* **2024**, *15*, 383. [CrossRef] [PubMed]
175. Timofticiuc, I.-A.; Caruntu, A.; Dragosloveanu, C.D.M.; Scheau, A.-E.; Badarau, I.A.; Periferakis, A.; Dragosloveanu, S.; Didilescu, A.C.; Caruntu, C.; Scheau, C. Head and Neck 3D Bioprinting—A Review on Recent Advancements in Soft Tissue 3D Bioprinting and Medical Applications. *J. Funct. Biomater.* **2025**, *16*, 240. [CrossRef]
176. Savulescu-Fiedler, I.; Mihalcea, R.; Dragosloveanu, S.; Scheau, C.; Baz, R.O.; Caruntu, A.; Scheau, A.-E.; Caruntu, C.; Benea, S.N. The Interplay between Obesity and Inflammation. *Life* **2024**, *14*, 856. [CrossRef] [PubMed]
177. Savulescu-Fiedler, I.; Dorobantu-Lungu, L.-R.; Dragosloveanu, S.; Benea, S.N.; Dragosloveanu, C.D.M.; Caruntu, A.; Scheau, A.-E.; Caruntu, C.; Scheau, C. The Cross-Talk Between the Peripheral and Brain Cholesterol Metabolisms. *Curr. Issues Mol. Biol.* **2025**, *47*, 115. [CrossRef] [PubMed]
178. Roman, I.I.; Constantin, A.M.; Marina, M.E.; Orasan, R.I. The role of hormones in the pathogenesis of psoriasis vulgaris. *Clujul Med.* **2016**, *89*, 11–18. [CrossRef] [PubMed]
179. Cassalia, F.; Lunardon, A.; Frattin, G.; Danese, A.; Caroppo, F.; Fortina, A.B. How Hormonal Balance Changes Lives in Women with Psoriasis. *J. Clin. Med.* **2025**, *14*, 582. [CrossRef] [PubMed]
180. Weber, G.; Klughardt, G.; Neidhardt, M.; Galle, K.; Frey, H.; Geiger, A. Treatment of psoriasis with Somatostatin. *Arch. Dermatol. Res.* **1981**, *272*, 31–36. [CrossRef] [PubMed]
181. Guilhou, J.J.; Boulanger, A.; Barneon, G.; Vic, P.; Meynadier, J.; Tardieu, J.C.; Clot, J. Somatostatin treatment of psoriasis. *Arch. Dermatol. Res.* **1982**, *274*, 249–257. [CrossRef] [PubMed]
182. Periferakis, A.; Tsigas, G.; Periferakis, A.-T.; Badarau, I.A.; Scheau, A.-E.; Tampa, M.; Georgescu, S.R.; Didilescu, A.C.; Scheau, C.; Caruntu, C. Antitumoral and Anti-inflammatory Roles of Somatostatin and Its Analogs in Hepatocellular Carcinoma. *Anal. Cell. Pathol.* **2021**, *2021*, 1840069. [CrossRef] [PubMed]
183. Periferakis, A.; Tsigas, G.; Periferakis, A.-T.; Tone, C.M.; Hemes, D.A.; Periferakis, K.; Troumpata, L.; Badarau, I.A.; Scheau, C.; Caruntu, A.; et al. Agonists, Antagonists and Receptors of Somatostatin: Pathophysiological and Therapeutical Implications in Neoplasias. *Curr. Issues Mol. Biol.* **2024**, *46*, 9721–9759. [CrossRef]
184. Rendon, A.; Schäkel, K. Psoriasis Pathogenesis and Treatment. *Int. J. Mol. Sci.* **2019**, *20*, 1475. [CrossRef] [PubMed]
185. Orzan, O.A.; Tutunaru, C.V.; Ianoși, S.L. Understanding the Intricate Pathophysiology of Psoriasis and Related Skin Disorders. *Int. J. Mol. Sci.* **2025**, *26*, 749. [CrossRef] [PubMed]
186. Hickmann, E.; Richter, P.; Schlieter, H. All together now—Patient engagement, patient empowerment, and associated terms in personal healthcare. *BMC Health Serv. Res.* **2022**, *22*, 1116. [CrossRef] [PubMed]
187. Varela, A.J.; Gallamore, M.J.; Hansen, N.R.; Martin, D.C. Patient empowerment: A critical evaluation and prescription for a foundational definition. *Front. Psychol.* **2025**, *15*, 1473345. [CrossRef] [PubMed]

medicina

MDPI

Article

Similarities and Differences Between Patients Diagnosed with ANCA-Associated Vasculitis Who Are Positive and Negative for ANCA: University Clinic Practice and Expertise

Giedre Deresevičiene [1,*], Jolanta Dadoniene [1,2] and Dalia Miltiniene [1,3]

1 State Research Institute Centre for Innovative Medicine, LT-08406 Vilnius, Lithuania
2 Department of Public Health, Institute of Health Sciences, Faculty of Medicine, Vilnius University, LT-03101 Vilnius, Lithuania
3 Orthopedics Traumatology and Reconstructive Surgery, Clinic of Rheumatology, Institute of Clinical Medicine, Faculty of Medicine, Vilnius University, LT-03101 Vilnius, Lithuania
* Correspondence: giedre.dereseviciene@imcentras.lt; Tel.: +370-66273602

Abstract

Background and objective. Anti-neutrophil cytoplasmic antibody (ANCA)-associated vasculitis (AAV) affects small- to medium-sized vessels and is characterized by the production of ANCAs. The ANCA-negative term is used if the patient otherwise fulfills the definition for AAV but has negative results on serologic testing for ANCAs. The objective of this study was to compare ANCA-positive and -negative vasculitis patients and to evaluate the main differences possibly related to the presence of ANCAs. *Material and methods.* A cross-sectional study of 73 patients treated at the tertiary Rheumatology Centre of University Hospital from the 1 January, 2001, to the 31August, 2023, with diagnoses of AAV was carried out. Clinical characteristics and laboratory data were collected at the onset or at the first year of the disease. *Results.* Forty-eight (65.8%) patients were ANCA-positive, while twenty-five (34.3%) were ANCA-negative. Distribution by gender was similar in both groups, with a female–male ratio of 2:1. C-reactive protein (CRP) and erythrocyte sedimentation rate (ESR) were elevated for all AAV patients, but values were higher in the ANCA-positive patients' group. The median hemoglobin was 106 g/L in the seropositive group and 127 g/L in the seronegative group. A higher prevalence of kidney involvement (60.4%) with elevated serum creatinine level (93.5 µmol/L) was observed in the ANCA-positive group compared with 24% and 70 µmol/l in the ANCA-negative group ($p < 0.05$). Neurological involvement was more frequently found in the ANCA-positive patient group, too: 29.2% compared to 20%. Among patients with ANCA-negative vasculitis, 88% had pulmonary; 92% ear, nose, throat (ENT); 48% joint; and 28% skin presentation. In comparison, involvement of these organs was less common in the ANCA-positive patients' group, at 79.2%, 60.4%, 31.3%, and 25 %, respectively. *Conclusions.* ANCA-positive patients appear to be in a more difficult clinical situation in terms of organ involvement and laboratory changes.

Keywords: ANCA-associated vasculitis; ANCA-positive; ANCA-negative

1. Introduction

Small vessel vasculitis is a rare disease affecting predominantly small- to medium-sized vessels, resulting in occlusive, stenotic, or aneurysmal changes that lead to ischemic or hemorrhagic events [1]. Anti-neutrophil cytoplasmic antibody (ANCA)-associated vasculitis (AAV) affects small- to medium-sized vessels and is characterized by the production of antibodies specific for myeloperoxidase (MPO-ANCA) or proteinase-3 (PR3-ANCA). The ANCA-negative term is used if the patient otherwise fulfills the definition for AAV but has negative results on serologic testing for ANCAs. The main AAV clinicopathologic types are granulomatosis with polyangiitis (GPA), microscopic polyangiitis (MPA), and eosinophilic granulomatosis with polyangiitis (EGPA) [2]. PR3-ANCA is mostly associated with GPA, whereas MPO-ANCA is predominantly found in MPA patients. MPO-ANCA-positive vasculitis mainly affects lungs and kidneys, less frequently eyes, ear, nose, and throat, while PR3-ANCA-positive vasculitis is characterized by predominant involvement of the upper respiratory tract [3]. Miloslavsky et al. reported that ANCA-negative patients with a lower Birmingham Vasculitis Activity Score for GPA than PR3-ANCA-positive patients have a lower prevalence of renal involvement [4]. EGPA is commonly associated with asthma, rhinosinusitis, and peripheral eosinophilia. Although EGPA is classified as AAV, only 30% to 40% of cases are ANCA (mostly MPO)-positive [5]. Furthermore, geographic location and ethnicity influence differences in clinical presentations of patients with AAV, and the predominant ANCA type also varies geographically [6–8]. Overall, AAV commonly causes life-threatening organ damage, with a reported 5-year mortality rate of 28% and significant long-term morbidity in survivors [9]. Although more recent studies show a significant improvement in survival, with a 5-year survival rate of 94.5% [10], mortality in AAV patients is still 2.7-fold increased compared to the general population [11]. ANCA seropositivity is one of the factors influencing unachieved remission, relapse, renal involvement, and overall survival [12]. Additionally, ANCA positivity is often used in AAV diagnostic algorithms. In 2022, the American College of Rheumatology (ACR)/European League Against Rheumatism (EULAR) developed and approved new classification criteria that increased the weight of ANCA seropositivity [13–15]. On the other hand, although ANCA is helpful in diagnosing AAV and in selecting a homogeneous population for clinical trials, according to the revised 2017 international consensus on ANCA testing, the diagnosis of AAV should be based primarily on clinicopathological features [16]. Furthermore, using newer criteria with higher ANCA weighting, classification of two AAVs may occur [17]. The goal of this study was to describe the similarities and differences between ANCA-positive and -negative patients who were treated at the tertiary Rheumatology Centre of the University clinic.

2. Materials and Methods

A cross-sectional study of patients treated at the tertiary Rheumatology Centre of University Hospital from the 1 January 2001, to the 31 August 2023, with diagnoses of AAV was carried out. Data for the study were collected from electronic documents in the Electronic Medical Record of the University Hospital and from the documentation in the Rheumatology Center. The diagnoses were confirmed by clinical evaluation, serological ANCA testing, and histological analysis and fulfilled the requirements of the GPA, MPO, and EGPA nomenclature according to the revised criteria of the Chapel Hill consensus 2012 [2]. The ANCA-negative term was used if the patient otherwise met the definition for AAV but had negative results on serologic testing for ANCAs. Data on demographics (gender, age at the time of diagnosis), clinical characteristics (organ involvement), and laboratory data (C-reactive protein, erythrocyte sedimentation rate, hemoglobin level, white blood cell count, ANCA test result, serum creatinine level, and the growth of Staphylococcus aureus in the nasopharynx) was collected. ANCA positivity in the first patients enrolled in the study was determined by indirect immunofluorescence (IFL) that indicated c-ANCA or p-

ANCA. Subsequently, enzyme-linked immunosorbent assays (ELISAs) showing anti-PR3 or anti-MPO ANCAs were also used together with IFL to determine ANCA positivity. Kidney involvement was defined as proteinuria, hematuria, elevated serum creatinine level, or by histopathological findings of pauci-immune necrotizing glomerulonephritis. Joint involvement was defined as arthralgia or arthritis, in some cases accompanied by myalgia. Lung or lower respiratory tract damage was determined if computed tomography (CT) or fiberoptic bronchoscopy (FBS) confirmed tracheal stenosis, bronchial stenosis, pleuritis, mucosal ulceration, granulomatous inflammation of the lower respiratory tract, signs of pulmonary hemorrhage, ground glass opacities, and/or foci in the lungs. Established bronchial asthma was also considered lung damage. Some cases of lower respiratory tract involvement were confirmed by histopathological findings of granulomatosis with polyangiitis or necrotizing granulomatous inflammation. ENT or upper respiratory tract involvement was assessed if rhinitis, sinusitis, otitis, epistaxis, hemoptysis, nasal septal ulcer, defect, perforation, or laryngeal stenosis was detected. Some cases of upper respiratory tract involvement were confirmed by histopathological findings of granulomatous or eosinophilic inflammation. Polyneuropathy or mononeuropathy was defined as neurological damage.

Clinical and laboratory data was collected at the onset or at the first year of the disease. We divided patients into two categories: seropositive (PR3-ANCA, c-ANCA, or MPO-ANCA, p-ANCA) and seronegative for ANCA. The patient was considered ANCA-positive if an ANCA-positive result was obtained at least once in cases where several tests were performed within the first year of diagnosis in order to rule out the influence of the immunosuppressive treatment on the ANCA positivity rate. Seroconversion later than 1 year from the date of diagnosis was not considered. For comparisons of numerical variables, we applied the Mann–Whitney U-test, and the Chi-square test was applied for associations of categorical variables. A p value < 0.05 was considered to be statistically significant. The study was approved by Vilnius Regional Bioethics Committee (approval number 158200-17-958-462). The study received a waiver for an informed consent form to be signed by participants.

3. Results

We analyzed 73 patients with a diagnosis of AAV: according to the 2012 Chapel Hill consensus criteria, GPA was diagnosed in 54.8% (40), MPA in 23.3% (17), and EGPA in 21.9% (16) of cases; 65.8% (48) had an ANCA-positive test, while in 34.3% (25) patients, ANCA was not detected. The distribution of ANCA-positive and ANCA-negative patients according to different AAV diagnoses was different in the study groups: according to the 2012 Chapel Hill consensus criteria, 48% (12) of ANCA-negative patients were diagnosed with GPA, 12% (3) with MPA, and 40% (10) with EGPA, while in the ANCA-positive group, 58.3% (28) of patients were diagnosed with GPA, 29.2% (14) with MPA, and only 12.5% (6) with EGPA. The distribution of study groups according to different AAV diagnoses and seropositive MPO-ANCA and PR3-ANCA patients in each AAV subgroup is shown in Table 1.

Considering the distribution of seropositive patients in each AAV disease group, PR3-ANCA was more prevalent in the GPA and EGPA groups, while MPO-ANCA was more prevalent in the MPA group

The mean age at the time of diagnosis was 48.8 years in the ANCA-positive group, similar to the ANCA-negative group—48.5 years, with MPA seronegative patients being the oldest at disease onset. Distribution by gender was similar in both groups, with a female-to-male ratio of 2:1. Interestingly, differences in the distribution of patients by gender were found in the AAV subgroups: all MPA-negative patients were female, while males were less likely to be seropositive than negative in the GPA group. The clinical and demographic characteristics of the studied groups are shown in Tables 2 and 3.

Table 1. Distribution of ANCA-positive and ANCA-negative patients according to different AVV diagnoses.

	ANCA+			ANCA−
	MPO+ or p-ANCA	**PR3+ or c-ANCA**	**Undifferentiated ANCA**	
GPA according to 2012 Chapel Hill consensus criteria, *n* = 40 (%)	3 (7.5)	24 (60)	1 (2.5)	12 (30)
MPA according to 2012 Chapel Hill consensus criteria, *n* = 17 (%)	8 (47.1)	5 (29.4)	1 (5.9)	3 (17.6)
EGPA according to 2012 Chapel Hill consensus criteria, *n* = 16 (%)	2 (12.5)	4 (25)	.	10 (62.5)

ANCA—anti-neutrophil cytoplasmic antibody, AAV—ANCA-associated vasculitis, GPA—granulomatosis with polyangiitis, MPA—microscopic polyangiitis, EGPA—eosinophilic granulomatosis with polyangiitis.

Table 2. The descriptive statistics of clinical and demographic patients' characteristics and laboratory test results at the onset of the disease.

	ANCA+ (PR3-ANCA, c-ANCA or MPO-ANCA, p-ANCA)	**ANCA−**	***p*-Value**
Demographic characteristics			
Female, *n* (%)	32 (66.7)	17 (68.0)	
Male, *n* (%)	16 (33.3)	8 (32.0)	
Mean age at diagnosis (±SD)	48.8 (±11.9)	48.5 (±14.4)	
Median age at the time of diagnosis	51	48	
Clinical manifestation			
Pulmonary involvement, *n* (%)	41 (85.4)	22 (88.0)	0.7607
Kidney involvement *n* (%)	29 (60.4)	6 (24.0)	0.0031
Kidney biopsies performed *n* (%)	25 (52.1)	5 (20)	0.0082
ENT involvement *n* (%)	37 (77.1)	23 (92.0)	0.1139
Skin involvement *n* (%)	12 (25.0)	7 (28.0)	0.7816
Joint involvement *n* (%)	19 (39.6)	11 (44.0)	0.7150
St. aureus from the swab n (%)	7 (14.6)	4 (16.0)	0.8724
Neurological involvement *n* (%)	14 (29.2)	5 (20)	0.3970
Laboratory tests			
Serum CRP level, mg/L			0.3457
Median	33.5	21.0	
Minimum	0.3	0.2	
Maximum	279.0	310.0	
ESR, mm/h			0.96
Median	51.5	42.5	
Minimum	2	5	
Maximum	120	120	
WBC			0.5226
Average (±SD)	11.24 (±8.5)	10.23 (±3.9)	
Median	9.1	9.6	
Minimum	2.9	4.6	
Maximum	45.7	18.6	
Hemoglobin, g/L			0.00007
Average (±SD)	106 (±18.2)	127 (±19.9)	
Median	106	130	
Minimum	70	81	
Maximum	137	167	
Serum creatinine level, μmol/L			0.058
Median	93.5	70.0	
Minimum	33	58	
Maximum	1058	493	

ANCA—anti-neutrophil cytoplasmic antibody; ENT—ear, nose, throat; CRP—C-reactive protein; ESR—erythrocyte sedimentation rate; WBC—white blood cell count; SD—standard deviation.

Table 3. Differences between AAV subgroups based on ANCA seropositivity in terms of demographics and organ involvement.

	GPA		MPA		EGPA	
	ANCA+	ANCA−	ANCA+	ANCA−	ANCA+	ANCA−
Demographic characteristics						
Female, *n* (%)	20 (71.4)	7 (58.3)	8 (57.1)	3 (100)	4 (66.7)	7 (70)
Male, *n* (%)	8 (28.6)	5 (41.6)	6 (42.9)	0 (0)	2 (33.3)	3 (30)
Mean age at diagnosis	48.14	48.89	47.45	56.52	54.84	45.63
Median age at the time of diagnosis	51	48	51	49	50	48
Clinical manifestation						
Pulmonary involvement, *n* (%)	27 (96.4)	11 (91.7)	9 (64.3)	2 (66.7)	5 (83.3)	9 (90)
Kidney involvement, *n* (%)	16 (57.1)	3 (25)	13 (92.9)	3 (100)	0 (0)	0 (0)
ENT involvement, *n* (%)	26 (92.9)	12 (100)	6 (42.9)	3 (100)	5 (83.3)	8 (80)
Skin involvement, *n* (%)	7 (25)	0 (0)	4 (28.6)	2 (66.7)	1 (16.7)	5 (50)
Joint involvement, *n* (%)	12 (42.9)	4 (33.3)	5 (35.7)	1 (33.3)	2 (33.3)	6 (60)
Neurological involvement, *n* (%)	6 (21.4)	2 (16.7)	4 (28.6)	1 (33.3)	4 (66.7)	2 (20)

GPA—granulomatosis with polyangiitis, MPA—microscopic polyangiitis, EGPA—eosinophilic granulomatosis with polyangiitis.

The difference in kidney involvement was statistically significant between the groups, with higher incidence in the ANCA-positive group; 60.4% (29) of patients with positive ANCA serology had signs of kidney involvement, whereas only 24.0% (6) of ANCA-negative patients featured with kidney damage (p-value—0.0031). The difference was most significant in the GPA patient subgroup (p-value—0.0621). Renal involvement was confirmed by histopathological findings of pauci-immune necrotizing glomerulonephritis in 52.1% (25) of ANCA-positive patients, compared to 20% (5) of ANCA-negative patients. On the contrary, upper and lower respiratory tract involvement was present more often in the seronegative group: 92.0% (23) of patients had ear, nose, and throat (ENT) involvement and 88.0% (22) had pulmonary involvement, compared with 77.1% (37) and 85.4% (41) in the seropositive group. However, in the GPA subgroup, lung involvement was slightly more frequently found among ANCA-positive patients: 96.4% (27) compared to 91.7% (11). In the seronegative group of patients, airway stenosis was also found more frequently: 16% (4) compared to 6.25% (3). Furthermore, more patients with bronchial asthma were found in the ANCA-negative patient group: 28% (7) compared to 10.4% (5) in the ANCA-positive patient group, reflecting the more frequent diagnosis of EGPA in this group. Overall, respiratory histopathological changes supporting the diagnosis of AAV were found in 40% (10) of ANCA-negative patients and 31.25% (15) of ANCA-positive patients, confirming that respiratory lesions were more common in the seronegative patient group. Due to the relatively small sample size, statistical significance was not found; however, clinical difference was noted. There was no clinical and statistical significance noted for other organ involvement: 28.0% (7) of the patients in the ANCA-negative group had skin involvement, similar to 25.0% (12) in the ANCA-positive group. Arthralgia/arthritis was more frequent in ANCA-negative patients: 44.0% (11) compared to 39.6% (19) in the ANCA-positive group, but the result was not statistically significant, either. On the contrary, polyneuropathy or mononeuritis, assessed as a neurological system disorder, was more frequently found in the ANCA-positive patient group: 29.2% (14) compared to 20% (5), but the difference was not statistically significant. In the subgroup of GPA patients, damage to all assessed organ systems, except for ENT, was more often found among seropositive patients. The trend was not observed in the MPA and EGPA patient groups; on the contrary, skin involvement in both groups, ENT involvement in MPA patients, and joint damage in EGPA patients were more prevalent in the ANCA-negative group.

Laboratory indicators of inflammatory activity were elevated in both groups, with higher levels in the ANCA-positive group. The CRP median was 33.5 mg/L and ESR median 51.5 mm/h in the seropositive patient group compared to 21.0 mg/L and 42.5 mm/h in the seronegative group. Moreover, WBC was equally elevated in both the ANCA-positive and ANCA-negative groups: 9.1×10^9/L and 9.6×10^9/L, respectively. The difference in decreased hemoglobin levels, indicative of anemia, was statistically significant between groups. The median hemoglobin was 106 g/L in the seropositive group, in comparison to 127 g/L in the seronegative group. Furthermore, the serum creatinine level was higher in the ANCA-positive patients' group, with a median of 93.5 µmol/L (minimum 33; maximum 1058) compared with a median of 70.0 µmol/L (minimum 58; maximum 493) in the ANCA-negative group; the difference was close to significance. Laboratory test results are also shown in Table 2.

4. Discussion

In 2022 ACR/EULAR developed and validated new classification criteria for GPA [13], MPA [14], and EGPA [15] that have improved sensitivity and specificity compared to previous criteria. According to the literature, the concordance rate between the new and previous criteria is 96.6% in the MPA group, 73.8% in the GPA, and 86.3% in the EGPA, with ANCA being the main discriminator [17]. However, newer criteria have been approved for the purpose of classifying vasculitis, which should be applied once the diagnosis is made to ensure that a homogeneous population is selected for clinical trials and research studies and that they are not appropriated for use in establishing a diagnosis of vasculitis [13].

This study was conducted to evaluate the similarities and differences between ANCA-positive and -negative patients with vasculitis, focusing on clinical characteristics and laboratory findings at the onset of the disease; therefore, we used the revised Chapel Hill consensus 2012 criteria for vasculitis nomenclature.

We found the most prominent differences in kidney damage were more likely in the ANCA-positive group, as well as lower hemoglobin levels found in this group. The patients were divided into two groups according to ANCA serology at the onset of the disease. Seroconversion was not taken into account. According to studies, either MPO-ANCAs or PR3-ANCAs are present in 90% of patients with GPA, MPA, or EGPA [18,19]; on the contrary, our cohort consists of 65.8% seropositive and 34.3% seronegative patients, indicating that more diagnoses were made based on clinicopathological features rather than a positive ANCA test. Although GPA was the most frequently detected AAV in both groups, accounting for 48% (12) in the ANCA-negative group of patients and 58.3% (28) in the ANCA-positive group of patients, there was a clear difference in the distribution of EGPA and MPA patients between the groups. In the group of seronegative patients, EGPA accounted for 40%, but in the group of seropositive patients, only 12.5%; on the contrary, MPA accounted for 12% and 29.2%, respectively. Our findings on the distribution of different AAVs in the groups support the findings of previous studies that patients diagnosed with EGPA are more likely to be ANCA-negative [5]. Overall, in our study, 37.5% of EGPA patients were ANCA-positive, while 70% of GPA patients and 82.4% of MPA patients were seropositive.

Although according to studies AAV is more common in men than in women, with a prevalence ratio between 1.07:1 and 1.48:1 and the peak incidence of vasculitis is at the age of 60–79 years [20,21], we estimated higher prevalence in women in both ANCA-positive and ANCA-negative groups: our estimated female-to-male prevalence ratio in both groups is 2:1. Moreover, we have found a younger age of the patients at the onset of the disease—48.8 years for ANCA-positive and 48.5 years for the ANCA-negative group.

As shown by others and confirmed by our data, ANCA positivity is related to higher disease activity characterized by elevated inflammatory markers, decreased hemoglobin, and higher prevalence of renal involvement [4,9,12]. Furthermore, elevated baseline CRP at the onset of AAV disease has been observed to be predictive of renal damage and poor long-term outcome, a trend particularly associated with MPO-ANCA seropositivity [22]. We have found that laboratory inflammatory indicators CRP and ESR are elevated for all AAV patients, but values are higher in the ANCA-positive patients' group. Due to the relatively small group, our estimated difference was not statistically significant. Higher prevalence of kidney involvement (60.4%) and elevated serum creatinine level (93.5 µmol/L) were observed in the ANCA-positive group, compared with 24.0% and 70.0 µmol/L in the ANCA-negative group.

On the contrary, ENT, pulmonary, skin, joint, and neurological involvement were not statistically different between the groups, confirming the results of previous studies and revealing that ANCA titers are more predictive of renal disease activity than nonrenal disease activity [23]. On the other hand, an inconspicuous difference in organ involvement between groups was established in our study. In our cohort, 88.0% of patients with ANCA-negative vasculitis had pulmonary, 92.0% ENT, 44.0% joint, and 28.0% skin presentation; in comparison, involvement of these organs was less common in the ANCA-positive patients' group: 85.4%, 77.1%, 39.6%, and 25.0%, respectively. ANCA-positive patients were more likely to experience neurological symptoms, as polyneuropathy or mononeuropathy was observed in 29% of this group of patients compared with 20% of ANCA-negative patients. Analyzing separate disease subgroups, we have noted that in the GPA patients' group, organ damage, except for ENT, was more prevalent among seropositive patients. The trend was not observed in MPA and EGPA patients' groups, although, due to the small number of patients in each group, the statistical significance of the trend was not noted.

However, we did not take into account other organ involvement; AAV can involve any organ system, such as orbital structures, genitals, gastrointestinal, or cardiovascular [24].

AAV has complex symptomatology, and the specificity of ANCAs is limited. This might be explained by studies revealing that some ANCAs are more pathogenic than others, depending on the epitope specificity of the antibody [25]. Therefore, not the presence of ANCAs but their specificity might help predict relapse of AAV [26]. Furthermore, in some of these patients, laboratory tests for ANCAs can give false-negative results because of fragments of ceruloplasmin binding to the ANCAs in the serum [27].

This study focused on seropositivity rather than ANCA type. Moreover, since the first included patients were diagnosed with AAV as early as 2001, and the study analyzed only data from disease onset, ELISA testing was not available at that time; therefore, we do not have MPO and PR3 test results for some patients. This is a rather significant limitation of our study because, as mentioned in the literature, the ANCA type is closely related to the clinical presentation and prognosis, as patients with PR3-ANCA have more organs involved compared to patients with MPO-ANCA, resulting in a faster deterioration of renal function and more frequent relapses of the disease [26,28]. Moreover, a recent review of AAV relapse prognostic factors defined low- and high-risk relapse subgroups: women who are anti-PR-3 negative, with high creatinine levels and no ENT involvement, have a lower risk of exacerbation compared with men who are PR-3 positive, with low creatinine levels and ENT involvement [26]. On the other hand, some studies have revealed the opposite, that the type of disease (GPA or MPA) rather than the type of ANCA is more closely associated with relapse [4,29].

Furthermore, our study was limited by its single-center, retrospective character, based on hospital records where not every single clinical feature may have been recorded.

5. Conclusions

Our results support that diagnosis should be based on clinical features rather than ANCA assay results, as the differences in involvement of most organ systems between ANCA-positive and -negative patient groups were not statistically significant. However, ANCA-positive patients appear to be in a more difficult clinical situation in terms of kidney involvement and laboratory changes. Renal involvement should be at the forefront of clinical attention from the onset of the disease, followed by careful monitoring and management.

Author Contributions: Conceptualization, J.D.; methodology, J.D.; software, J.D.; validation, J.D.; formal analysis, G.D., J.D. and D.M.; investigation, J.D., G.D. and D.M.; resources, J.D. and D.M.; data curation, J.D. and G.D.; writing—original draft preparation, G.D. and D.M.; writing—review and editing, J.D.; visualization, G.D.; supervision, J.D.; project administration, J.D.; funding acquisition, J.D. All authors have read and agreed to the published version of the manuscript.

Funding: This research received no external funding.

Institutional Review Board Statement: The study was conducted according to the guidelines of the Declaration of Helsinki and approved by the Vilnius Regional Bioethics Committee (approval number 158200-17-958-462, 7 November 2017).

Informed Consent Statement: This study received a waiver for an informed consent form to be signed by participants. The document granting permission to conduct the study without informed consent may be added upon request.

Data Availability Statement: The participants of this study did not give written consent for their data to be shared publicly. This study received a waiver for an informed consent form to be signed by participants. The document granting permission to conduct the study without informed consent may be added upon request.

Conflicts of Interest: The authors declare no conflicts of interest.

References

1. Mukhtyar, C.; Guillevin, L.; Cid, M.C.; Dasgupta, B.; de Groot, K.; Gross, W.; Hauser, T.; Hellmich, B.; Jayne, D.; Kallenberg, C.G.M.; et al. EULAR recommendations for the management of primary small and medium vessel vasculitis. *Ann. Rheum. Dis.* **2009**, *68*, 310–317. [CrossRef]
2. Jennette, J.C.; Falk, R.J.; Bacon, P.A.; Basu, N.; Cid, M.C.; Ferrario, F.; Flores-Suarez, L.F.; Gross, W.L.; Guillevin, L.; Hagen, E.C.; et al. 2012 revised International Chapel Hill Consensus Conference Nomenclature of Vasculitides. *Arthritis Rheum.* **2013**, *65*, 1–11. [CrossRef] [PubMed]
3. Millet, A.; Pederzoli-Ribeil, M.; Guillevin, L.; Witko-Sarsat, V.; Mouthon, L. Republished: Antineutrophil cytoplasmic antibody-associated vasculitides: Is it time to split up the group? *Postgrad. Med. J.* **2014**, *90*, 290–296. [CrossRef] [PubMed]
4. Miloslavsky, E.M.; Lu, N.; Unizony, S.; Choi, H.K.; Merkel, P.A.; Seo, P.; Spiera, R.; Langford, C.A.; Hoffman, G.S.; Kallenberg, C.G.; et al. Myeloperoxidase-Antineutrophil Cytoplasmic Antibody (ANCA)-Positive and ANCA-Negative Patients with Granulomatosis with Polyangiitis (Wegener's): Distinct Patient Subsets. *Arthritis Rheumatol.* **2016**, *68*, 2945–2952. [CrossRef] [PubMed] [PubMed Central]
5. Fijolek, J.; Radzikowska, E. Eosinophilic granulomatosis with polyangiitis—Advances in pathogenesis, diagnosis, and treatment. *Front. Med.* **2023**, *10*, 1145257. [CrossRef] [PubMed] [PubMed Central]
6. Pearce, F.A.; Craven, A.; Merkel, P.A.; Luqmani, R.A.; Watts, R.A. Global ethnic and geographic differences in the clinical presentations of anti-neutrophil cytoplasm antibody-associated vasculitis. *Rheumatology* **2017**, *56*, 1962–1969. [CrossRef] [PubMed]
7. Furuta, S.; Chaudhry, A.N.; Hamano, Y.; Fujimoto, S.; Nagafuchi, H.; Makino, H.; Matsuo, S.; Ozaki, S.; Endo, T.; Muso, E.; et al. Comparison of phenotype and outcome in microscopic polyangiitis between Europe and Japan. *J. Rheumatol.* **2014**, *41*, 325–333. [CrossRef] [PubMed]
8. Furuta, S.; Chaudhry, A.N.; Arimura, Y.; Dobashi, H.; Fujimoto, S.; Homma, S.; Rasmussen, N.; Jayne, D.R. Comparison of the Phenotype and Outcome of Granulomatosis with Polyangiitis Between UK and Japanese Cohorts. *J. Rheumatol.* **2017**, *44*, 216–222. [CrossRef] [PubMed]

9. Flossmann, O.; Berden, A.; de Groot, K.; Hagen, C.; Harper, L.; Heijl, C.; Höglund, P.; Jayne, D.; Luqmani, R.; Mahr, A.; et al. European Vasculitis Study Group. Long-term patient survival in ANCA-associated vasculitis. *Ann. Rheum. Dis.* **2011**, *70*, 488–494. [CrossRef] [PubMed]
10. Jardel, S.; Puéchal, X.; Le Quellec, A.; Pagnoux, C.; Hamidou, M.; Maurier, F.; Aumaitre, O.; Aouba, A.; Quemeneur, T.; Subra, J.F.; et al. French Vasculitis Study Group (FVSG). Mortality in systemic necrotizing vasculitides: A retrospective analysis of the French Vasculitis Study Group registry. *Autoimmun. Rev.* **2018**, *17*, 653–659. [CrossRef] [PubMed]
11. Tan, J.A.; Dehghan, N.; Chen, W.; Xie, H.; Esdaile, J.M.; Avina-Zubieta, J.A. Mortality in ANCA-associated vasculitis: Ameta-analysis of observational studies. *Ann. Rheum. Dis.* **2017**, *76*, 1566–1574. [CrossRef]
12. Mukhtyar, C.; Flossmann, O.; Hellmich, B.; Bacon, P.; Cid, M.; Cohen-Tervaert, J.W.; Gross, W.L.; Guillevin, L.; Jayne, D.; Mahr, A.; et al. European Vasculitis Study Group (EUVAS). Outcomes from studies of antineutrophil cytoplasm antibody associated vasculitis: A systematic review by the European League Against Rheumatism systemic vasculitis task force. *Ann. Rheum. Dis.* **2008**, *67*, 1004–1010. [CrossRef] [PubMed]
13. Robson, J.C.; Grayson, P.C.; Ponte, C.; Suppiah, R.; Craven, A.; Judge, A.; Khalid, S.; Hutchings, A.; Watts, R.A.; Merkel, P.A.; et al. DCVAS Investigators. 2022 American College of Rheumatology/European Alliance of Associations for Rheumatology classification criteria for granulomatosis with polyangiitis. *Ann. Rheum. Dis.* **2022**, *81*, 315–320. [CrossRef] [PubMed]
14. Suppiah, R.; Robson, J.C.; Grayson, P.C.; Ponte, C.; Craven, A.; Khalid, S.; Judge, A.; Hutchings, A.; Merkel, P.A.; Luqmani, R.A.; et al. DCVAS INVESTIGATORS. 2022 American College of Rheumatology/European Alliance of Associations for Rheumatology classification criteria for microscopic polyangiitis. *Ann. Rheum. Dis.* **2022**, *81*, 321–326. [CrossRef] [PubMed]
15. Grayson, P.C.; Ponte, C.; Suppiah, R.; Robson, J.C.; Craven, A.; Judge, A.; Khalid, S.; Hutchings, A.; Luqmani, R.A.; Watts, R.A.; et al. DCVAS Study Group. 2022 American College of Rheumatology/European Alliance of Associations for Rheumatology Classification Criteria for Eosinophilic Granulomatosis with Polyangiitis. *Ann. Rheum. Dis.* **2022**, *81*, 309–314. [CrossRef] [PubMed]
16. Bossuyt, X.; Cohen Tervaert, J.W.; Arimura, Y.; Blockmans, D.; Flores-Suárez, L.F.; Guillevin, L.; Hellmich, B.; Jayne, D.; Jennette, J.C.; Kallenberg, C.G.M.; et al. Revised 2017 international consensus on testing of ANCAs in granulomatosis with polyangiitis and microscopic polyangiitis. *Nat. Rev. Rheumatol.* **2017**, *13*, 683–692. [CrossRef]
17. Pyo, J.Y.; Lee, L.E.; Park, Y.B.; Lee, S.W. Comparison of the 2022 ACR/EULAR Classification Criteria for Antineutrophil Cytoplasmic Antibody-Associated Vasculitis with Previous Criteria. *Yonsei Med. J.* **2023**, *64*, 11–17. [CrossRef] [PubMed] [PubMed Central]
18. Eisenberger, U.; Fakhouri, F.; Vanhille, P.; Beaufils, H.; Mahr, A.; Guillevin, L.; Lesavre, P.; Noël, L.H. ANCA-negative pauci-immune renal vasculitis: Histology and outcome. *Nephrol. Dial. Transplant.* **2005**, *20*, 1392–1399. [CrossRef] [PubMed]
19. Jennette, J.C.; Nachman, P.H. ANCA Glomerulonephritis and Vasculitis. *Clin. J. Am. Soc. Nephrol.* **2017**, *12*, 1680–1691. [CrossRef] [PubMed] [PubMed Central]
20. Watts, R.; Lane, S.; Bentham, G.; Scott, D. Epidemiology of systemic vasculitis: A ten-year study in the united kingdom. *Arthritis Rheum.* **2000**, *43*, 414–419. [CrossRef]
21. Zhao, W.M.; Wang, Z.J.; Shi, R.; Zhu, Y.Y.; Zhang, S.; Wang, R.F.; Wang, D.G. Environmental factors influencing the risk of ANCA-associated vasculitis. *Front. Immunol.* **2022**, *13*, 991256. [CrossRef] [PubMed] [PubMed Central]
22. Korsten, P.; Baier, E.; Hakroush, S.; Tampe, B. C-Reactive Protein Levels Are Associated with Complement C4 Deposits and Interstitial Arteritis in ANCA-Associated Renal Vasculitis. *Int. J. Mol. Sci.* **2023**, *24*, 3072. [CrossRef] [PubMed] [PubMed Central]
23. Kemna, M.J.; Damoiseaux, J.; Austen, J.; Winkens, B.; Peters, J.; van Paassen, P.; Cohen Tervaert, J.W. ANCA as a predictor of relapse: Useful in patients with renal involvement but not in patients with nonrenal disease. *J. Am. Soc. Nephrol.* **2015**, *26*, 537–542. [CrossRef] [PubMed] [PubMed Central]
24. Almaani, S.; Fussner, L.A.; Brodsky, S.; Meara, A.S.; Jayne, D. ANCA-Associated Vasculitis: An Update. *J. Clin. Med.* **2021**, *10*, 1446. [CrossRef] [PubMed] [PubMed Central]
25. Houben, E.; Bax, W.A.; van Dam, B.; Slieker, W.A.T.; Verhave, G.; Frerichs, F.C.P.; van Eijk, I.C.; Boersma, W.G.; de Kuyper, G.T.M.; Penne, E.L. Diagnosing ANCA-associated vasculitis in ANCA positive patients: A retrospective analysis on the role of clinical symptoms and the ANCA titre. *Medicine* **2016**, *95*, e5096. [CrossRef] [PubMed] [PubMed Central]
26. Wawrzycka-Adamczyk, K.; Korkosz, M.; Musiał, J.; Wójcik, K. Relapse Predictors in Antineutrophil Cytoplasmic Antibody (ANCA)-Associated Vasculitis. *Diagnostics* **2024**, *14*, 1849. [CrossRef]
27. Roth, A.J.; Ooi, J.D.; Hess, J.J.; van Timmeren, M.M.; Berg, E.A.; Poulton, C.E.; McGregor, J.; Burkart, M.; Hogan, S.L.; Hu, Y.; et al. Epitope specificity determines pathogenicity and detectability in ANCA-associated vasculitis. *J. Clin. Investig.* **2013**, *123*, 1773–1783. [CrossRef] [PubMed] [PubMed Central]

28. FijoŁek, J.; Wiatr, E. Antineutrophil cytoplasmic antibodies (ANCA)—Their role in pathogenesis, diagnosis, and treatment monitoring of ANCA-associated vasculitis. *Cent. Eur. J. Immunol.* **2020**, *45*, 218–227. [CrossRef] [PubMed] [PubMed Central]
29. Deshayes, S.; Martin Silva, N.; Khoy, K.; Yameogo, S.; Mariotte, D.; Lobbedez, T.; Aouba, A. Clinical impact of subgrouping ANCA-associated vasculitis according to antibody specificity beyond the clinicopathological classification. *Rheumatology* **2019**, *58*, 1731–1739. [CrossRef] [PubMed]

MDPI AG
Grosspeteranlage 5
4052 Basel
Switzerland
Tel.: +41 61 683 77 34

Medicina Editorial Office
E-mail: medicina@mdpi.com
www.mdpi.com/journal/medicina

www.ingramcontent.com/pod-product-compliance
Lightning Source LLC
Chambersburg PA
CBHW061627210926
51850CB00009B/2461
* 9 7 8 3 7 2 5 8 5 9 0 5 4 *